Aktuelle Probleme
aus dem Gebiet der Cancerologie II

Aktuelle Probleme aus dem Gebiet der Cancerologie II

Zweites Heidelberger Symposion

Herausgegeben von

H. Lettré und G. Wagner

Mit 96 Abbildungen

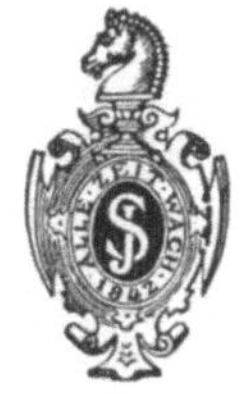

Springer-Verlag Berlin Heidelberg New York 1968

ISBN-13: 978-3-540-04036-1   e-ISBN-13: 978-3-642-85519-1
DOI: 10.1007/ 978-3-642-85519-1

Vorwort

Aus Anlaß des 75. Geburtstages von Prof. Dr. Karl Heinrich Bauer fand im September 1965 das erste Symposion des Deutschen Krebsforschungszentrums in Heidelberg statt. Damals wurde beschlossen, in zweijährigem Abstand weitere Symposien zu veranstalten. Der vorliegende Band – der zweite in der als Fortsetzungsfolge geplanten Reihe „Aktuelle Probleme aus dem Gebiet der Cancerologie" – bringt die Vorträge, die außer von eingeladenen Rednern im wesentlichen von Wissenschaftlern des Deutschen Krebsforschungszentrums bei dem zweiten Symposion im September 1967 gehalten wurden. Der Band gibt so zugleich einen Einblick in die Tätigkeit der Institute des Deutschen Krebsforschungszentrums von 1965 bis 1967.

Die Veranstaltung des Symposions und die Drucklegung der Vorträge wurden durch den „Verein zur Förderung der Krebsforschung in Deutschland e. V." ermöglicht, wofür auch an dieser Stelle gedankt sei.

Heidelberg, Juli 1968 H. Lettré G. Wagner

Inhaltsverzeichnis

A.

1. wissenschaftliche Sitzung am Montag, den 25. 9. 1967

(Vorsitz: H. Lettré)

C.

3. wissenschaftliche Sitzung am Dienstag, den 26. 9. 1967

(Vorsitz: E. Boyland)

D.

4. wissenschaftliche Sitzung am Mittwoch, den 27. 9. 1967

(Vorsitz: G. Wagner)

Liste der Referenten

ADAM, W. E., Dr. med.
Nuklearmedizinische Sektion des
Zentrums für Innere Medizin der Universität
Ulm

ARNSTADT, K. I., cand. chem.
Institut für experimentelle Geschwulsterzeugung und -behandlung
am Deutschen Krebsforschungszentrum
Heidelberg

BALLWEG †, H., Priv. Doz. Dr. rer. nat.
Institut für experimentelle Geschwulsterzeugung und -behandlung
am Deutschen Krebsforschungszentrum
Heidelberg

BARTSCH, H., Dr. rer. nat.
Biochemisches Institut
am Deutschen Krebsforschungszentrum
Heidelberg

BAUER, K. H., Prof. Dr. med.,
Dr. med. h. c., Dr. jur. h. c., Dr. med. h. c.,
Deutsches Krebsforschungszentrum
Heidelberg

BOYLAND, E., Prof. D. Sc.
The Chester Beatty Research Institute,
Dept. of Biochemistry, Royal Cancer Hospital
London

BRÜMMER, W., Dr. med.
Institut für Virusforschung
am Deutschen Krebsforschungszentrum
Heidelberg

BÜHLER, W. J., Ph. D.
Institut für Dokumentation, Information und Statistik
am Deutschen Krebsforschungszentrum
Heidelberg

FISCHER, H., Dr. med.
Institut für Virusforschung
am Deutschen Krebsforschungszentrum
Heidelberg

FITZGERALD, TH. J., Ph. D.
Institut für experimentelle Krebsforschung
am Deutschen Krebsforschungszentrum
Heidelberg

GOERTTLER, KL., Prof. Dr. med.
Institut für experimentelle Pathologic
am Deutschen Krebsforschungszentrum
Heidelberg

GSCHWENDT, M., Dr. rer. nat.
Biochemisches Institut
am Deutschen Krebsforschungszentrum
Heidelberg

HECKER, E., Prof. Dr. rer. nat.
Biochemisches Institut
am Deutschen Krebsforschungszentrum
Heidelberg

HOCHBERG, K., Dr. med.
Chirurgische Universitätsklinik
Heidelberg

IMMICH, H., Priv. Doz. Dr. med.
Institut für Dokumentation, Information und Statistik
am Deutschen Krebsforschungszentrum
Heidelberg

KINZEL, V., Dr. med.
Institut für experimentelle Pathologie
am Deutschen Krebsforschungszentrum
Heidelberg

KÖHLER, C., Dipl. Volksw.
Institut für Dokumentation, Information und Statistik
am Deutschen Krebsforschungszentrum
Heidelberg

KREIBICH, G., Dr. rer. nat.
Biochemisches Institut
am Deutschen Krebsforschungszentrum
Heidelberg

KRÜGER, F. W., Dr. rer. nat.
Institut für experimentelle Geschwulsterzeugung und -behandlung
am Deutschen Krebsforschungszentrum
Heidelberg

LETTRÉ, H., Prof. Dr. phil.
Institut für experimentelle Krebsforschung
am Deutschen Krebsforschungszentrum
Heidelberg

LETTRÉ, R., Priv. Doz. Dr. med.
Institut für experimentelle Krebsforschung
am Deutschen Krebsforschungszentrum
Heidelberg

LORENZ, W. J., Dr. rer. nat.
Institut für Nuklearmedizin
am Deutschen Krebsforschungszentrum
Heidelberg

MACDONALD, E. J., A. B.
Department of Epidemiology
The University of Texas
M. D. Anderson
Hospital and Tumor Institute
Houston/Texas

MACPHERSON, I., Prof. M. D.
Institute of Virology
University of
Glasgow/Schottland

MAZIA, D., Prof. Ph. D.
Dept. of Zoology,
University of California
Berkeley/California

MOHR, U., Priv. Doz. Dr. med.
Institut für experimentelle Pathologie
am Deutschen Krebsforschungszentrum
Heidelberg

MOPPERT, J., Dr. med.
Pathologisches Institut
der Universität
Basel/Schweiz

MUNK, K., Prof. Dr. med.
Institut für Virusforschung
am Deutschen Krebsforschungszentrum
Heidelberg

NURI, M., Dr. med.
Chirurgische Universitätsklinik
Heidelberg

OSSWALD, H., Priv. Doz. Dr. med.
Institut für experimentelle Geschwulsterzeugung und -behandlung
am Deutschen Krebsforschungszentrum
Heidelberg

OTT, G., Dr. med.
Chirurgische Universitätsklinik
Heidelberg

PAWELETZ, N., Dr. rer. nat.
Institut für experimentelle Krebsforschung
am Deutschen Krebsforschungszentrum
Heidelberg

PROCHOTTA, L., cand. med.
Institut für experimentelle Geschwulsterzeugung und -behandlung
am Deutschen Krebsforschungszentrum
Heidelberg

SCHEER, K. E., Prof. Dr. med.
Institut für Nuklearmedizin
am Deutschen Krebsforschungszentrum
Heidelberg

SCHIEMER, H. G., Priv. Doz. Dr. med.
Pathologisches Institut
der Universität
Heidelberg

SCHLEICH, A., Dr. med.
Institut für experimentelle Krebsforschung
am Deutschen Krebsforschungszentrum
Heidelberg

SCHLOSSER, M., Priv.-Doz. Dr. rer. nat.
Institut für experimentelle Krebsforschung
am Deutschen Krebsforschungszentrum
Heidelberg

SCHMÄHL, D., Prof. Dr. med.
Institut für experimentelle Geschwulsterzeugung und -behandlung
am Deutschen Krebsforschungszentrum
Heidelberg

SEIDEL, H. J., cand. med.
Institut für experimentelle Pathologie
am Deutschen Krebsforschungszentrum
Heidelberg

WAGNER, G., Prof. Dr. med.
Institut für Dokumentation, Information und Statistik
am Deutschen Krebsforschungszentrum
Heidelberg

WERNER, D., Dr. rer. nat.
Institut für experimentelle Krebsforschung
am Deutschen Krebsforschungszentrum
Heidelberg

WIESER, O., Priv. Doz. Dr. med.
Institut für experimentelle Pathologie
am Deutschen Krebsforschungszentrum
Heidelberg

WOLF, P. F., B. S.
Department of Epidemiology
The University of Texas
M. D. Anderson
Hospital and Tumor Institute
Houston/Texas

A.

1. wissenschaftliche Sitzung am Montag, den 25. 9. 1967

Vorsitz: H. Lettré

The Causes of Cancer

By

E. BOYLAND

Cancer is not only a disease of civilisation or modern times. It was known to the ancients, and tumours have been seen in the bodies of Egyptian mummies which were embalmed four thousand years ago. Tumours occur in animals and bone cancers have been observed in fossils of animals which lived a hundred million years ago. At one time such tumours might have been considered as spontaneous, but we now consider that they could have been induced by external factors. Bone tumours seen in fossil dinosaurs, for example, may have been caused by local concentration of radioactive material, such as strontium from the environment.

Table 1. *Standardized Mortality at Ages 20–65 Years of all Occupied and Retired Civilian Males and of the Five Social Classes from Cancer of the Stomach, 1921–23* (From HUEPER & CONWAY, 1964)

Social Class	Gastric Cancer Mortality Ratio
I. Professional and well-to-do individuals	60
II. Intermediates between classes I and III	82
III. Skilled artisans and analogous workers	100
IV. Intermediates between classes III and V	106
V. Laborers and unskilled workers	130

That some cancer is caused by external agents has been known since the observations of Sir Percival Pott on scrotal cancer in chimney sweeps almost two hundred years ago. The number of recognised carcinogenic agents is increasing so that the causes of many types of cancer are now known. The incidence of cancer at some sites including tongue, mouth, jaw, penis and scrotum is decreasing due to reduction in exposure to carcinogens. Improvements in nutrition, hygiene and cleanliness associated with improved standards of living often reduce exposure to carcinogenic factors. Cancer of the stomach is less common in Britain and some European countries than it used to be. It is also less common in richer people (Table 1) and the decrease in this disease is probably due to the improvement in standards of living during the present century. It is not possible to say whether the change that is responsible for the decrease in gastric cancer is in hygiene or in nutrition.

Cancer like all natural phenomena has causes which may be biological, chemical or physical. It is unlikely that more than 5% of cancer in man is caused by viruses when one includes the Burkitt tumour and leukaemia that may be of viral origin. Not more than 5% of cancer in man is due to radiation including ionising radiations and ultra-violet light. Some 90% of human cancer is therefore caused by chemical substances, but we do not know what proportion of the disease is due to endogenous and how much to environmental agents because most of the causes of cancer have still to be discovered and identified.

Many experts in cancer research, however, consider that most cancer in man is caused by external factors, which are theoretically avoidable. I consider that the most hopeful approach to the cancer problem is to seek out the causes and remove them. The difficulty of this approach is, however, illustrated by lung cancer which is caused largely by cigarette smoking. Last year almost 40% of all deaths from cancer in men in Britain were due to lung cancer and as 90% of these could be attributed to cigarette smoking and air pollution, a third of all cancer deaths in the British male is therefore due to these causes. The difficulties of reducing cigarette smoking and air pollution are, however, very great.

Even if the causes were found and removed cancer would continue to occur for fifty years, because of the long latent period between exposure to a carcinogen and the occurrence of the disease. There are still some cancers such as tumours of the breast in women of which as yet we have little idea of the causes. Research into the treatment of cancer as well as investigation into the causes will therefore be necessary for a long time.

The causes of cancer in man could be found by epidemiological studies but the detection of carcinogens by such studies is difficult because of the long latent period necessary for cancer induction and the low incidence of the disease. An effective way of reducing the incidence of cancer is by preventing the use of carcinogenic substances in human food, cosmetics and other materials with which human beings come in contact.

Indications of substances which may be carcinogenic might be obtained by knowledge of the mechanisms by which known carcinogens act. The study of the mechanisms of carcinogenesis could also lead to reduction of the disease as understanding the mechanisms might enable the defence processes to be increased and this should also make prevention possible.

Carcinogenesis and Cancer Chemotherapy

Basic research into carcinogenesis and therapy of cancer are linked because many of the agents used in the treatment of cancer are themselves carcinogenic. This was recognised with radiotherapy many years ago, but it applies to chemotherapy with many different agents. Thus oestrogens, used for treatment of cancer of the breast and of cancer of the prostate, induce cancer of several different organs in animals.

The alkylating agents are used extensively in the treatment of leukaemia, reticuloses and other malignant conditions. Most of these alkylating agents can be considered as derivatives of the vesicant poison gases, mustard gas and the nitrogen mustards. It was recognised that the active vesicants produced many of the biological effects of ionising radiation and they were therefore called radiomimetic. Almost 20 years ago we thought that nitrogen mustard could be carcinogenic, because it had other radiomimetic properties, and showed that it induced tumours in mice (BOYLAND & HORNING, 1949). The leucopenic, the leukaemogenic, the growth inhibiting, the carcinogenic actions, the effects on fertility and immune processes are produced by some carcinogens and by radiation.

In many cases of treatment of cancer the risk of cancer must be taken because the therapy with a carcinogenic drug produces benefits that outweigh the disadvantage of the cancer risk. One alkylating agent, *2-naphthyl-bis(2-chloroethyl)amine* (Chlornafthazine, Erysan) has induced bladder cancer in many patients who have been treated with it. There are alternative drugs that do not have this effect so that this drug should no longer be used.

Other Carcinogenic Medicinal Products

Some drugs used for other conditions, however, are also known to cause cancer in animals. Thus the vermifuge *carbon tetrachloride* induces liver damage and hepatomas in rodents. The use of carbon tetrachloride in treatment of helminth infections is not justified in view of the risk and the availability of other remedies.

Griseofulvin is an antibiotic which is very effective in treatment of fungal infections such as ringworm. It has, however, been shown to induce liver tumours when administered orally to mice (HURST & PAGET, 1963). Griseofulvin is such a valuable drug that the carcinogenic hazard must be accepted if no other remedy is available. It should not, however, be used for conditions where a safer drug would be effective.

Imferon or *iron dextran* is an effective form of iron for use by intramuscular injection in patients in whom orally administered iron is not absorbed. This and some other forms of iron have induced tumours on injection into animals (HADDOW & HORNING, 1960). As it is injected in the patients in relatively small doses the hazard to man is perhaps small. Nevertheless it should only be used in patients who fail to respond to other iron preparations given by mouth.

Sometimes a carcinogenic drug is extremely difficult to replace. Thus *isoniazid* (isonicotinic hydrazide), an invaluable drug in the treatment of tuberculosis, has induced lung tumours in mice. The carcinogenic action might be due to impurities in the product as tests with isoniazid in at least one laboratory have failed to induce tumours. The problem is complicated because administration of isoniazid has also reduced the incidence of mammary tumours in mice (TOTH & SHUBIK, 1966). Isoniazid is such a useful and well established drug that it is difficult to see how it can be replaced, because patients with tuberculosis should not be deprived of the benefits of the certainly effective treatment to allow an unproved replacement to be tried.

The experience with isoniazid indicates that new drugs should be tested for carcinogenic activity before they are widely used in clinical practice. A successful example of this is in the β-adrenergic blocking agents introduced for the treatment of heart diseases by Imperial Chemical Industries. One of them, *Alderlin* [Pronethalol, 2-isopropyl-amino-1-(2-naphthyl-ethanol-hydrochloride)] was found to be carcinogenic in mice but a related compound *Inderal* [Propanolol, 1-isopropyl-amino-3-(1-naphthyloxy)-propan-2-ol] produced no tumours. The non-carcinogenic drug Inderal has since been marketed and has in fact been found to be a more effective drug in clinical use.

Causes of Cancer of the Bladder

Bladder cancer has been known as an industrial disease in the chemical industry since the discovery by Rehn in Germany 70 years ago. Workers exposed to *2-naphthylamine*, *1-naphthylamine*, *benzidine* and *4-aminobiphenyl* or concerned in the manufacture of the dyestuffs *auramine* and *magenta* have an increased incidence of bladder cancer. CASE (1966) points out how the incidence of bladder cancer increases with increase in exposure, so that all men engaged in the distillation of 2-naphthylamine developed bladder cancer. Thus if the stimulus is great enough resistance to cancer is overcome (Fig. 1).

Dogs, but in general not other species, develop this disease when treated with 2-naphthylamine, 4-aminobiphenyl, 2-acetylaminofluorene or 4-dimethylaminoazobenzene. The appearance of tumours at sites remote from that of application of the carcinogen indicates that the action is due to metabolites. The local action on the bladder could be due to slow release of an active compound from an inactive conjugated metabolite excreted in the urine. Of the 25 known metabolites of 2-naphthyl-amine, 5 are carcinogenic when applied to the bladder of mice so that there is no simple explanation of the mechanisms of action of aromatic amines (BOYLAND, 1965).

Since the description of bladder cancer in chemical workers the risk has been seen in men making rubber (CASE & HOSKER, 1954) and electri-cal cables (CASE, 1966) in which aromatic amines were used. An excess of

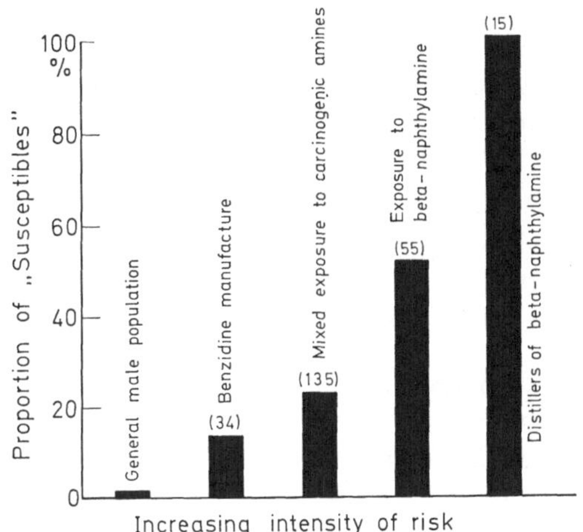

Fig. 1. Bladder cancer "susceptibles" in dyestuff intermediate workers. The "final incidence" in different occupational groups. (Data of CASE et al. 1954 and CASE unpublished)

bladder cancer is still occuring in the rubber industry although the known bladder carcinogens are no longer used in Britain. It seems remarkable that the increased incidence of bladder cancer in rubber workers has, up till now, been seen only in Britain. A risk of bladder cancer is also present in rat catchers who used the rodenticide *α-naphthylthiourea* (Antu) which is a derivative of 1-naphthylamine and has been withdrawn in Britain. The raised incidence of bladder cancer in coal gas workers could be due to *2-naphthylamine* which is present in coal tar and in the atmosphere near retort houses (BATTYE, 1966). 2-Naphthylamine is formed on pyrolysis of amino acids.

Some of the metabolites of tryptophan are *ortho*-aminophenols similar to known metabolites of the carcinogenic aromatic amines. *3-Hydroxyanthranilic acid* and *3-hydroxykynurenine* are carcinogenic when implanted in the mouse bladder. Bladder cancer could therefore be caused by such metabolites. BENASSI [2] has found that a proportion of patients with bladder cancer excrete increased amounts of 3-hydroxykynurenine and some patients with renal cancer excrete increased 3-hydroxyanthranilic acid. Bilharzia infection in Egypt is associated with bladder cancer and bilharzia infection is reported to increase excretion of 3-hydroxyanthranilic acid and 3-hydroxykynurenine.

Bladder cancer is higher in smokers than in non-smokers. This could be due to either excretion of *cotinine* or other carcinogenic metabolites of nicotine or to increased excretion of active tryptophan metabolites.

We know more about the causes of cancer of the bladder than of cancer at other sites. This could be due in part to the disease being relatively rare so that differences in incidence are more easily recognised. Perhaps if Rehn had seen three cases of cancer of the stomach instead of cancer of the bladder in his chemical workers he would not have deduced the relationship between exposure and the disease.

Other Industrial Cancers

Many other causes of cancer have been found because of increased incidence of some particular form of the disease in specific industries. Some of the materials known to cause cancer in man are listed in Table 2. It is possible to control and prevent the use of cancer-producing substances in certain products such as food, drink and cosmetics. We know that some of these products produce cancer in animals, and it is prudent to assume that a substance which causes cancer in animals could be dangerous for man.

The induction of cancer differs from most other toxic or poisonous effects. There is a long latent period between exposure to a cancer-

Table 2. *Some Industrial Human Carcinogens*

Carcinogen	Site in Man	Latent Period Years
Arsenite	Skin	18–25
Asbestos	Lung	18
Chromium Ore	Lung	15
Nickel	Nose	22
Benzene	Blood?	3–19
β-Naphthylamine	Bladder	11–20
Coal Tar	Skin and Lung	16–24
Isopropyl Oil	Nose and Lung	10
Radium	Bone	10–25
Bilharzia	Bladder	7–15
X-Rays	Skin	7–30
Oil	Scrotum and Skin	?
Tobacco Smoke	Lung	?

inducing agent and the recognition of the disease. In many cases the delay has been shown to be as much as 30 years in man. For this reason it is important to test materials – in food, cosmetics or other products – which come in contact with the body.

The only way to test such a substance is by animal experiments, which are difficult, expensive and time consuming. The requirements for such experiments have been defined in Britain (by the Ministry of Health) and in some other countries. Attempts are being made to obtain worldwide agreement on the regulation of food additives.

Two new industrial cancers have been described this year. One is cancer of the nasal sinuses that is more common among men making furniture from wood. It is not known whether the active carcinogen is derived from wood, varnish, adhesives or other materials used in the factories. This form of cancer may be similar to that seen in men who were occupied in nickel manufacture by the Mond process which involves formation of the volatile nickel carbonyl. By improving the conditions in nickel plant this form of cancer has been prevented and it is hoped that the cause of the furniture makers nasal cancer will be found and controlled.

An increased incidence of cancer of the prostate has been seen among men exposed to *cadmium* in factories in Birmingham, England (Table 3).

Table 3. *Cancer Incidence in Men Exposed to Cadmium Oxide*
(From KIPLING and WATERHOUSE, 1967)

Site of Cancer	No. of Cases		Probability of Occurrence
	Expected	Observed	
All Sites	13.13	12	0.660
Bronchus	4.40	5	0.449
Bladder	0.51	1	0.398
Prostate	*0.58*	*4*	*0.003*
Testis	0.11	0	0.898

ROE, DUKES, CAMERON, PUGH and MITCHLEY (1964) had induced neoplasia of the Leydig cells of the testis in rats by administration of cadmium salts. This provides an interesting example of the different site of action of a carcinogen in different species, which is frequently seen in carcinogenesis.

Most substances, with the exception of arsenical compounds, which cause cancer in man have induced cancer in at least one species when they have been adequately tested in animals. There is, however, considerable species variation: 2-naphthylamine, which causes cancer of the bladder in man and in dogs, induces liver tumours in mice. The colouring matter Butter Yellow induces liver tumours more readily in rats than in mice and causes bladder cancer in dogs. For this reason at least two species of animal should be used in tests because of the variation in response of different species.

More research is needed to develop and improve the methods of testing for carcinogenic activity. The attitude to this kind of work has changed during the past decades. Workers on carcinogenesis were more interested in demonstrating activity; now many of us are anxious to show that materials are safe. The proof of the negative–of absence of carcinogenic activity–is difficult and needs careful consideration and work.

Naturally Occurring Carcinogens

Although most of the compounds known to cause cancer are synthetic, products of combustion or materials associated with industry, some natural products are carcinogenic. *Oestrogens* are present in some clovers and other plants in sufficient concentration to cause disturbances of reproduction in sheep. Oestrogens have been shown to be carcinogenic in several species of animals and it is a reasonable assumption that they present a carcinogenic hazard to women. Even small amounts of oestrogen might facilitate the growth of oestrogen dependent mammary tumours in menopausal women (BOYLAND, 1967). It is doubtful whether any vegetables with high oestrogenic activity are consumed by Europeans. In some Eastern countries, however, the plant *Pueravia mirifica* (or *Butea superba*) is taken for its reputed aphrodisiac and rejuvenating properties. This plant contains miroestrol, which is more potent than stilboestrol or oestradiol. The possible occurrence of potent oestrogens in other plants that are consumed as food or herbal remedies require investigation.

Some *pyrrolizidine alkaloids* present in plants of the *Crotalaria, Heliotropium* and *Senecio* species are potent liver carcinogens (COOK, DUFFY & SCHOENTAL, 1950). Preparations of these plants have been widely used as herbal remedies and might well cause the liver cancer which is much more common in Bantus in Africa than it is among Europeans or coloured people in Britain or the U.S.A.

An exciting development in carcinogenesis of natural products has been the discovery of the potent carcinogenic mould products. In an investigation of the toxicity of some Brazilian ground nut meal, which had caused the death of some 100,000 turkeys in 1960, LANCASTER, JENKINS & PHILP (1961) found that the material produced multiple hepatomata when fed to rats. The toxic factor was shown to be the product of the common mould *Aspergillus flavus* growing on the ground nuts and was called *Aflatoxin*. Two closely related chemical substances Aflatoxin B and Aflatoxin G were isolated. These substances are extremely toxic to young birds and both produce liver tumours in animals in very small doses. It is difficult to assess the danger to man of the Aflatoxins and other mould products but they probably cause some cancer among people living in the tropics and possibly elsewhere.

Another natural carcinogen which has not yet been isolated is present in the fern, *bracken (Pteridium aquilinium)* which is all too common in the hills of Britain and many other parts of the world. Bracken contains an enzyme, thiaminase, which destroys the vitamin thiamine, and also a factor which causes leucopenia and increased capillary fragility similar to the symptoms produced by radiation (EVANS, EVANS & HUGHES, 1951). Bracken is therefore radiomimetic. EVANS & MASON (1965) showed that rats fed on a diet containing dried bracken developed tumours of the intestine. These tumours were similar to those which WALPOLE, WILLIAMS & ROBERTS (1954) had induced in rats with derivatives of 4-amino-biphenyl.

PAMUKCU, GÖKSOY & PRICE (1967) have found that cancer of the bladder develops in cattle fed on diets containing bracken (Table 4). PAMUKCU, OLSON & PRICE (1966) had previously shown that the urine of cattle fed on bracken contains a carcinogen that induces bladder cancer when applied to the bladder of mice.

One problem which has intrigued me for many years is the high incidence of cancer of the stomach in North Wales, which had been shown by STOCKS (1936). The distribution of the incidence of this disease was such that the cause could be waterborn, as the areas where

Table 4. *Bladder Tumours in Cows fed Bracken Supplements*
(From PAMUKCU, GÖKSOY and PRICE, 1967)

Group	No. of Cows	Bracken consumed g. per Day		Survival Time (Days)	Bladder Tumours
		Dried	Fresh		
I	7	600	1000	360–395	2 Papillomas
II	4	500	600	276–327	1 Papilloma 1 Haemangioma 1 Fibroma
III	4	400	500	374–936	1 Papilloma 2 Transitional Cell Carcinomas
IV	3	300	400	978–1192	1 Squamous Cell Carcinoma 1 Haemangioma

                E. Boyland

the disease is most common have peaty water (Fig. 2). The water supplies
in the areas of Wales where gastric cancer is most frequent could sometimes be extracts of bracken. When the active compound in bracken is
known it will be of great interest to see if it occurs in any water supplies.

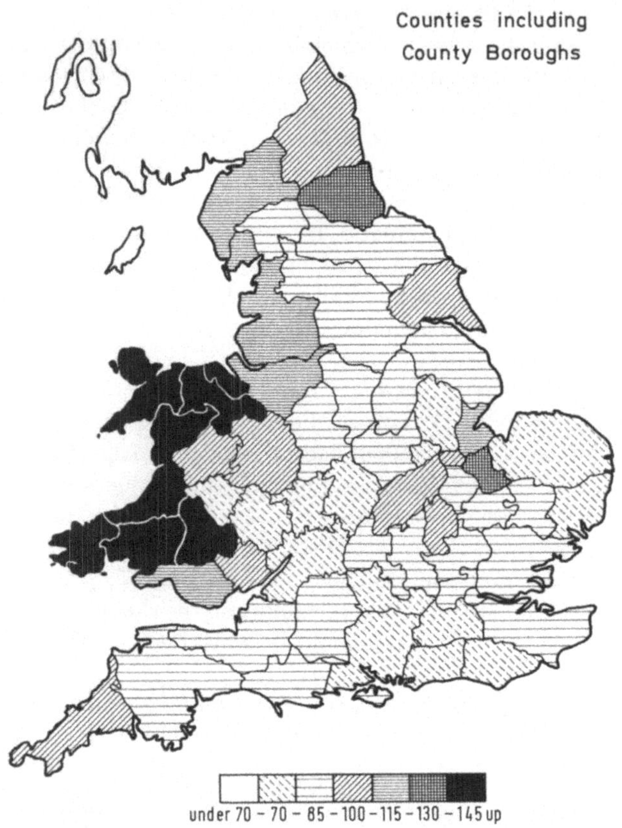

Fig. 2. Cancer of stomach 1921–1930 in persons aged 25–65. Actual mortality per
cent of that expected from the distribution of population by sex, age and class of
district

These examples of carcinogenic agents in natural products support the
contention that most cancer is due to external carcinogenic factors. The
naturally occurring carcinogens may be more difficult to identify and
more difficult to control than the synthetic compounds which are used as
food additives and for other purposes.

In addition to the colouring matters, preservatives, flavouring agents
and other materials added intentionally, food may contain unintentional

contaminants such as pesticide residues. Many of the *pesticides* used to control insect and other pests that are carcinogenic and persistent occur in small amounts in food. Aldrin, Dieldrin and DDT are examples of such pesticide contaminants and they have been found not only in food but in the fat of men and women in Britain and Europe and in even higher concentrations in the fatty tissues of subjects in the U.S.A.

Some hundreds of such materials may be used such as *insecticides, herbicides, fungicides* and for other purposes. Some are not persistent so that they are not present in food and many are probably harmless. Control of these materials, which improve the quality of crops, is a complicated and difficult problem.

The risk of cancer from one particular food additive or contaminant to one individual is perhaps small; but millions of people are exposed to these materials. It is therefore important to prevent exposure to any substance likely to cause cancer in order to prevent the incidence of cancer increasing.

References

1. BATTYE, R.: Bladder carcinogens occuring during the production of town gas by coal carbonisation. 15th International Congress on Occupational Health. Vol. III. BV-9, 153 (1966).
2. BENASSI, C. A., B. PERISSINOTTO, and G. ALLEGRI: The metabolism of tryptophan in patients with bladder cancer and other urological diseases. Clin. chim. Acta **8**, 822 (1963).
3. BOYLAND, E.: Natural oestrogens and the safe level of oestrogen intake. Tumori **53**, 9 (1967).
4. — The biochemistry of bladder cancer. Springfield, Ill.: C. C. Thomas Publ. 1963.
5. — and E. S. HORNING: The induction of tumours with nitrogen mustards. Brit. J. Cancer **3**, 118 (1949).
6. CASE, R. A. M.: Tumours of the urinary tract as an occupational disease in several industries. Ann. Roy. Coll. Surg. **39**, 213 (1966).
7. — and M. E. HOSKER: Tumours of the urinary bladder as an occupational disease in the rubber industry in England and Wales. Brit. J. prev. soc. Med. **8**, 39 (1954).
8. COOK, J. W., E. DUFFY, and R. SCHOENTAL: Primary liver tumours in rats following feeding with alkaloids of Senecio Jacobaea. Brit. J. Cancer **4**, 405 (1950).
9. EVANS, W. C., E. T. R. EVANS, and L. E. HUGHES: Studies on bracken poisoning in cattle. I. Brit. Vet. J. **110**, 295 (1954).
10. EVANS, I. A. and J. MASON: Carcinogenic activity of bracken. Nature **208**, 913 (1965).
11. HADDOW, A. and E. S. HORNING: On the carcinogenicity of an iron-dextran complex. J. nat. Cancer Inst. **24**, 109 (1960).
12. HUEPER, W. C. and W. D. CONWAY: Chemical carcinogenesis and cancers. Springfield, Ill.: C. C. Thomas 1964.
13. HURST, E. W. and G. E. PAGET: Protoporphyrin, cirrhosis and hepatomata in the livers of mice given griseofulvin. Brit. J. Dermat. **75**, 105 (1963).

14. KIPLING, M. D. and J. A. H. WATERHOUSE: Cadmium and prostatic carcinoma. Lancet I, 730 (1967).
15. LANCASTER, M. C., F. P. JENKINS, and J. McL. PHILP: Toxicity associated with certain samples of groundnuts. Nature **192**, 1095 (1961).
16. PAMUKCU, A. M., S. K. GÖKSOY, and J. M. PRICE: Urinary bladder neoplasms induced by feeding bracken fern. Cancer Res. **27**, 917 (1967).
17. —, C. OLSON, and J. M. PRICE: Assay of fractions of bovine urine for carcinogenic activity after feeding bracken fern (Pteris aquilina). Cancer Res. **26**, 1745 (1966).
18. ROE, F. J. C., C. E. DUKES, K. M. CAMERON, R. C. B. PUGH, and B. C. V. MITCHLEY: Cadmium neoplasia: testicular atrophy and Leydig cell hyperplasia and neoplasia in rats and mice following the subcutaneous injection of cadmium salts. Brit. J. Cancer **18**, 674 (1964).
19. STOCKS, P.: Comment on Dr. Stocks' maps and investigations by Professor Major Greenwood, F.R.S., F.R.C.P. Brit. Empire Cancer Campaign **13**, 239 (1936).
20. TOTH, B. and P. SHUBIK: Mammary tumor inhibition and lung adenoma induction by isonicotinic acid hydrazide. Science **152**, 1376 (1966).
21. WALPOLE, A. L., M. H. C. WILLIAMS, and D. C. ROBERTS: Tumours of the urinary bladder in dogs after ingestion of 4-aminodiphenyl. Brit. J. industr. Med. **11**, 105 (1954).

Untersuchung über den Wirkungsmechanismus cancerogener Nitrosamine

Von

H. Ballweg †, F. W. Krüger und K. I. Arnstadt

Seit der Entdeckung der cancerogenen Wirkung des Dimethyl-nitrosamins durch Magee [11] im Jahre 1956 ist vor allem durch die Arbeitsgruppen von Druckrey und Schmähl gezeigt worden, daß viele Nitrosamine starke cancerogene Eigenschaften besitzen [7].

Untersuchungen über diese Verbindungen sind vom Standpunkt der Präventivmedizin aus wichtig, weil Nitrosamine immer dann entstehen können, wenn sekundäre Amine und Nitrosegase zusammen auftreten, wie dies bei Industrieabgasen häufig der Fall sein kann. Nitrosamine haben nicht nur große praktische Bedeutung im Rahmen der Ursachenforschung des Krebses, sondern verfügen auch über einige Besonderheiten, die sie für den experimentellen Krebsforscher interessant machen.

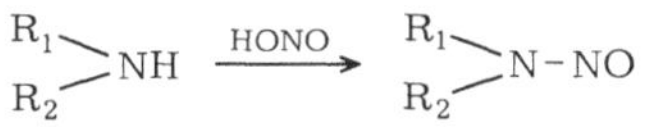

$$\begin{array}{c}R_1 \\ \diagdown \\ R_2 \diagup\end{array}\!\!NH \xrightarrow{\ \text{HONO}\ } \begin{array}{c}R_1 \\ \diagdown \\ R_2 \diagup\end{array}\!\!N-NO$$

$R_1 = R_2 = -CH_3$: Dimethylamin $\qquad$ $R_1 = R_2 = -CH_3$: Dimethylnitrosamin
$R_1 = R_2 = -C_2H_5$: Diäthylamin $\qquad$ $R_1 = R_2 = -C_2H_5$: Diäthylnitrosamin

Abb. 1. Schema der Umsetzung eines sekundären Amins mit salpetriger Säure

Nitrosamine sind synthetisch leicht zugänglich. Sie entstehen allgemein durch Umsetzung eines sekundären Amins mit salpetriger Säure nach dem in Abb. 1 gegebenen Schema. Verglichen mit anderen cancerogenen Substanzen handelt es sich um relativ einfach gebaute Verbindungen mit unterschiedlicher organotroper Wirkung. Dadurch wird es möglich, durch Wahl einer geeigneten Substanz, Dosierung und Applikationsart selektiv autochthone Organtumoren zu erzeugen, die als Modelle für die Prüfung chemotherapeutisch wirksamer Substanzen besser geeignet sind als Transplantationstumoren [19, 22, 23, 24].

Als Ursache für die cancerogene Wirkung der Nitrosamine nimmt man heute allgemein eine Veränderung der Bestandteile der Nukleinsäuren an, die entweder durch direkte Reaktion oder durch Umsetzung biologischer Abbauprodukte der Nitrosamine mit den Nucleinsäurebestandteilen erklärt wird [8, 12, 13, 14]. Die dadurch bedingte Änderung an genetischer Information soll schließlich zur Cancerisierung führen.

In Untersuchungen von LINGENS [10] konnte gezeigt werden, daß bei der Umsetzung von Adenin mit 1-Nitroso-3-nitro-1-methylguanidin die Bildung von Hypoxanthin zu 20% und von 6-(Nitroguanidino)-adenin zu beobachten ist. Bei der Umsetzung von Cytosin mit der gleichen Verbindung läßt sich die Bildung der entsprechenden Nitroguanidinoverbindung des Cytosins feststellen. Eine Desaminierung zum Uracil erfolgt in diesem Fall nicht.

Nach FAHR und Mitarb. [8] reagieren Cytosin, Cytidin und Cytidylsäure in wäßriger Lösung, bei pH 3–4, in Gegenwart eines Überschusses an Dimethylnitrosamin, bei 37 °C, während Adenin und Guanin nicht umgesetzt werden (Tab. 1). Die an unserem Institut von ARNSTADT [1] durchgeführte Untersuchung (Tab. 2) mit dem Ziel, Reaktionsprodukte dieser Umsetzung zu isolieren, zeigte jedoch, daß ein solcher Abbau nicht stattfindet. Dies gilt auch, wenn an Stelle von Dimethylnitrosamin Diäthylnitrosamin verwendet wird. FAHR nimmt an, daß die abweichenden Befunde auf Verunreinigungen des von ihm verwendeten Nitrosamins zurückzuführen sind.

Tabelle 1. *Die Umsetzung von Cytosin mit Dimethyl-nitrosamin im molaren Verhältnis 1:200 bei 30° (nach KLEBER, s. [8])*

a) *Konzentration an nicht umgesetztem Cytosin (%) bei der Umsetzung im pH 4,2*
b) *Konzentration an nicht umgesetztem Cytosin (%) bei der Umsetzung im pH 3,0*

t (Std)	a	b
9	98	95
24	93	89
33	89	87
54	85	81
76	79	74
101	72	66

Tabelle 2. *Die Umsetzung von Cytosin mit Dimethyl-nitrosamin im molaren Verhältnis 1:200 bei 30°*

Konzentration an nicht umgesetztem Cytosin (%) bei der Umsetzung im pH 4,2

Zeit (Std)	Konz. (γ/ml)	Konz. (%)
0	4,80	100
16,5	4,65	97
40	4,70	98
340	4,90	100,2

(Fehler der Methodik ∼ 3%)

Grundlegende Untersuchungen über den biologischen Wirkungsmechanismus, der zur Cancerisierung führen soll, sind von MAGEE u. Mitarb. durchgeführt worden [12, 13, 14]. Nach Gabe von markiertem Dimethylnitrosamin isolierten sie RNS und DNS aus Rattenleber, -niere und -milz und konnten nach Hydrolyse im Hydrolysat 7-Methylguanin

nachweisen. In der Milz wurde ein großer Teil der Aktivität im Adenin
und Guaninanteil gefunden. Auf Grund dieser Ergebnisse wird allgemein
der in Abb. 2 dargestellte Mechanismus für die biologische Wirkung der
Nitrosamine und Nitrosamide angenommen, und zwar zunächst Oxydation am α-C Atom durch eine Hydroxylase, dann Hydrolyse unter

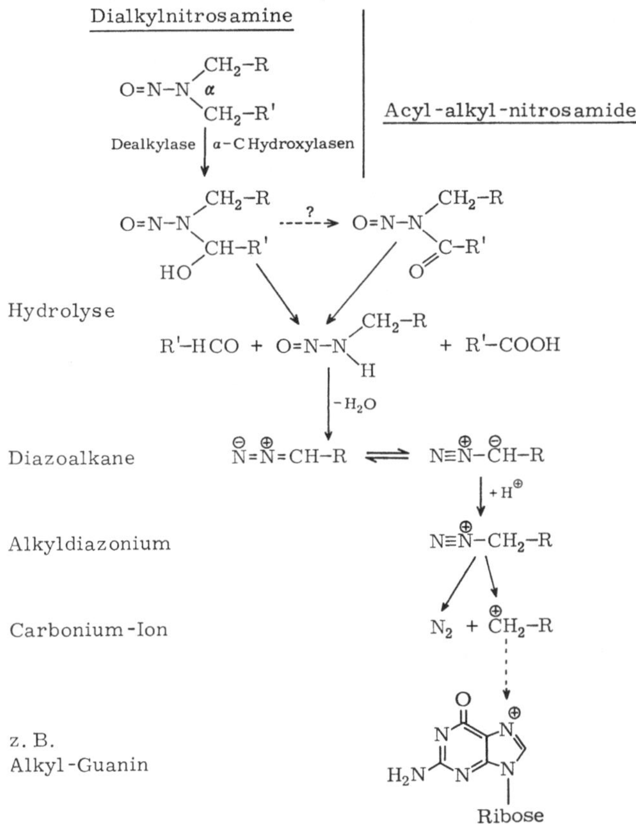

Abb. 2. Schema für den Reaktionsablauf bei der Aktivierung von Dialkylnitrosami-
nen und Alkylnitrosamiden zu alkylierend wirkenden Diazoalkanen

Abspaltung von Carbonsäure bzw. Aldehyd, Bildung von Diazoalkan,
Alkyldiazoniumverbindung und Reaktion des Carboniumions mit Guanin
in 7-Stellung. Bei der Verwendung von Dimethylnitrosamin sollte nach
diesem Schema neben 7-Methylguanin auch Formaldehyd als Reaktionsprodukt entstehen und ist auch in in-vitro-Versuchen nachgewiesen
worden [5].

Im Arbeitskreis von SCHMÄHL wurde in den letzten Jahren vor allem
das Diäthylnitrosamin auf seine cancerogene Wirkung untersucht. Die

Verbindung erzeugt Leberkrebs bei Mäusen, Ratten, Hamstern, Meerschweinchen, Kaninchen, Hunden, Affen, Schweinen, Fischen und Vögeln [20, 21]. Beim Frosch gelang die Tumorerzeugung indessen noch nicht. Hinsichtlich des breiten Tierspektrums ist Diäthylnitrosamin damit das am besten untersuchte Cancerogen.

Aus Untersuchungen mit Dimethylnitrosamin ist bekannt, daß der Abbau dieser Verbindung vorwiegend in der Leber erfolgt, und zwar in erster Linie durch die Mikrosomen. BALLWEG versuchte, durch in-vitro-

Tabelle 3. *Abbau von Diäthylnitrosamin durch Rattenleberhomogenate am Licht und im Dunkeln*

	nach	1	3	5 Std
Zurückerhaltenes Diäthylnitrosamin	Dunkel	99,5	98,6	99,8
(in %)	Licht	97,3	89,7	76,8

Untersuchungen zu klären, ob Diäthylnitrosamin durch Leberhomogenate und die Mikrosomenfraktion der Leber von Ratte und Frosch unterschiedlich abgebaut wird, da die Verbindung bei Ratten sehr stark, beim Frosch hingegen nicht cancerogen wirkt. Zunächst wurden Rattenleberhomogenate mit 200 γ Diäthylnitrosamin pro Gramm Leber inkubiert. Dabei ließ sich ein Abbau von Diäthylnitrosamin feststellen (Tab. 3), allerdings nur, wenn die Versuche bei Licht durchgeführt wurden. Im Dunkeln erfolgte ein Abbau unter sonst gleichen Bedingun-

Tabelle 4. *Abbau von Diäthylnitrosamin durch verschiedene Organhomogenate und durch Mikrosomen aus Rattenlebern am Licht und im Dunkeln bei Zusatz von TPNH nach 1 Std*

	Leber (dunkel)	(hell)	Milz (hell)	Niere (hell)	Lebermikrosomen (dunkel)	(hell)
Zurückerhaltenes Diäthylnitrosamin (in %)	98,1	85,3	89,8	91,9	98,8	88,7

gen nicht [2]. Dies traf auch zu, wenn an Stelle von Homogenaten Leberschnitte, die Mikrosomenfraktion der Leber, oder Homogenate von Niere und Milz verwendet wurden (Tab. 4). Auffallend war, daß jedes Organhomogenat unter sonst gleichen Bedingungen am Licht einen unterschiedlichen Abbau des Diäthylnitrosamins bewirkte. Der stärkste Abbau erfolgt durch die Leber, dann folgen Milz und schließlich Niere.

Wir haben uns daher auf Grund dieser Befunde zunächst mit der Photolyse von Nitrosaminen befaßt, einmal, weil in der Literatur Hinweise fehlen, ob entsprechende in-vitro-Versuche am Licht und im

Dunklen durchgeführt wurden, zum anderen, um zu untersuchen, ob zwischen photolytischem und biologischem Abbau Parallelen bestehen, die nach dem unterschiedlichen Abbau des Diäthylnitrosamins durch Organhomogenate am Licht vermutet werden könnten. Ich darf vielleicht noch einmal darauf hinweisen, daß der stärkste Abbau am Licht durch die Leber erfolgt, deren RNS auch in in-vivo-Versuchen nach Verabreichung von ^{14}C-Dimethylnitrosamin die höchste spezifische Aktivität zeigt [12].

Die Photolyse von Nitrosaminen ist bekannt. Bereits 1939 beschrieb BAMFORD [4] die photolytische Spaltung des Dimethylnitrosamins in der Gasphase. Auf der photolytischen Spaltung des Nitrosamins und dem Nachweis des entstandenen Nitrits beruhen zwei Verfahren zur Bestimmung dieser Verbindungen mit Hilfe der Dünnschichtchromatographie [17, 18]. Nach PREUSSMANN [16] erfolgt eine photolytische Spaltung in wäßriger Lösung durch UV-Licht unter Bildung des sekundären Amins und von Nitrit. CHOW [6] beschrieb kürzlich die photolytische Spaltung von Nitrosamin in wäßrig-methanolischer HCl.

Bei der Untersuchung des photolytischen Abbaus der Nitrosamine am Tageslicht konnten wir feststellen, daß die Geschwindigkeit des Abbaus durch Verschiebung des pH-Wertes zu niederen Werten beschleunigt wird, ebenso wie durch Zusatz von Wasserstoffperoxyd. Um unter standardisierten Bedingungen und mit höheren Konzentrationen arbeiten zu können, verwendeten wir bei unseren weiteren Untersuchungen eine 260 Watt Quecksilberdampftauchlampe. Alle Untersuchungen wurden bei einer Temperatur von 25 °C ausgeführt.

Die Bestrahlung einer 4%igen wäßrigen Lösung von Diäthylnitrosamin unter den angegebenen Bedingungen führte zu einer Verschiebung des pH-Wertes in den alkalischen Bereich unter starker Dunkelfärbung der Lösung. Nach Eindampfen des Reaktionsgemisches im Vakuum erhielten wir einen schwarzen, teerartigen Rückstand, dessen Zusammensetzung wir noch nicht kennen. Nach Zusatz einer äquimolaren Menge HCl ließ sich, wie nach den Versuchen am Tageslicht zu erwarten war, die Umsetzungsgeschwindigkeit wesentlich steigern. Das Reaktionsgemisch blieb farblos.

Nach CHOW [6] verläuft die photolytische Spaltung von Nitrosaminen im ultravioletten Licht, in wäßriger methanolischer Salzsäure, nach dem in Abb. 3 gegebenen Schema: Abspaltung von Nitroxyl unter Beteiligung der Protonen des Lösungsmittels, intermediäre Bildung einer „Schiffschen Base", nucleophile Anlagerung des Nitroxyls an den positivierten Kohlenstoff und Stabilisierung des Reaktionsproduktes unter Abspaltung eines Protons zum entsprechenden Amidoxim. Die Umsetzung des Diäthylnitrosamins in wäßrig salzsaurer Lösung verläuft offensichtlich ebenfalls nach diesem Schema. Als Reaktionsprodukt konnten wir Essigsäureäthylamidoxim isolieren (Abb. 4). Die Verbindung zeigt im Gegensatz

zum Diäthylnitrosamin keine akute hepatotoxische Wirkung. Nach
Gabe von 500 mg/kg konnten bei der Ratte keine histologischen Veränderungen der Leber festgestellt werden, während Diäthylnitrosamin
nach Verabreichung von 300 mg/kg zu schweren Leberparenchym-
nekrosen führt, die für 50% der Tiere tödlich verlaufen (DL_{50}). Chronische

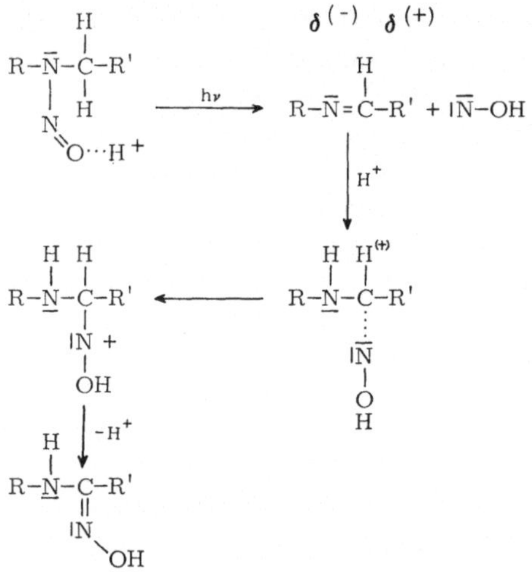

Abb. 3. Photolytische Spaltung von Nitrosaminen (nach Chow [6])

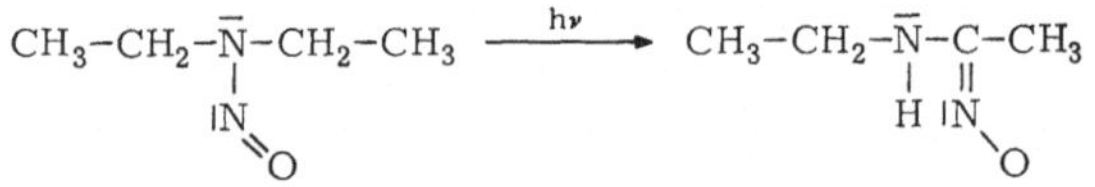

Abb. 4. Reaktionsschema für die photolytische Zersetzung von Nitrosaminen in
wäßrig-methanolischer HCl (nach Chow [6])

Versuche mit dieser Verbindung auf cancerogene Wirkung werden zur
Zeit durchgeführt. Eine am Tageslicht photolysierte Lösung von Diäthylnitrosamin erwies sich im chronischen Versuch im Vergleich zum un-
gespaltenen Diäthylnitrosamin jedoch als nicht cancerogen [3].

Bei der Photolyse von Dimethylnitrosamin in wäßriger Lösung unter
Zusatz einer äquimolaren Menge HCl gelang die Isolierung des zu
erwartenden Methylformamidoxims jedoch nicht. Vielmehr entstanden
hier Monomethylamin und, interessanterweise, Formaldehyd als Reaktionsprodukte. Methylamin wurde als Hydrochlorid, Formaldehyd als
2,4-Dinitro-phenylhydrazon und als Dimedonderivat isoliert. Außerdem
gelang der Nachweis beider Verbindungen im Photolysat durch Zugabe
von KOH und Abtrennung des 1,3,5-N-Trimethyl-perhydro-triazins.
Alle Verbindungen wurden u. a. durch IR-spektroskopischen Vergleich
mit den authentischen Verbindungen identifiziert. Die Photolyse des

Dimethylnitrosamins verläuft unter Gasentwicklung. Im entstandenen Gas ließ sich IR-spektroskopisch nur N_2O nachweisen. Auf Grund dieser Ergebnisse halten wir die Umsetzung nach folgendem Reaktions-mechanismus für wahrscheinlich (Abb. 5):

Abspaltung eines Protons und Nitroxyls unter intermediärer Bildung der Schiffschen Base, die hier nicht unter Addition von Nitroxyl sondern von Wasser zum Methylaminomethanol reagiert, das in saurer Lösung zu Formaldehyd und Methylamin gespalten wird. Dimerisierung des Nitroxyls zu untersalpetriger Säure, Zerfall dieser Verbindung zu N_2O

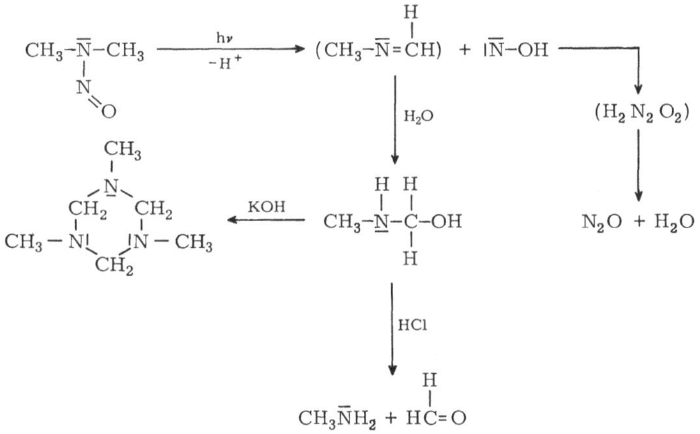

Abb. 5. Reaktionsmechanismus der Photolyse des Dimethylnitrosamins

und Wasser. Dabei ist nochmals hervorzuheben, daß Formaldehyd, der bei Inkubationsversuchen von Organschnitten mit Dimethylnitrosamin nachgewiesen wurde und nach der Diazoalkantheorie als biologisches Abbauprodukt gefordert wird, auch durch photolytische Zersetzung im sauren Medium aus Dimethylnitrosamin entsteht.

Es soll jetzt noch auf einige Versuche eingegangen werden, die mit ^{14}C-markierten Verbindungen unternommen wurden*. Zunächst wollten wir feststellen, ob eine in der vorher beschriebenen Weise photolytisch zersetzte Lösung von Dimethylnitrosamin noch alkylierende Eigenschaften besitzt.

Außerdem wollten wir untersuchen, ob äquitoxische Mengen von Dimethylnitrosamin und Diäthylnitrosamin zu einer vergleichbaren Alkylierung der RNS führen (Tab. 5). In der ersten Spalte der Tab. 5 ist

* Diese Versuche wurden in Zusammenarbeit mit dem Institut für Nuklear-medizin durchgeführt. Für die uns zuteil gewordene Hilfe möchten wir uns bei Herrn Dr. MAIER-BORST, Frl. GLÖKLE und Herrn JÜNGER bedanken.

die spezifische Aktivität der RNS aus Rattenleber nach Gabe von 30 mg
und μCi Dimethylnitrosamin angegeben. Sie wurde als 100% angenommen. Die zweite Spalte zeigt die spezifische Aktivität der RNS nach Gabe
derselben Menge photolytisch zersetzter Dimethylnitrosaminlösung. Eine

Tabelle 5. *Aktivität in 5 mg RNS aus Rattenleber nach Gabe äquitoxischer Mengen*
verschiedener Nitrosamine

	Imp/min	DMNA = 100%
[14]C-DMNA		
30 mg/30 μ Ci/kg	433	100
[14]C-DMNA-Photolys.		
30 mg/30 μ Ci/kg	13	3
[14]C-DÄNA		
300 mg/300 μ Ci/kg	82	19
[14]C-PNDA		
100 mg/200 μ Ci/kg	197	—

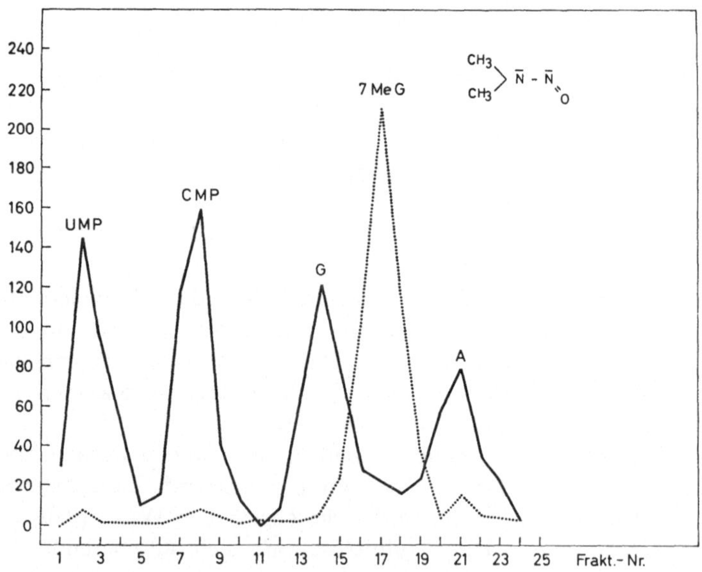

Abb. 6. Auftrennung eines RNS-Hydrolysates aus Rattenleber nach Gabe von
30 mg u. 30 μCi/kg ^{14}C-Dimethylnitrosamin ip. 16 h nach Applikation.
—— Ext.   ... Imp./min/ml × 2,5

Alkylierung erfolgt hier offensichtlich nicht mehr. Dimethylnitrosamin
und Diäthylnitrosamin unterscheiden sich in der akuten Toxizität etwa
um eine Größenordnung. Die zur Tumorerzeugung benötigten Mengen
und die Induktionszeiten liegen bei beiden Verbindungen jedoch in der

gleichen Größenordnung. Wir haben uns an der akuten Toxizität orientiert und eine, bezogen auf Dimethylnitrosamin, 10-fach höhere Dosis gleicher spezifischer Aktivität Diäthylnitrosamin injiziert. Wie aus Zeile 3 der Tab. 5 zu entnehmen ist, beträgt die spezifische Aktivität der RNS aber nur 19%, bezogen auf Dimethylnitrosamin, in der in der Zeile 1 angegebenen Dosierung. In Abb. 6 und 7 ist die Auftrennung dieser RNS-Hydrolysate dargestellt, wie sie auch von MAGEE beschrieben

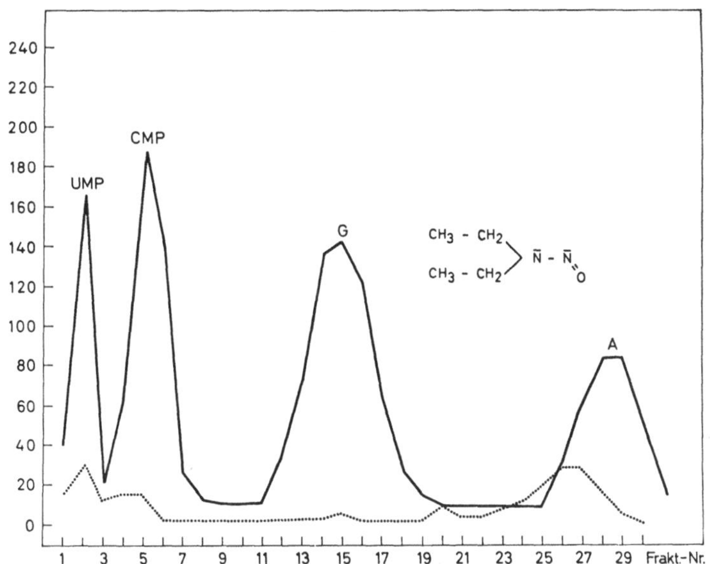

Abb. 7. Auftrennung eines RNS-Hydrolysates aus Rattenleber nach Gabe von 300 mg und 300 μCi/kg 1-^{14}C-Diäthylnitrosamin ip. 16 h nach Applikation. —— Ext. ... Imp./min/ml × 5,0

wurde. Abb. 6 zeigt die Auftrennung eines RNS-Hydrolysates nach Gabe von 30 mg und 30 μCi Dimethylnitrosamin mit dem ausgeprägten Maximum des 7-Methylguanins (gepunktete Linie). Die Abb. 7 zeigt die Auftrennung des RNS-Hydrolysates nach Gabe von 300 mg und 300 μCi Diäthylnitrosamin. Nach MAGEE handelt es sich bei der durch die gepunktete Linie angedeuteten Verbindung um 7-Äthylguanin, wie er durch papierchromatographischen und UV-spektroskopischen Vergleich folgerte [14].

Nach Untersuchungen von LEE und LIJINSKY [9] findet man in der RNS der Rattenleber nach Applikation von mit Tritium markiertem N-Nitrosomorpholin ebenfalls 7-Methylguanin. Hier tritt also eine Methylierung der RNS ein, obgleich nach dem Mechanismus der Diazoalkantheorie eine Alkylierung stattfinden sollte. Eine plausible Erklärung dieser Befunde ist zur Zeit noch nicht möglich (Abb. 8). Nach neueren Untersuchungen wird die Struktur der Nitrosamine allgemein nicht

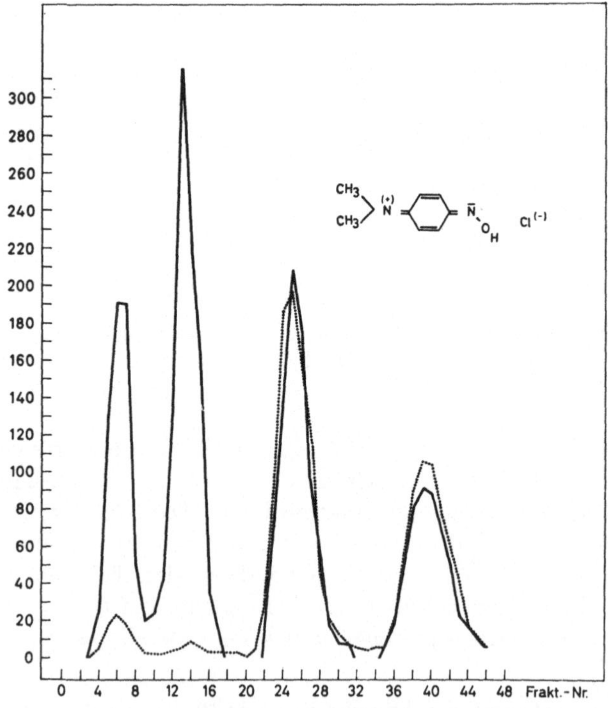

Abb. 8. Formelvorschläge für die Struktur der Nitrosamine

Abb. 9. Auftrennung eines RNS-Hydrolysates aus Rattenleber nach Gabe von
150 mg und 300 μCi/kg-p-Nitroso-^{14}C-dimethylanilinhydro-chlorid.
—— Ext.   ... Imp./min/ml
(Wegen der hohen Toxizität der Substanz wurde die Verbindung in einstündigem
Abstand in Dosen von 5 mg/kg iv. injiziert)

durch die hier für Dimethylnitrosamin angegebene Formel links in Abb. 8, sondern besser durch die rechte Formel wiedergegeben. Diese Annahme wird durch Untersuchungen von MANNSCHRECK, MÜNSCH und MATHEUS [15] gestützt, denen es gelang, bei ungleich substituierten Nitrosaminen Konformationsisomere zu isolieren. Außerdem erfolgt nach SCHMIDPETER [25] die Alkylierung von Nitrosaminen nicht am Stickstoff, sondern am Sauerstoff.

Die Positivierung des Stickstoffs ließ es möglich erscheinen, daß beim Dimethylnitrosamin die Methylierung des Guanins nicht nach dem Diazoalkanmechanismus, sondern als Transmethylierung erfolgt. Um diese Frage zu klären, haben wir Untersuchungen mit ^{14}C-markiertem p-Nitroso-dimethylanilin durchgeführt. Diese Verbindung ist als benzyloges Dimethylnitrosamin aufzufassen. Die Stickstoffatome sind jedoch durch den Benzolring getrennt, so daß eine Diazoalkanbildung nicht möglich ist (Abb. 9). Abb. 9 zeigt die Auftrennung eines RNS-Hydrolysates aus Rattenleber nach Gabe von p-Nitroso-^{14}C-Dimethylanilin. Im wesentlichen erfolgt hier ein Einbau in die Adenin- und Guaninfraktion. Eine Alkylierung findet nicht statt. Die Substanz wird zur Zeit im chronischen Versuch geprüft.

Zusammenfassend läßt sich sagen: Die Untersuchungen von FAHR u. Mitarb. [8] über die direkte Reaktion von Dimethylnitrosamin mit Cytosin, Cytidin und Cytidylsäure konnten nicht bestätigt werden. Diäthylnitrosamin wird am Licht in Gegenwart verschiedener Organhomogenate unterschiedlich abgebaut, während im Dunkeln kein Abbau erfolgt. Zwischen biologischem und photolytischem Abbau läßt sich eine Parallele vermuten. Der beim biologischen Abbau von Dimethylnitrosamin entstehende Formaldehyd entsteht auch unter den Bedingungen der Photolyse dieser Verbindung. Photolytisch gespaltenes Dimethylnitrosamin zeigt keine alkylierende Wirkung. Eine am Tageslicht photolysierte Diäthylnitrosaminlösung erwies sich im chronischen Versuch als nicht cancerogen. Die Alkylierung der RNS aus Rattenleber nach Gabe von Diäthylnitrosamin ist, verglichen mit der Alkylierung durch Dimethylnitrosamin, außerordentlich gering. Eine Parallele zwischen carcinogener und alkylierender Wirkung besteht bei diesen Verbindungen nicht. Das als benzyloges Dimethylnitrosamin aufzufassende p-Nitrosodimethylanilin zeigt keine alkylierende Wirkung.

Literatur

1. ARNSTADT, K. I.: Diplomarbeit Heidelberg 1967/68.
2. BALLWEG, H. u. D. SCHMÄHL: Über Photolyse bei Nitrosaminen. Naturwissenschaften **54**, 116–117 (1967).
3. —, F. W. KRÜGER u. D. SCHMÄHL: Fehlen einer carcinogenen Wirkung von photolysiertem Diäthylnitrosamin. Naturwissenschaften **54**: 591 (1967).
4. BAMFORD, D. H.: A study of the photolysis of organic nitrogen compounds. Part I. Dimethyl- and Diethylnitrosamines. J. chem. Soc. **1939**, 12–26.

5. Brouwers, J. A. J. and P. Emmelot: Microsomal N-demethylation and the effect of the hepatic carcinogen Dimethylnitrosamine on amino acid incorporation into the proteines of rat-livers and hepatomas. Exper. Cell Research **19**, 467–474 (1960).

6. Chow, J. and A. C. H. Lee: Photochemistry of nitroso compounds in solution. V. Photolysis of N-nitrosodialkylamines. Canad. J. Chem. **45**, 53–62 (1967).

7. Druckrey, H., R. Preussmann, S. Ivankovic u. D. Schmähl: Organotrope cancerogene Wirkungen bei 65 verschiedenen N-Nitrosoverbindungen an BD-Ratten. Z. Krebsforsch. **69**, 103–201 (1967).

8. Fahr, E., R. Kleber u. E. Boeblinger: Einwirkung von UV-Strahlung und von cancerogenen Nitrosaminen auf Nucleinsäurebestandteile. Angew. Chem. **77**, 1091 (1965).

9. Lee, K. Y. and J. Lijinsky: Alkylation of rat liver RNA by cyclic N-Nitrosoamines in vivo. J. nat. Cancer Inst. **37**, 401–407 (1966).

10. Lingens, F.: Wirkungsmechanismus einiger chemischer Mutagene. Verhandlungen Deutsch. Pharmakol. Ges. Naunyn-Schmiedebergs Arch. exper. Path. **253**, 116–131 (1966).

11. Magee, P. N. and J. M. Barnes: The production of malignant primary hepatic tumours in the rat by feeding Dimethylnitrosamin. Brit. J. Cancer **10**, 114–122 (1956).

12. — and E. Faber: Toxic liver injury and carcinogenesis. Methylation of rat-liver nucleic acids by Dimethylnitrosamin in vivo. Biochem. J. **83**, 114–124 (1962).

13. — and T. Hultin: Toxic liver injury and carcinogenesis. Methylation of Proteines of rat-liver slices by Dimethylnitrosamine in vitro. Biochem. J. **83**, 106–114 (1962).

14. — and K. Y. Lee: Cellular injury and Carcinogenesis. Alkylation of Ribonucleic acid of rat-liver by Diethylnitrosamine and N-butyl-methylnitrosamine in vivo. Biochem. J. **91**, 35–42 (1964).

15. Mannschreck, A., H. Münsch u. A. Matheus: Trennung der Konformationsisomere eines Nitrosamins. Angew. Chem. **78**, 751 (1966).

16. Preussmann, R.: Zum oxydativen Abbau von Nitrosaminen mit enzymfreien Modellsystemen. Arzneimittel-Forsch. **14**, 769–774 (1964).

17. —, D. Daiber, and H. Hengy: A sensitiv colour reaction for Nitrosamines in thin layer chromatograms. Nature **201**, 502–503 (1964).

18. —, G. Neurath, G. Wulf-Lorentzen, D. Daiber u. H. Hengy: Anfärbemethoden und Dünnschichtchromatographie von organischen N-Nitrosoverbindungen. Z. analyt. Chem. **202**, 187–192 (1964).

19. Schmähl, D.: Die heutige Situation in der experimentellen Chemotherapie von Tumoren. Dtsch. med. Wschr. **91**, 2132–2135 (1966).

20. — and H. Osswald: Carcinogenesis in different animal species by Diethylnitrosamine. Experientia **23**, 297–299 (1967).

21. — — u. U. Mohr: Hepatotoxische Wirkung von Diäthylnitrosamin bei Schweinen. Naturwissenschaften **54**, 341 (1967).

22. — — u. H. Brune: Chemotherapie-Versuche mit Endoxan an autochthonen Benzpyren-Sarkomen bei Ratten und Mäusen. Z. Krebsforsch. **68**, 293–302 (1966).

23. — u. G. Schrick: Chemotherapie-Versuche an authochthonen Gehörgangscarcinomen bei Ratten. Arzneimittel-Forsch. **14**, 72–73 (1964).

24. — — u. K. König: Chemotherapie-Versuche an Hepatomen. Arzneimittel-Forsch. **13**, 370–371 (1963).

25. Schmiedpeter, A.: Reaktionen von Nitrosaminen mit Elektrophilen. I. Die Alkylierung von Nitrosaminen. Tetrahedron Letters **1963**, 1421–1424.

Über die Resistenz verschiedener Organe
gegen inoculierte Tumorzellen

Von

H. Osswald, L. Prochotta und D. Schmähl

Die Metastasenbildung stellt ein charakteristisches Merkmal bösartiger Tumoren dar. Die mechanische Vorstellung des Metastasierungsvorganges geht von einer ausschließlich hämodynamischen Verteilung [2, 17, 18] der Metastasen aus. Die in die Blutbahn gelangenden Tumorzellen werden in den Organen wie von Filtern abgefangen und beginnen unter bestimmten Voraussetzungen ein erneutes Wachstum. Die Tatsache, daß es bei einer Reihe von Tumoren im nächstgelegenen „Filterorgan", z. B. der Lunge, nicht zur Metastasenbildung kommt, wird durch das Vorhandensein arteriovenöser Anastomosen erklärt [1]. Trotz dieser bestechend einfachen Deutung des Metastasierungsvorganges bleiben eine Reihe klinischer und experimenteller Beobachtungen ungeklärt. Bestimmte Tumorarten besitzen ein fast spezifisches Metastasierungsmuster. Gallertcarcinome des Magens neigen zur Metastasierung in die Ovarien. Das Bronchuscarcinom bildet vorwiegend Absiedlungen in der Leber, den Nebennieren, den Knochen und im Gehirn. Hingegen metastasieren Mamma-, Prostata- und Schilddrüsencarcinome vorwiegend in das Skelettsystem [4, 7, 8]. Ebenso weisen eine Anzahl von Transplantationstumoren [3, 5, 6, 9, 12, 15] charakteristische Metastasierungsmuster auf. Die Tatsache der elektiven Metastasierung führt zu der Frage, auf welchen Faktoren die Resistenz eines Organs gegen einen bestimmten Tumor beruht. Als Deutungsmöglichkeit könnte eine organtypische Abwehr gegen bestimmte Tumorarten angenommen werden. Jedoch bleibt die Frage offen, inwieweit es sich um eine Leistung des Organs handelt. In gleicher Weise könnten manche Organe für bestimmte Tumoren einen ungeeigneten Mutterboden darstellen.

Zur weiteren Untersuchung dieser Fragestellung haben wir in Modellversuchen Zellen von zwei verschiedenen Transplantationstumoren der Ratte quantitativ mit unterschiedlichen Zellzahlen in verschiedene Organe und Gewebe implantiert und die Angangsrate an den Inoculationsorten kontrolliert. Vorwiegend interessierten dabei die Fragen, ob sich beide Tumorarten bei diesem Verfahren gleichsinnig verhalten und ob sich Unterschiede zwischen den verschiedenen Organen hinsichtlich der für eine erfolgreiche Verimpfung benötigten Zellzahl ergeben.

Methodik

Zur Anwendung kamen das Yoshida-Sarkom und das DS-Carcino-sarkom der Ratte in Ascitesform. Die biologischen Eigenschaften der Tumoren sind bekannt [9, 19]. Nach der Methode von SCHMÄHL u. MECKE [10] erfolgte die Bestimmung der Anzahl der Tumorzellen im Ascites. Vor der Implantation wurde der Tumorascites mit Ringer-Lösung verdünnt, zentrifugiert und in Ringer-Lösung resuspendiert. (Der Glucosezusatz der verwendeten Ringer-Lösung betrug 200 mg%). Nach Bestimmung des Gehaltes an Tumorzellen erfolgte eine weitere Ver-dünnung mit Ringer-Lösung in der Form, daß die zur Implantation gewünschte Zellzahl in 0,05 ml der Suspension enthalten war.

Für die Versuche wurden insgesamt 1160 junge männliche Wistar-Ratten (Koloniezucht IVANOVAS) im Gewicht von 100 g verwendet.

Folgende Implantationsorte wählten wir:

1. Großhirn	8. Niere
2. Glaskörper (Auge)	9. Blasenschleimhaut
3. Pleuraraum	10. Testes
4. Äußere Magenwand	11. Markraum des Femur
5. Milz	12. Muskulatur (Oberschenkel)
6. Leber	13. Subcutis
7. Dünndarmschleimhaut	14. Peritonealraum

Außerdem wurden die Tumorsuspensionen oral bzw. intravenös appliziert.

Für jeden Einzelversuch wurden die Tumorzellen nur von einem Spendertier entnommen, entsprechend verdünnt und auf die Empfänger-tiere (10 Ratten pro Lokalisation) übertragen. Die Implantation in Magenwand, Milz, Leber, Niere, Dünndarm- und Blasenschleimhaut, Glaskörper sowie Markraum des Femur erfolgte in Nembutal-Äther-Narkose. Die Organe des Bauchraumes wurden dabei operativ freigelegt. Die Implantation in die Schleimhäute des Darmes und der Blase erfolgte mit einer kurzgeschliffenen Kanüle Nr. 20. Es konnte gut verfolgt werden, ob die Infiltrationen der Schleimhäute gelungen waren. Die nicht schon vorher an Tumoren gestorbenen Ratten wurden 6 Wochen nach der Impfung getötet und seziert. Als Beurteilungskriterium diente das *makroskopische* Geschwulstwachstum in den einzelnen Organen.

Da die Tumorübertragung für das jeweils zu beimpfende Tierkollektiv ca. 4 Std benötigte, wurde die Tumorzell-Suspension auf einem mit gerin-ger Umdrehungszahl eingestellten Magnetrührer unter Eiskühlung auf-bewahrt. Um das Wachstumsverhalten der verwendeten Tumorzellen zu prüfen, injizierten wir jeweils 5 Ratten mit 10^7 Zellen intraperitoneal, wie es der routinemäßigen Implantation entspricht, und bestimmten die Angangsraten und Angangszeiten, welche stets in der Norm lagen.

Ergebnisse

Die Angangsraten des Yoshida-Ascites-Sarkoms und des DS-Carcinosarkoms nach Verimpfung in verschiedene Organe und Gewebe in Abhängigkeit von der Zellzahl finden sich in Tab. 1. Als positiv wurden nur diejenigen Tiere gewertet, bei denen es am Implantationsort zu einem makroskopisch nachweisbaren Tumorwachstum kam. Einige Ratten starben an Geschwulstmanifestationen, welche entfernt vom Implantationsort (in anderen Organen) auftraten. Diese Tiere wurden in Tab. 1

Tabelle 1. *Angangsraten des Yoshida-Sarkoms (Yo.-Sa.) und des DS-Carcinosarkoms (DS-CS) in verschiedenen, mit Tumorzellen geimpften Organen bei Ratten in Abhängigkeit von der inoculierten Zellmenge*
(— = Versuch nicht durchgeführt)

Beimpftes Organ	Tumorangang bei Zellzahl							
	10^1		10^2		10^3		10^4	
	Yo.-Sa.	DS-CS	Yo.-Sa.	DS-CS	Yo.-Sa.	DS-CS	Yo.-Sa.	DS-CS
Gehirn	0/10	0/10	0/10	0/10	3/10	3/10	6/10	—
Auge	0/10	0/10	2/10	8/10	3/10	—	9/10	—
Pleuraraum	1/20	2/10	9/40	13/30	6/20	—	—	—
Magenwand	0/10	0/10	2/10	0/20	1/20	5/10	6/10	—
Milz	0/10	0/10	2/10	2/20	4/20	2/10	2/10	—
Leber	0/10	0/20	2/10	7/10	1/20	—	1/10	—
Dünndarm	0/10	0/10	1/10	4/20	2/20	7/10	5/10	—
Niere	0/20	1/20	10/30	9/10	10/10	—	10/10	—
Blase	0/10	2/10	3/20	8/30	8/20	—	—	—
Hoden	3/10	0/10	3/10	3/10	4/10	5/20	10/10	8/10
Knochen	0/10	0/10	0/10	0/10	0/10	0/10	0/10	—
Muskel	0/10	0/10	2/10	1/10	1/10	8/10	6/10	—
Subcutis	0/10	0/10	1/10	8/10	1/10	—	5/10	—
Peritonealraum	2/10	0/10	2/10	0/10	4/10	9/10	7/10	10/10
intravenös	0/10	0/10	0/10	0/10	0/10	0/10	0/10	6/10
peroral	0/10	0/10	0/10	0/10	0/10	0/10	1/20	—

nicht als positiv bewertet. Eine Diskussion dieser Befunde erfolgt weiter unten. Aus der Tabelle geht hervor, daß zwischen der Zahl der implantierten Zellen und der Häufigkeit des Tumorangangs eine deutliche Relation besteht. Das DS-Carcinosarkom weist insgesamt eine höhere Angangsrate auf als das Yoshida-Sarkom. Nach Transplantation von 10^2 DS-Tumorzellen unter Berücksichtigung aller Transplantationsorte kam es bei 27% (63/230) Ratten zu einem Tumorwachstum. Nach Transplantation von 10^3 DS-Tumorzellen ergab sich bei 36% (39/110) ein positives Ergebnis. Hingegen liegen die entsprechenden Werte für das Yoshida-Sarkom bei 18% (39/220) resp. 22% (48/220).

Die bessere Transplantabilität des DS-Carcinosarkoms zeigte sich auch, wenn man die mittlere Zellzahl (D_{50}) berücksichtigt, die in den einzelnen Organen und Geweben notwendig war, um bei 50% der Tiere einen Geschwulstangang zu erreichen. Diese lag für das DS-Carcinosarkom bei Beimpfung des Glaskörpers bei etwa 50 Tumorzellen; hingegen benötigte das Yoshida-Sarkom bei der gleichen Lokalisation 5×10^3 Zellen. Für die Magenwand ergab sich ein Unterschied der D_{50} von 10^3 beim DS-Carcinosarkom zu 10^4 beim Yoshida-Sarkom, während sich bei intramuskulärer Implantation noch größere Unterschiede (5×10^2 zu 10^4) zeigten. Hingegen ergaben sich zwischen beiden Tumorarten bei Implantation in die Testes und in das Gehirn keine deutlichen Unterschiede. Hieraus läßt sich ein Einfluß des Implantationsortes auf das Wachstumsverhalten des Tumors erkennen.

In die gleiche Richtung wiesen weitere Befunde. Die Niere bildete den geeignetsten Implantationsort. Es genügten 10^2 Tumorzellen des Yoshida-Sarkoms, um eine Angangsrate von 33% zu erreichen, während beim DS-Carcinosarkom nach 10^2 Tumorzellen die Angangsrate bei 90% lag. Hingegen kam es auch nach Implantation von 10^4 Tumorzellen in den Markraum des Femurs bei beiden Tumorarten zu keiner Geschwulstentwicklung. Ähnliche Resultate ergaben sich beim Vergleich der intravenösen oder intralienalen Implantation mit den Ergebnissen der Angangsrate in der Niere oder im Auge.

Insbesondere weisen die Ergebnisse der Implantationsversuche in die Leber auf eine Wechselwirkung zwischen der Leber und dem Yoshida-Sarkom hin. Schon in früheren Versuchen [11, 12] fiel auf, daß der von uns verwendete Stamm des Yoshida-Sarkoms in der Leber niemals zu einem soliden Geschwulstwachstum führt. Sogar die intraportale Injektion großer Mengen des Yoshida-Ascites-Sarkoms [12] erweist sich als wirkungslos. In gleicher Weise besitzt eine Leberschädigung durch verschiedene hepatotoxische Agentien keinen Einfluß auf den Tumorangang in der Leber [11, 13, 14]. Die Ergebnisse der direkten Implantation in die Leber bestätigen die früheren Beobachtungen. Obwohl durch diesen Eingriff am Implantationsort ein zusätzliches Trauma gesetzt wird, kommt es nur ausnahmsweise zur Tumorentwicklung. Histologisch ließen sich in diesen Fällen in der Leber zahlreiche Tumorzellen nachweisen; jedoch bestand keine Wachstumstendenz. Im Gegensatz hierzu führte beim DS-Carcinosarkom die Transplantation von 10^2 Tumorzellen bei mehr als der Hälfte der Tiere zu einem ausgedehnten Geschwulstwachstum in der Leber, das sich in zahlreichen erbs- bis bohnengroßen Tumorknoten manifestierte. Es bestehen somit grundsätzliche Unterschiede im Verhalten des Tumorwachstums in der Leber zwischen beiden Tumorzellarten. Es ergibt sich zwischen Implantationserfolg und Metastasierungsverhalten eine Parallelität. Das DS-Carcinosarkom bildet häufig Lebermetastasen, während das verwendete Yoshida-Sarkom nie in die Leber metastasiert.

Die Latenzzeiten vom Tage der Implantation bis zum Tod der Tiere lagen zwischen 14 und 42 Tagen und zeigten keine Abhängigkeit vom verwendeten Tumortyp. Außerdem ergab sich keine deutliche Abhängigkeit von der Anzahl der implantierten Tumorzellen. Die kürzeste Latenzzeit beobachteten wir nach Implantation in die Niere oder in die Bauchhöhle. Am langsamsten entwickelten sich die Geschwülste in der Magenwand und in der Skelettmuskulatur.

Eine ausführliche Darstellung der makroskopischen Befunde der entstandenen Tumoren übersteigt den Rahmen der Arbeit. Daher seien nur einige charakteristische Befunde hervorgehoben. Die Geschwülste konnten in den beimpften Organen eine enorme Größe erreichen. Dieses Verhalten zeigte sich besonders nach Implantation in die Niere. Häufig metastasierten die Primärtumoren in die regionalen Lymphdrüsen und in parenchymatöse Organe, wobei das Yoshida-Sarkom vorwiegend im Mesenterium, in den Nebennieren, im Thymus und im Pankreas Absiedlungen bildete. Hingegen bevorzugte das DS-Carcinosarkom Leber, Mesenterium und Nieren. Bei Geschwulstabsiedlungen im Bauchraum entstand häufig blutiger Ascites. Ebenso kam es bei einer Tumorentwicklung in Lunge oder Pleura zu einem Hämothorax.

Eine interessante Variante stellen die Ratten dar, bei welchen es entfernt vom Implantationsort zum Tumorwachstum kam. Beim Yoshida-Sarkom beobachteten wir nach Übertragung von 10^2 Zellen in die Milz nur bei 2 von 10 Tieren eine Tumorentwicklung am Implantationsort. Bei weiteren zwei Tieren bildeten sich Geschwülste im Milzmesenterium, in den Nebennieren, im Thymus und in der Lunge. Nach Inoculation von 10^3 oder 10^4 Yoshida-Ascites-Tumorzellen in die Milz entstanden neben den Organtumoren (4/10 resp. 2/10 Tiere) noch bei zwei resp. fünf weiteren Tieren Absiedlungen, die vorwiegend im Mesenterium, den Nebennieren und im Pankreas lokalisiert waren. Nach Implantation des DS-Carcinosarkoms in die Milz wuchsen bei 17 Ratten Absiedlungen außerhalb des Implantationsortes (1 Tier nach intralienaler Injektion von 10 DS-Tumorzellen, 10 Tiere nach 10^2 DS-Tumorzellen und 6 Tiere nach 10^3 DS-Tumorzellen). Prädilektionsstellen bildeten Mesenterium, Leber und Lunge. Auch nach Übertragung von 10^2 (5 Tiere), 10^3 (4 Tiere) und 10^4 (4 Tiere) Yoshida-Sarkomzellen in die Leber traten bei insgesamt 13 Tieren Geschwülste im Mesenterium, den abdominalen Lymphknoten und den Nebennieren auf. Bei insgesamt 5 Ratten kam es nach Übertragung des Yoshida-Sarkoms in ein Organ des Bauchraumes zu Tumoren in der Operationsnarbe. Da ein Teil der Bauchwandtumoren mit dem Tumor der Implantationsstelle verbunden war, dürfte es sich vorwiegend um eine direkte Einbringung in das Wundbett handeln.

Diskussion

Das wesentliche Ergebnis der Untersuchungen besteht in der Beobachtung, daß die Vermehrungsfähigkeit von Tumorzellen im Empfänger nicht nur eine Funktion ihrer Transplantabilität darstellt, sondern auch entscheidend vom Implantationsort (Mutterboden) mitbestimmt wird. Daher müssen Wechselwirkungen zwischen Tumorart und Mutterboden angenommen werden. Dafür sprechen die enormen Unterschiede der Tumorangangsrate in Abhängigkeit vom Implantationsort und der Art der Geschwulst. Die Unterschiede zwischen dem Transplantationserfolg nach intraperitonealer und intravenöser Gabe erklären sich möglicherweise u. a. aus der Tatsache, daß es im strömenden Blut zu einer raschen Verdünnung der Tumorzellen kommt und somit die für einen positiven Tumorangang kritische Zellzahl unterschritten wird. Ähnliche Beobachtungen bestehen auch beim Vergleich des Transplantationserfolges nach Übertragung von Tumorzellen in die Lymph- oder Blutbahn [16].

Zwar zeigten frühere Beobachtungen am Yoshida-Sarkom [10, 12], daß dieser Tumor in relativ hoher Ausbeute mit einer Zelle übertragbar war, in den vorliegenden Versuchen wurden jedoch etwa 10^3 Tumorzellen benötigt. Einerseits bleibt kein Transplantationstumor in seinen biologischen Eigenschaften stabil, da ständig innerhalb einer Zellpopulation Mutationen ablaufen. Andererseits können geringfügige genetische Unterschiede der Spender- und Empfängertiere eine Veränderung der Transplantabilität hervorrufen. Außerdem existieren 50 verschiedene Stämme des Yoshida-Sarkoms [19], welche erhebliche Unterschiede im Wachstumsverhalten und in der Metastasierung aufweisen. Die Ergebnisse gelten daher nur für die bei uns verwendeten Tumorstämme. Für die grundsätzlichen Befunde besitzen diese Einzelheiten allerdings keine Bedeutung.

Die Ergebnisse stehen in einem engen Zusammenhang mit dem Metastasierungsvorgang. Die Wechselwirkungen zwischen Tumorzellen und Organ entscheiden das Zustandekommen, die Entwicklung und die Lokalisation der Metastasen. Weitere Untersuchungen dieser Frage sollen nähere Einblicke in das Phänomen der Metastasierung ermöglichen.

Zusammenfassung

Zellen des Yoshida-Sarkoms (Ascitesform) und des DS-Carcinosarkoms (Ascitesform) wurden mit unterschiedlichen Zellzahlen (10^1–10^4) in 16 verschiedene Organe und Gewebe von Ratten implantiert. Vor allem in der Niere kam es nach Übertragung bereits kleiner Zellzahlen zur Tumorentwicklung. Hingegen kam es auch bei Verwendung von 10^4 Tumorzellen im Markraum des Femur zu keinem Tumorangang. Die Yoshida-

Sarkomzellen wuchsen bei Implantation in die Leber nur ausnahmsweise, während die DS-Carcinosarkomzellen in der Leber in hoher Ausbeute Tumoren bildeten. Für das Zustandekommen des metastatischen Tumorwachstums ist neben der Transplantabilität auch das Organmilieu entscheidend, in welches die Tumorzellen hineingelangen.

Literatur

1. CAIN, H.: Hämatogene Geschwulstzellenentwicklung in der Lunge, unter besonderer Berücksichtigung sog. regelwidriger Fälle. Z. Krebsforsch. **62**, 323 (1958).
2. COMAN, D. R., R. P. DE LONG, and MC. CUTCHEON: Studies on the Mechanisms of Metastasis. The Distribution of Tumors in Various Organs in Relation to the Distribution of Arterial Emboli. Cancer Res. **11**, 648 (1951).
3. DRUCKREY, H., H. HAMPERL, H. HERKEN u. B. BAREI: Chirurgische Behandlung von Tiergeschwülsten. Z. Krebsforsch. **48**, 451 (1939).
4. FANFANI, M., E. PIERAGNOLI e A. MORETTINI: Richerchi sulla patogenesis delle metastasi e critica della doltrina dei filtri ablogati. Arch. De Vecchi Anat. pat. **18**, 937 (1952).
5. LUCKÉ, B., C. BREEDIS, Z. P. WOO, L. BERWICK, and P. NOWELL: Differential Growth of Metastatic Tumors in Liver and Lung. Experiments with Rabbit V_2 Carcinoma. Cancer Res. **12**, 734 (1952).
6. SCHAIRER, E.: Über die Resistenz der Rattenleber gegen das Jensen-Sarkom. Z. Krebsforsch. **50**, 329 (1940).
7. SCHINZ. H, R.: Die elektive hämatogene Metastasierung bei Malignomen. Bull. Schweiz. Akad. med. Wiss. **6**, 448 (1950).
8. SCHMÄHL, D.: Krebsmetastasen: Ihre Entstehung und Prophylaxe. Medizinische **9**, 1847 (1959).
9. — Entstehung, Wachstum und Chemotherapie maligner Tumoren. Aulendorf: Editio Cantor 1963.
10. — u. R. MECKE: Quantitative Transplantationsversuche mit dem Yoshida-Ascites-Sarkom der Ratte. Z. Krebsforsch. **60**, 711 (1955).
11. —, H. OSSWALD u. C. THOMAS: Experimentelle Untersuchungen über die Metastasierung des Yoshida-Sarkoms. Z. Krebsforsch. **67**, 141 (1965).
12. — u. TH. RIESEBERG: Experimentelle Untersuchungen an Ratten über die Metastasierung von Tumoren. Z. Krebsforsch. **62**, 456 (1958).
13. — u. W. SATTLER: Der Einfluß der Vorbehandlung von Ratten mit alkylierenden Substanzen und anderen Giften auf das Geschwulstwachstum des Yoshida-Sarkoms. Arzneimittel-Forsch. **14**, 746 (1964).
14. — u. E. STUTZ: Abhängigkeit der Tumorentwicklung bei Ratten nach intravenöser Injektion des Yoshida-Ascites-Sarkoms von vorausgegangener Ganzkörperbestrahlung. Naturwissenschaften **49**, 424 (1962).
15. SUGARBAKER, E. D.: The Organ Selectivity of Experimentally Induced Metastasis in Rats. Cancer **5**, 382 (1954).
16. WALLACE, A. C.: Metastasis as an Aspect of Cell Behaviour. Canad. Cancer Conf. **4**, 139 (1961).
17. WALTHER, H. E.: Untersuchungen über Krebsmetastasen. Z. Krebsforsch. **46**, 313 (1937).
18. — Krebsmetastasen. Bern: Verlag B. Schwabe & Co. 1948.
19. YOSHIDA, T.: Zelluläre Multizentrizität der Krebsentstehung. Dtsch. med. Wschr. **88**, 2229 (1963).

Experimentell-teratologische Aspekte zur Onkologie

Von

KL. GOERTTLER

Jeder Pathologe kann aus der langjährigen Anregung durch den Sektionssaal über Fälle berichten, bei denen die dysgenetische Wurzel einer Neubildung offensichtlich war. Wir wissen auch von der verhältnismäßig seltenen Kombination Tumor und Mißbildung. Die Frage nach dem inneren Zusammenhang bleibt meist dunkel, was eine etwas spöttische Bemerkung von RUDOLF VIRCHOW [18] über den *Mystizismus des Embryonalen* zu bestätigen scheint, zumindest nicht zurückweist.

Es soll geprüft werden, wie weit heute teratologische und onkologische Experimente schlüssige Antwort über die Beziehung zwischen Dysontogenese und Geschwulstwachstum geben können, wo wir noch immer auf Hilfshypothesen angewiesen sind, endlich, in welchem Lichte uns die an die Namen COHNHEIM [4], RIBBERT [16, 17] und ALBRECHT [1] geknüpften Vorstellungen jetzt erscheinen (s. auch K. H. BAUER [2]). Das Problem ist theoretisch, praktisch und prognostisch gleichermaßen bedeutsam; im National Institute of Health in Bethesda beschäftigt sich eine Arbeitsgruppe mit der Materialsichtung und Prüfung möglicher Zusammenhänge.

FRANZ BÜCHNER [3] hat ein einfaches Grundschema abgebildet, das wenig verändert an den Anfang der Diskussion gestellt werden soll (Abb. 1). Danach stehen Differenzierung und Wachstum während des Lebens, also von der Befruchtung bis zum Tod in einer gewissen Wechselbeziehung, indem reziprok mit der Abnahme der plastischen Potenzen eine formale Ausgestaltung erfolgt. Gegen Ende des Lebens bedingen Alterungsvorgänge einen gewissen Differenzierungsabfall, der mit einem Anstieg der einfachen Wachstumsfähigkeit verbunden sein kann. Hier fragen wir nach der Mechanik dieser Koppelung beider Grundvorgänge. Vorzeitiges Altern als Überlastungsfolge durch überbeanspruchte Regeneration infolge wie auch immer beschaffener Schädigung soll Entdifferenzierung, Metaplasie und neoplastische Potenzen freisetzen. Konsequenterweise müßte auch die vorgeburtliche Schädigung ein vorzeitiges Altern und eine weitere Vorverlegung des Zeitpunktes neoplastischer Wachstumsfähigkeit begünstigen. In der Tat lassen sich die in den letzten beiden Jahrzehnten in Amerika und in Deutschland durchgeführten Experimente mit ein- oder mehrmaliger pränataler Schädigung durch Carcinogene als Bestätigung dieser bestechenden These interpretieren.

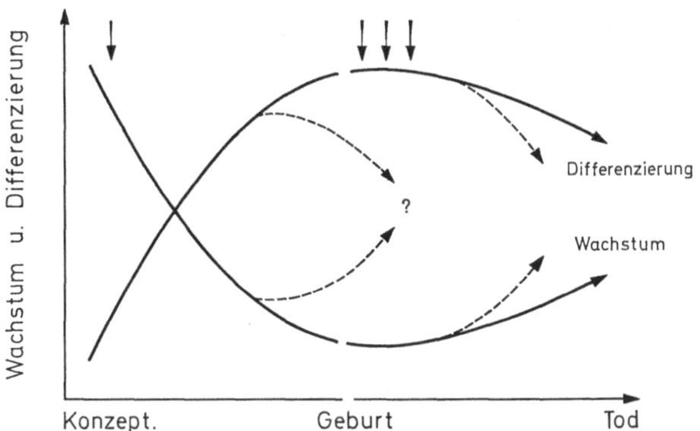

Abb. 1. Wachstum und Differenzierung in ihrem gegenläufigen Verhalten während des Lebens. Gestrichelte Pfeile deuten Differenzierungsverlust (bzw. Entdifferenzierung) und erneute Wachstumstendenz an; abwärts gerichtete Pfeile = prä- bzw. postnatale Belastung oder Schädigung

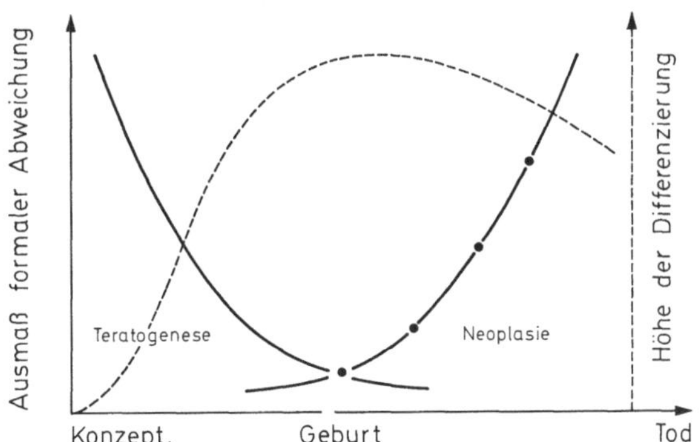

Abb. 2. Teratogenese und neoplastisches Wachstum im Laufe des Individualzyklus zwischen Befruchtung und Tod. Durchgezogene Linie = Determinationsperiode sowie Häufigkeit der Entstehung von Mißbildungen; durch Punkte unterbrochene Linie = Sichtbarwerden bzw. Häufigkeit von Neoplasmen. Höhe und Ablauf der Differenzierung (s. Abb. 1) sind als gestrichelte Linien zur Übersicht miteingetragen

Bei empirischem Vorgehen bringen uns einfache Überlegungen in gewisse Schwierigkeiten. In Abb. 2 ist das Ausmaß möglicher Deformation zum sichtbaren Anstieg neoplastischen Wachstums und zur Lebenszeit eines Individuum in Beziehung gesetzt. Zur Übersicht ist auch noch der Differenzierungsablauf aus Abb. 1 hinzugefügt. Mißbildungen werden nur im ersten Drittel der Pränatalzeit induziert, Neoplasien sind dagegen meist erst viele Jahrzehnte später nachweisbar. Dies zwingt zu Überlegungen, ob durch den Mißbildungsvorgang eine Veränderung der Grundsituation erzeugt und hierdurch der Startpunkt für neoplastisches Wachstum in eine frühere Lebensperiode vorverlegt wurde. Dazu müssen wir wissen, mit welchen formalen Möglichkeiten während der Teratogenese zu rechnen ist. Man kann mit verschiedenen Carcinogenen Mißbildungen erzeugen (instruktive Zusammenfassung: DI PAOLO u. KOTIN [7]). Auf eine dabei wirksame *Substratspezifität* soll nicht näher eingegangen werden, sie hängt mit unterschiedlichen Wirkungsmechanismen zusammen. Eine *Phasenspezifität* bestimmt innerhalb gewisser Grenzen, zu welchem Zeitpunkt eine Noxe eingewirkt haben muß, um ein abgrenzbares Spektrum von Mißbildungen zu erzeugen. Einzelne Organe mit hoher Wachstumsintensität sind besonders empfindlich.

Im Gefolge der Schädigung des Embryo kommt es kurze Zeit später zu Nekrosen, die wir besonders am embryonalen ZNS beobachten konnten, dabei auch zu Blutungen (GOERTTLER [8]). Wartet man mit der Untersuchung etwas länger, ist das noch sichtbare Ausmaß der Zerstörung oft überraschend gering. Selbst schwere Schäden werden narbenlos im Sinne einer Restitutio ad integrum beseitigt. Wenn das Ausmaß des gesetzten Schadens besonders groß ist, bleiben minimale bis erhebliche Restzustände zurück, unter Umständen bis zum Zusammenbruch der bereits gebildeten Struktur. Auch dann bemüht sich das noch zur Regeneration fähige Gewebe um eine möglichst nahe an den alten Formbildungsauftrag heranreichende Formgebung. Das Resultat ist zwar eine Mißbildung, zugleich aber auch ein Versuch des Organismus, nach Zerstörung der Kontinuität mit einem Defizit an verfügbarer Zellmasse die alte Form, so gut es irgend geht, wieder aufzubauen. Hier steht die Mißbildung im scharfen Gegensatz zur Geschwulst, in deren Pathogenese gerade das Bestreben nach gehöriger Einpassung fehlt. Damit werden Äußerungen verständlich, nach denen man eher adultes als embryonales Gewebe mit Geschwulstgewebe vergleichen könne, schon gar nicht eine Mißbildung und eine Geschwulst. Die eine steht am Anfang, die andere am Ende der Entwicklungsreihe eines Blastemes; beide sind Antipoden des Wachstums; hier Differenzierung bei meist verminderter Masse, dort mangelnde Differenzierung bei unbeschränktem Massenwachstum.

Wir kehren zur Frage zurück, ob eine deformative Entwicklungsstörung als Basis für neoplastisches Wachstum zu werten ist. In Abb. 3 wurde der normale Differenzierungsablauf eines Individualzyklus mit Anstieg und Abfall eingezeichnet und die Determinationsperioden deformativer Störungen, und zwar sowohl die dysgenetische als auch die neoplastische Formabweichung, senkrecht schraffiert. Die durch Cancerogene oder andere Substanzen erzeugte Schädigung bedeutet kurzzeitig oder definitiv eine Abweichung vom normalen Entwicklungsprozeß. Dann wird der Normalwert nicht mehr erreicht, nur noch ein quasi-stationärer Defektzustand, also eine Pathie. Dürfen wir unterstellen, daß hiermit eine Einschränkung der regenerativen Kapazität verbunden ist? Bisher gibt es keine systematischen Untersuchungen, die eine schlüssige Antwort erlauben. Hier müßte die am postnatalen Organismus nach gesetzter Schädigung durchgeführte Technik der autoradiographischen Untersuchung weiterhelfen. Einige Indizien sprechen für unsere Annahme: Das

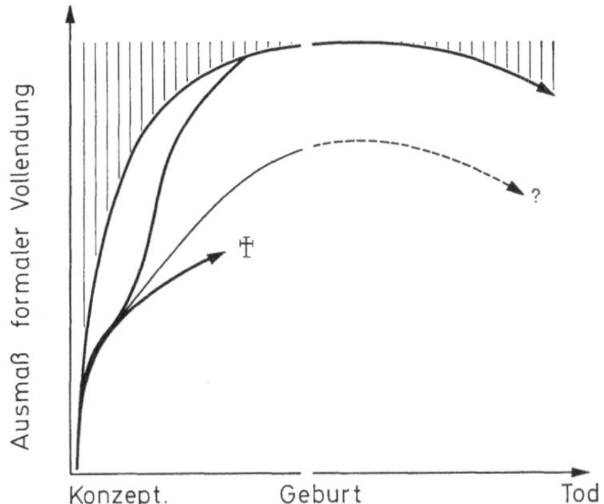

Abb. 3. Der Differenzierungsablauf unter normalen und pathologischen Bedingungen in Beziehung zu teratologischer und neoplastischer Deformation (Einzelheiten s. Text)

Schädigungsexperiment zeigt bei normal erscheinenden Individuen in der Lupendimension oder im histologischen Detail eine Fülle von Mikroläsionen, die sich z. B. an der Wirbelsäule durch Reduktion der Spongiosa-Strukturen zu erkennen geben. Ähnliche oder vergleichbare Bilder sahen wir nach Thalidomid-Applikation, z. T. mit einer Fülle von Abnormitäten an anderen Wirbelkörpern kombiniert, die uns den Gedanken nahelegten, daß hier auch die Strukturerhaltung gestört sein dürfte, also die physiologische Regeneration. Wir beobachteten entsprechende Schäden an der Wirbelsäule eines Kindes mit Thalidomid-Embryopathie und konnten damit den viele Jahre zuvor (GOERTTLER [8]) theoretisch geforderten Zusammenbruch des unterwertigen Organes auch für die menschliche Pathologie bestätigen.

Wir dürfen die unzureichende Formerhaltung als Indiz für Störungen der regenerativen Kapazität einsetzen. Wie steht es aber mit der Frage, ob der nächste Schritt vom Absinken der Differenzierungshöhe zur Fehlregeneration und der darauf folgende von dieser in das neoplastische Wachstum führt? Vor einigen Jahren erzeugten wir mit dem Mesenchymgift Beta-amino-propio-nitril, der Wirksubstanz des Lathyrusfaktors, embryonale Blutungen bis zur Verblutung aus Herz und Gefäßen (GOERTTLER u. HARTMANN [9]). In einigen Fällen wurde die Schädigung überstanden, und es kam erst während des Schlupfes der Küken zum Tod. Wir fanden bei einem Keim eine polycystische Nierenmißbildung, also eine Störung an der Grenze zwischen Mißbildung und Geschwulst.

In unsere Überlegungen, wie man sich den Übergang vorstellen soll, fiel eine Beobachtung aus der menschlichen Pathologie. Wir erhielten Gewebe aus der Oberschenkelcyste eines 4jährigen Thalidomid-geschädigten Kindes, dachten zuerst an eine einfache Knochencyste, klassifizierten später nach einigem Zögern das Bild als Osteoid-Fibrom. Der Tumor entstand auf dem Boden einer gesicherten Vorschädigung und in Verbindung mit manifesten Mißbildungen. Wir sind damit aber unserem Problem nur einen Teilschritt näher gekommen. Der von uns beobachtete Fall blieb bisher der einzige, und die Kürze der Beobachtungszeit erlaubt noch keine weitere Stellungnahme. Immerhin fällt bei Kindern mit Thalidomid-Embryopathie eine Neigung zur Keloidbildung auf, also eine Tendenz zu überschüssigem, über die Notwendigkeit der Wundheilung hinausgehendem, nicht ganz eingepaßtem Regenerationswachstum.

Zusammenfassend ist festzustellen, daß eine Schädigung gleichwelcher Art, ob durch Carcinogene und Teratogene oder Substanzen ohne bekannte Carcinogenität einen Schaden an einem kompetenten, empfindlichem Blasten erzeugt. Dieser kann ausheilen. Gelingt das nicht, bleibt eine Wachstumsarretierung oder ein locus minoris resistentiae zurück oder eine echte Mißbildung. Jene können zum sekundären Zusammenbruch und über eine unvollkommene Regeneration zum Fehlregenerattumor führen. Wir bleiben verpflichtet, unsere an Hand von Indizien gestellte Arbeitshypothese weiter zu prüfen.

Wir fragen nunmehr, ob die experimentelle Geschwulstforschung, ergänzende Angaben liefern kann. 1940 berichtete LAW [11] über die experimentelle Erzeugung von Tumoren durch Injektion eines Carcinogens in die Amnionflüssigkeit, und 1947 konnte LARSEN [10] Lungentumoren durch transplacentare Exposition gegen Urethan erzeugen. 1962 beobachteten DRUCKREY u. STEINHOFF [5] bei ihren Experimenten mit Diäthylnitrosamin ein Jungtier mit Leberkrebs, dessen Mutter 100 Tage nach Behandlungsbeginn Junge geworfen hatte, diskutierten einen Übertritt der leichtlöslichen Substanz durch die Placenta und die Milch. Hiervon unabhängig haben MOHR u. Mitarb. [12, 13, 14] bei systematischen Versuchen am Goldhamster Tumoren durch transplacentare Induktion entstehen sehen und konnten durch Ammenversuche den Übertritt der Substanz mit der Milch ausschließen. Sie fanden in der Niere der Jungtiere neben adenomatösen Regeneratwucherungen an den Tubuli contorti I. Ordnung auch Nierenpapillome, weiterhin Tumoren des

Respirationstraktes. DRUCKREY u. Mitarb. [6] haben 1967 in ihrer Sammelarbeit über die carcinogene Wirkung von Nitroso-Verbindungen ein Kapitel über diaplacentare Geschwulstentstehung, sogar nach einmaliger Applikation der Substanz eingefügt und bilden in dieser Arbeit eine Extremitätenmißbildung ab. Also auch hier Fehlregenerate, manifeste Schäden, Mißbildungen, gut- und bösartige Tumoren, wobei die sonst selten beobachteten Geschwülste der Neuroglia in überraschender Anzahl nachweisbar waren.

Schädigung, Zerstörung, mangelhafter Ersatz sind als Teile einer Reihe verständlich und gut begründbar. Der erste Sprung in die Metaplasie und in den Differenzierungsverlust und der zweite in die echte Neoplasie bleiben nach wie vor problematisch. Auf die Mutationstheorie soll hier nicht eingegangen werden. Wir benötigen weitere Hinweise über den Nucleoproteidstoffwechsel und Kerngrößenbestimmungen.

Vielleicht ist aber die geschädigte Zelle gar nicht allein und direkt, sondern erst auf einem Umweg für die Neoplasie verantwortlich. COHN-HEIM (1877) und ALBRECHT (1967) beschuldigten bekanntlich liegengebliebene, pluripotente Blasteme, und nach RIBBERT (1904, 1906) genügten sogar traumatisch abgesprengte, in ein zwar ernährendes, aber nicht kompetentes Blastem verlagerte Epithelkomplexe. Welche Anhaltspunkte ergeben sich hierfür aus dem teratologischen und dem onkologischen Experiment? Nach Einwirkung von Cytostatica kann man mitunter eine komplette Zersprengung des Rückenmarkes beobachten, Röntgenstrahlen erzeugen das gleiche Bild. Statt eines einzigen sehen wir mehrere Zentralkanäle. Zu einem Zeitpunkt, der sonst eine deutliche Differenzierung erkennen läßt, bleibt ein primitives, pluripotentes Blastem zurück. Auch die Ursegmentseitenplatten haben sich – wohl bei fehlender Induktion – nicht mehr ausgebildet: Der Kairos, der günstige Zeitpunkt zum Aufbau einer Struktur, ist verstrichen. Also eine Geschwulstkeimanlage im Sinne der alten Autoren. Der Schritt in die Neoplasie ist natürlich leichter zu verstehen, wenn man (wie auch bei den Retinarosetten im Augapfel mikrophthalmer menschlicher Neugeborenen) mit einem bereits partiell aus dem Gewebsverband herausgesprengten Blastem bei noch vorhandener regenerativer Potenz rechnen kann.

Auch die experimentelle Onkologie gibt uns einen interessanten Hinweis: NOTHDURFT [15] implantierte bei Ratten chemisch inerte Alloplastiken mit unterschiedlicher Wölbung in die Subcutis. Er sah Sarkome am schnellsten dort entstehen, wo sich durch die Gestalt des Implantates ein lockeres Füllgewebe zwischen straff gespannter Narbenkapsel und Fremdkörper eingelagert hatte, also an der Konkavität von Krümmungen. Hier bewirkte die Form des Implantates Persistenz eines lockeren, für die narbige Differenzierung offenbar nicht gebrauchten, aber dennoch wachstumsbereiten Blastems.

Wir fragen nach den Beziehungen zwischen pränataler Zersprengung und Ablagerung eines nicht für Differenzierungsprozesse benötigten Gewebes. Beiden gemeinsam ist die vorausgehende Gewebsstörung und eine auf verschiedene Ursachen beziehbare Aussonderung aus dem normalen Bauplan. Zellen, die nicht differenziert, d. h. zu „vernünftiger" Arbeit eingesetzt werden oder eingesetzt werden können, betreiben Mikrorevolutionen oder – um einen Vergleich aus unserem staatlichen Leben zu verwenden: Soziale Unruhen und Rassenkrawalle im Organismus des Körpers entstehen durch dessen Unfähigkeit, die Kapazität der Zellindividuen zu nutzen und ihre Aktivitäten in sinnvolle Arbeit zu transformieren. Das Narbenneurom ist eine Regenerationsgeschwulst. Werden schon während der Markreifung Leitungsbahnen unterbrochen, dann ist es gar nicht so verwunderlich, wenn viel später einmal Gliome des Zentralnervensystemes auf einem solchermaßen vorbereiteten Boden bei vorhandenem wachstumsbereiten Material entstehen.

Mißbildungen sind in den Organismus eingegliederte Deformationen auf dem Boden einer pränatalen Schädigung. Die Schädigung, nicht die Mißbildung ist Voraussetzung für neoplastisches Wachstum. Auch wenn keine Mißbildung entstand, könnte eine nicht mehr nachweisbare embryonale oder fetale Krankheit abgelaufen sein, die zu einer Erschöpfung der regenerativen Kapazität oder auch zu einer Bereitstellung von Material führte, das durch örtliche Narbenbildungen oder andere Behinderung nicht sinnvoll eingebaut werden kann und dann als Geschwulstkeimanlage zur Verfügung steht. Betrachtet man aus dieser Sicht die menschliche Carcinogenese, dann kann die Ursache eines noch gar nicht abschätzbaren Anteiles von Tumoren auch in einer Alteration während der plastischen Phase des betroffenen Organes gesucht werden.

Aus meiner Sicht ist die alte Alternative Dysontogenese oder postnatale Geschwulstentstehung kein logischer Gegensatz. Sie bezieht sich vielmehr auf ein unterschiedliches Spektrum von Folgeerscheinungen durch Änderung der Reaktionsbereitschaft des Organismus oder eines Organes zwischen Befruchtung und Tod. Ich sehe keine „Mystik des Embryonalen", dafür aber viele unbeantwortete Fragen und ein noch weitgehend unerforschtes Arbeitsgebiet. Für mich ist der alte Streit zwischen VIRCHOW und COHNHEIM reduziert auf einen mehr statischen und einen mehr dynamischen Aspekt des gleichen Grundvorganges. Die Regeln, nach denen der Organismus reagiert, sind die gleichen, auch die pathogenetischen Mechanismen, während das Resultat verschieden sein kann. Die Beziehungen zwischen Anlagestörung und Geschwulstwachstum sind einer logischen Bearbeitung zugänglich.

Der Streit um Meinungen behindert erfahrungsgemäß die Erkundung von Tatsachen. Sicherer Besitz der Wissenschaft sind aber nie Meinungen, sondern nur Tatsachen.

Literatur

1. ALBRECHT, F.: Grundprobleme der Geschwulstlehre. Frankfurt. Z. Path. **1**, 221, 377 (1907).
2. BAUER, K. H.: Das Krebsproblem. 2. Aufl. Berlin-Göttingen-Heidelberg: Springer 1963.
3. BÜCHNER, F.: Allgemeine Pathologie. Pathologie als Biologie und als Beitrag zur Lehre vom Menschen. 5. Aufl. München-Berlin-Wien: Urban & Schwarzenberg 1966.
4. COHNHEIM, J.: Vorlesungen über allgemeine Pathologie. Ein Handbuch für Ärzte und Studirende. Bd. I. Berlin: August Hirschwald 1877.
5. DRUCKREY, H. u. D. STEINHOFF: Erzeugung von Leberkrebs an Meerschweinchen. Naturwissenschaften **49**, 497 (1962).
6. —, R. PREUSSMNAN, S. IVANKOVIC u. D. SCHMÄHL: Organotrope carcinogene Wirkungen bei 65 verschiedenen N-Nitroso-Verbindungen an BD-Ratten. Z. Krebsforsch. **69**, 103 (1967).
7. DI PAOLO, J. and P. KOTIN: Teratogenesis-Oncogenesis. A Study of Possible Relationships. Arch. Path. **81**, 3 (1966).
8. GOERTTLER, KL.: Die Ätiopathogenese angeborener Entwicklungsstörungen vom Standpunkt des Pathologen. Verh. 1. Europ. Anatomenkongreß Straßburg 1960. Anat. Anz. Erg. Heft zu Bd. **109**, (1960/61).
9. — u. F. HARTMANN: Histopathologische Befunde am Hühnchenkeim nach Applikation von Beta-Aminopropionitril (BAPN; Lathyrusfaktor). Klin. Wschr. **39**, 1077 (1961).
10. LARSEN, C. D.: Pulmonary-Tumor Induction by Transplacental Exposure to Urethane. J. nat. Cancer Inst. **8**, 63 (1947).
11. LAW, L. W.: The Production of Tumors by Injection of a Carcinogen into the Amniotic Fluid of Mice. Science **91**, 96 (1940).
12. MOHR, U.: Die Cancerogenese durch Diäthylnitrosamin beim Goldhamster. Untersuchungen zur diaplacentaren Wirkung. Habil. Schrift Univ. Heidelberg 1967.
13. — u. J. ALTHOFF: Mögliche diaplacentar-carcinogene Wirkung von Diäthylnitrosamin beim Goldhamster. Naturwissenschaften **51**, 515 (1964).
14. — — Die diaplacentare Wirkung des Cancerogens Diäthylnitrosamin bei der Maus. Z. Krebsforsch. **67**, 152 (1965).
15. NOTHDURFT, H.: Sarkomerzeugung bei Ratten durch implantierte Fremdkörper. Therap. Monat **1961**, 262.
16. RIBBERT, H.: Geschwulstlehre für Ärzte und Studierende. Bonn: Cohen 1904.
17. — Beiträge zur Entstehung der Geschwülste. Ergänzung zur Geschwulstlehre für Ärzte und Studierende. Bonn: Cohen 1906.
18. VIRCHOW, R.: Krankheitswesen und Krankheitsursachen. Virchows Arch. path. Anat. **79**, 1, 185 (1880).

Untersuchungen an einem Plasmocytom des Goldhamsters

a) Morphologie und Verhalten dieses Transplantationstumors in vivo*

Von

U. Mohr

Transplantationstumoren auf Ratten und Mäusen zeigen gewöhnlich einen relativ schnellen Wechsel der biologischen, morphologischen und genetischen Eigenschaften (Lettré [5], Wrba u. Rabes [9] und Eicke, Meiners u. Wrba [2]). Für immunologische und genetische Untersuchungen müssen isogenetische Systeme, d. h. reine Inzuchtstämme, zur Verfügung stehen.

Auf die Sonderstellung des Verhaltens syrischer Goldhamster gegenüber isologen Hauttransplantaten haben Adams, Patt u. Lutz [1], Hildemann u. Walford [3] sowie Schöne [8] hingewiesen. Das Problem der Transplantation in die Backentasche des Hamsters wird dadurch nicht berührt. Die aufgeworfenen Fragen werden z. T. nach Hildemann [4] durch die dem syrischen Goldhamster eigene Schwäche, Isoantigene zu bilden, erklärt. Isologe Hauttransplantate werden, wenn überhaupt, vom syrischen Goldhamster sehr spät abgestoßen. Das bedeutet für den speziellen Fall eines Transplantationstumors einen relativ geringen immunologischen Selektionsdruck auf die Tumortransplantate. Das Wirtstier wird bereits lange vor der möglichen Transplantationsreaktion durch den Tumor getötet. Dementsprechend finden sich weder spontan resistente Tiere, noch lassen sich durch geeignete Maßnahmen resistente Tiere gegen Nicht-Virus-Tumoren erzeugen. Diese besonderen Bedingungen erklären auch die Tumorangehrate mit 100%. Ausdruck der ungewöhnlich biologischen Konstanz des KG-13-Plasmocytoms ist darüber hinaus sein gleichgebliebenes morphologisches und genetisches Verhalten, sowie die regelmäßige pathologische Proteinbildung. Bei Kenntnis der Eigenschaften des untersuchten Tumors kann angenommen werden, daß trotz jahrelanger Transplantation auf Nicht-Inzucht-Hamster ein recht einheitliches System zur Verfügung steht.

---

* Für die freundliche Unterstützung danken wir der Strebel-Stiftung Mannheim.

Der solide Tumor erreicht 2–3 Wochen nach Transplantation etwa Walnußgröße. Seine Oberfläche ist knollig; auf dem Schnitt erkennt man einen grauweißen, in den Randpartien rötlichen Tumor mit häufig zentralen Nekrosen. Die Tumorzellen liegen in einem lockeren Gewebsverband und sind von einer bindegewebigen Kapsel umgeben. Sie haben ovale Formen und eine Größe von 10–13 μ. Ihre Zellkerne sind rundlich bis oval, sie liegen meist exzentrisch. Am Kernrand ist das Chromatin

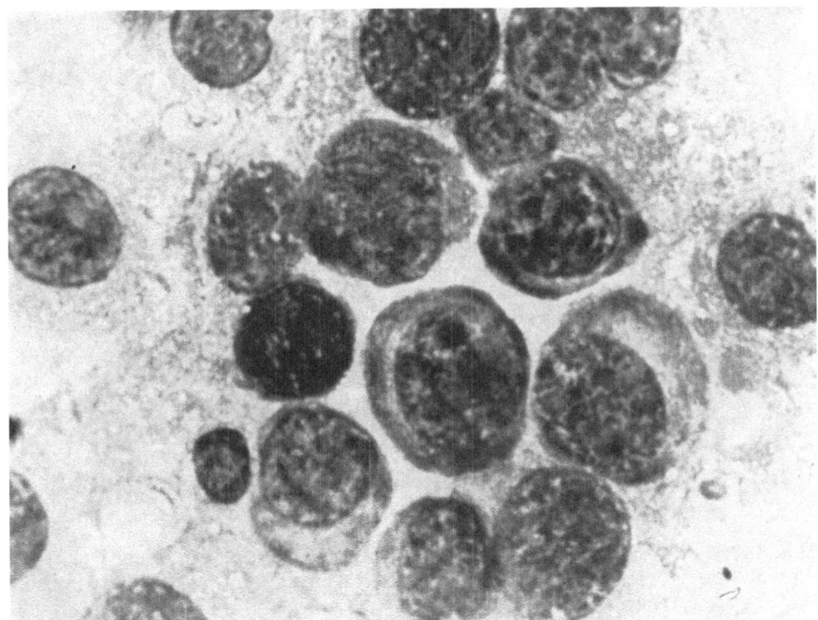

Abb. 1. Knochenmarkausstrich eines Hamsters mit KG-13-Plasmocytom. Zwei Wochen nach Tumorstrangulation diffuse Durchsetzung mit Plasmocytomzellen

verdichtet und schollig. Nucleolen sind erkennbar. Die bekannte Radspeichenstruktur wird kaum gefunden. Histologisch und histochemisch zeigt das Cytoplasma Granulaanhäufungen mit deutlich positiver Reaktion bei Methylgrün-Pyronin-Färbung.

Die Nieren der plasmocytomtragenden Hamster zeigen z. T. schwere Eiweißnephrosen. Dabei sind die Tubulusepithelien geschwollen, das Protoplasma erscheint hyalintropfig entartet. Im Glomerulum zwischen den beiden Blättern der Bowman'schen Kapsel und in den Lumina der Tubuli finden sich schollige und homogene Eiweißzylinder. Das Ausmaß des Nierenbefundes ist direkt proportional der Überlebenszeit der Tiere.

10–14 Tage nach Tumortransplantation zeigt die Leber eine positive Fettreaktion. Mit zunehmender Überlebenszeit wird die anfangs zentral feintropfige Verfettung diffus und grobtropfig.

Die Überlebenszeit der Hamster nach Transplantation des soliden
Tumors beträgt durchschnittlich 25, die der mit Tumorascites beimpften
Tiere im Mittel 12 Tage. Die Hamster sterben an dem Tumor bzw. an
sekundären Organveränderungen. Metastasen sind selten. Durch
Operation oder Strangulation des Tumors bei Hamstern mit der soliden

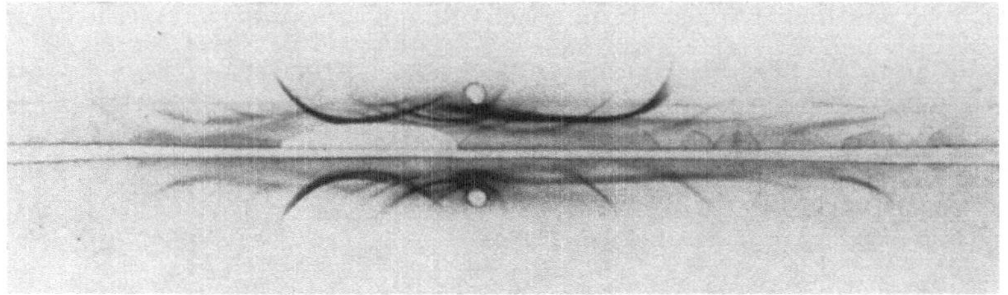

Abb. 2. 1963 durchgeführte Immunelektrophorese. Oben: Auftrennung von Serum
eines plasmocytomtragenden Hamsters. Unten: Auftrennung von Normal-Hamster-
Serum

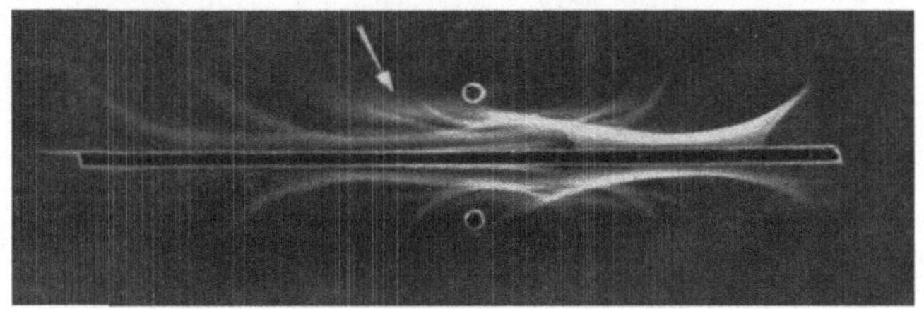

Abb. 3. 1967 durchgeführte Immunelektrophorese. Oben: Auftrennung von Serum
eines plasmocytomtragenden Hamsters. Unten: Auftrennung von Normal-Hamster-
Serum

Geschwulst erreicht man eine Überlebenszeit von durchschnittlich
45 Tagen. Dabei wurden jetzt häufiger Metastasen im Bereich der axillären
oder inguinalen Lymphknoten, im Retroperitonealgewebe und in den
Knochen gefunden. Abb. 1 zeigt eine diffuse Durchsetzung des Knochen-
markes mit Plasmocytomzellen.

Die Bluteiweißveränderungen zeigen einen charakteristischen Befund.
In der Papier- und Agar-Gel-Elektrophorese wurde ein pathologisches
Protein mit Beweglichkeit im beta-2-Bereich gefunden. In der Immun-
elektrophorese gelang zunächst der Nachweis einer sehr intensiv ab-
gebogenen Präzipitationslinie, die dem Verlauf des gamma-M_1 entsprach
(Abb. 2). Neueste Ergebnisse (Medizinische Poliklinik der Universität
Heidelberg) lassen vermuten, daß ein Eiweißprodukt vom Typ des
gamma-A vorliegt (Abb. 3). Für diese Annahme spricht auch der seiner-
zeit ermittelte Wert in der Ultrazentrifuge von 14,6 Svedberg-Einheiten.
Die Klärung dieser Befunde und die Auftrennung der Uroproteine bei der

wir früher einen Gradienten im beta-gamma-Bereich gefunden haben, ist Gegenstand weiterer Untersuchungen.

Die zusammen mit DONTENWILL u. SCHAUER [6] und DONTENWILL [7] beobachteten Befunde haben sich bis heute bei wiederholten Kontrollen der Morphologie und Serologie nicht geändert. Das KG-13-Plasmocytom zeigt eine Konstanz seiner Eigenschaften. Dieser Tumor ist daher für die verschiedensten Fragestellungen auf Zeit geeignet.

Literatur

1. ADAMS, R. A., D. I. PATT, and B. R. LUTZ: Long Term Persistence of Skin Homografts in Untreated Hamsters. Transpl. Bull. **3**, 41 (1956).
2. EICKE, J., M. L. MEINERS u. H. WRBA: Veränderungen der Stammlinie von Walker-Carcinom-Zellen durch Umweltfaktoren. Z. Krebsforsch. **66**, 193 (1964).
3. HILDEMANN, W. H. and R. L. WALFORD: Chronic Skin Homograft Rejection in the Syrian Hamster. Ann. N.Y. Acad. Sci. **87**, 56 (1960).
4. — Diskussionsbemerkung. In: Ciba Foundation, Symposium on Transplantation, S. 116. London: Churchill 1962.
5. LETTRÉ, H.: Eigenschaftsänderungen von Tumorzellen. Z. Krebsforsch. **59**, 568 (1953).
6. MOHR, U., W. DONTENWILL u. A. SCHAUER: Experimentelle Untersuchungen an einem spontanen Plasmocytom des Goldhamsters. Klin. Wschr. **41**, 25 (1963).
7. — — Organ- und Bluteiweißveränderungen beim KG-13-Plasmocytom des Goldhamsters. Z. Krebsforsch. **66**, 29 (1964).
8. SCHÖNE, G.: Transplantation und Genetik. Die Sonderstellung des Laboratoriumsgoldhamsters. Bruns' Beitr. klin. Chir. **202**, 129 (1961).
9. WRBA, H. u. H. RABES: Spontane und induzierte Wandlungen in Biologie und Wachstum von Geschwülsten. Z. Krebsforsch. **65**, 316 (1963).

Untersuchungen an einem Plasmocytom des Goldhamsters

b) Vorläufige elektronenoptische Befunde an Nierenglomerula plasmocytomtragender Hamster

Von

J. Moppert*

Wir hatten in den letzten Monaten Gelegenheit, Nierengewebe plasmocytomtragender Goldhamster elektronenoptisch zu untersuchen. Unser Augenmerk richtete sich dabei hauptsächlich auf die Glomerula, da über die Ultrastruktur dieses Nephronabschnittes bei Paraproteinämie noch recht wenig bekannt ist. Der Umfang unseres Beobachtungsgutes ist noch klein. Der folgende Bericht muß daher als vorläufig bezeichnet werden.

Glomeruläre Alterationen sind am versilberten Semidünnschnitt bereits lichtoptisch faßbar. Dies vor allem bei Tieren, deren Überlebenszeit durch die Entfernung des Primärtumors (mit nachfolgendem Recidiv) auf ca. 10 Wochen verlängert werden konnte (Mohr u. Dontenwill [6]). Es handelt sich um Veränderungen an der glomerulären Basalmembran. Diese verläuft, im Gegensatz zur Norm bei Kontrolltieren, unregelmäßig, bald mäanderartig, bald in engen Schleifen, scheint aber nicht verdickt zu sein. An den intrakapillären und epithelialen Zellen sind lichtoptisch keine Besonderheiten sichtbar, vor allem erscheinen sie zahlenmäßig nicht vermehrt (Abb. 1). Auf die tubulären Veränderungen soll hier nicht weiter eingegangen werden.

An Glomerula mit lichtoptisch leichten Veränderungen findet sich ultrastrukturell in einzelnen Lobuli wiederum der abnorme Verlauf der Basalmembran, meist kenntlich an ungewöhnlich engen Schleifen. In diesen Bereichen kann dabei aber die typische Dreischichtung der Lamina basalis vollkommen erhalten sein. Dagegen werden nunmehr Alterationen der Begleitzellen faßbar. Auf der Lumenseite ist die endotheliale Cytoplasmatapete oft geschwollen und läßt kaum mehr Fenestrae erkennen. Die gegenüberliegenden epithelialen Fußfortsätze sind dabei meist ausgesprochen plump oder, infolge von Fusion, über kurze Strecken durch eine kontinuierliche Cytoplasmaschicht ersetzt (Abb. 2).

---

* Stipendiat der Forschungskommission der Universität Basel.

Parallel zur Intensität der lichtoptischen Befunde stößt man zunehmend häufiger auf Glomerulumabschnitte, wo nun auch die Basalmembran selbst morphologische Alterationen aufweist. Es finden sich alle Übergänge von einzelnen, meist epithelwärts gerichteten Ausbuchtungen bis zu multiplen, korallenstockartigen Aufsplitterungen. Diesen Basal-

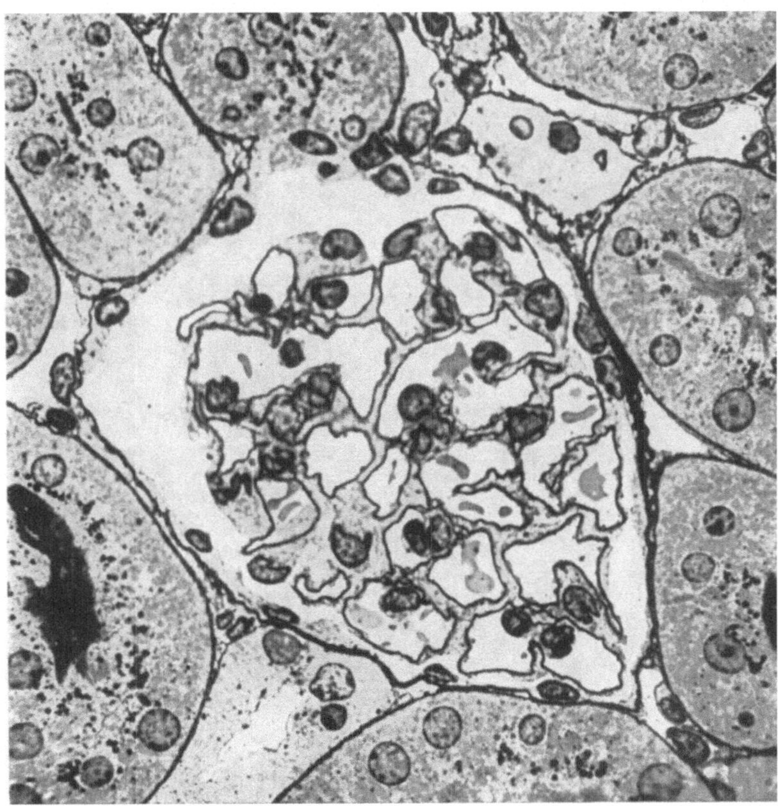

Abb. 1. Glomerulum eines Goldhamsters bei Plasmocytom. Großes Recidiv nach Entfernung des Primärtumors. Bizarr-eckiger Verlauf der Basalmembran. Keine sicheren Veränderungen an den zahlenmäßig nicht vermehrten Begleitzellen. Versilberter Semidünnschnitt; 800×

membranabschnitten liegen die Epithelzellen unter Wegfall der füßchenförmigen Fortsätze flach auf (Abb. 3). Ihr Cytoplasma erscheint geschwollen und enthält meist zahlen- und größenmäßig vermehrte Organellen, wie Golgifelder oder Ergastoplasmabezirke. Ihr Kern ist oft mehrfach eingebuchtet und weist viele Poren auf.

Zusammenfassend sind die beobachteten Veränderungen als unspezifische Glomerulonephrose (Lit. s. ZOLLINGER [7]) anzusprechen, die,

zum mindesten zu Beginn herdförmig, vor allem die Glomerulum-
peripherie, das heißt, die eigentliche Filterbarriere, in Mitleidenschaft
zieht. Ebenfalls fokale Glomerulumveränderungen finden sich auch beim
menschlichen Plasmocytom (ZOLLINGER [7]; FISHER et al. [3]; ABRA-
HAMS et al. [1]).

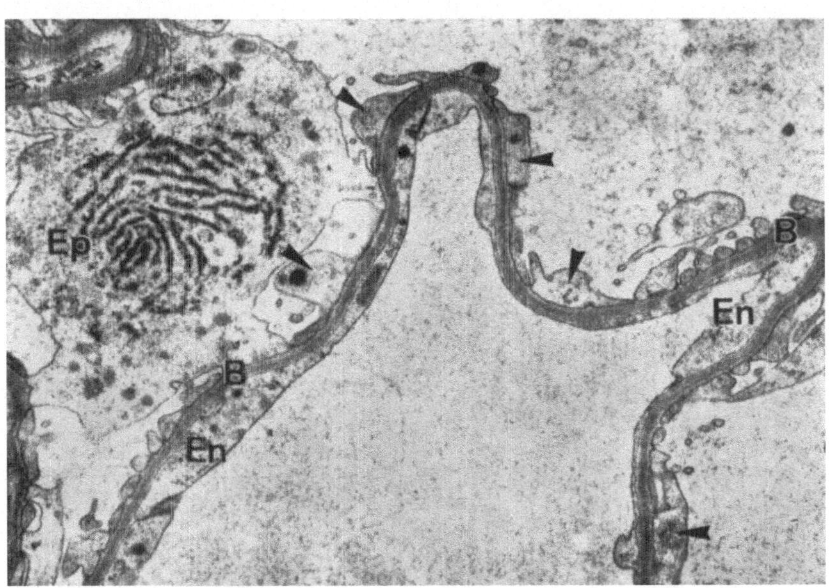

Abb. 2. Material wie Abb. 1. Ungewöhnlich enge Schleifen der morphologisch nicht
veränderten, typisch dreigeschichteten Basalmembran (B). Mehrere, ausgesprochen
plumpe epitheliale Fußfortsätze (▶). Schwellung der endothelialen Cytoplasmatapete (En) bei weitgehend fehlenden Fenestrae. Ep = Epithelzelle. Kombinierte
Bleicitrat-Uranylacetatkontrastierung; 10 500×

Aussagen über die Pathogenese dieser Glomerulonephrose oder deren
funktionelle Bedeutung bereiten erhebliche Schwierigkeiten. Vieles
spricht dafür, daß vom Tumor gebildete Paraproteine das Glomerulum
direkt schädigen, indem sie hier vielleicht teilweise abgelagert werden
oder auch nur über längere Zeit das Ultrafilter passieren (ZOLLINGER [7]).
An unserem Modell, wie auch an menschlichem Material (FISHER et
al. [3]), finden sich aber auch elektronenoptisch keine sicheren Anhaltspunkte für solche Ablagerungsprozesse; andererseits können glomeruläre
Läsionen auch dann beobachtet werden, wenn Paraproteine lediglich im
Serum, dagegen nicht im Urin auftreten, ihre Filtrationsrate somit in
diesen Fällen zum mindesten sehr klein ist (FISHER et al. [3]). Ferner läßt
sich aus einer neueren, sehr eingehenden Analyse der Nierenfunktion
beim Myelom des Menschen entnehmen, daß bisher keine logische
Relation zwischen Dauer, Ausprägung und Art einer gegebenen Para-

proteinämie einerseits und einer etwaigen Störung der Filterfunktion andererseits aufgestellt werden kann (HARRISON et al. [4]), Befunde, denen Beobachtungen an plasmocytomtragenden Inzuchtmäusen zu entsprechen scheinen (COLEMAN et al. [2]; McINTYRE and POTTER [5]).

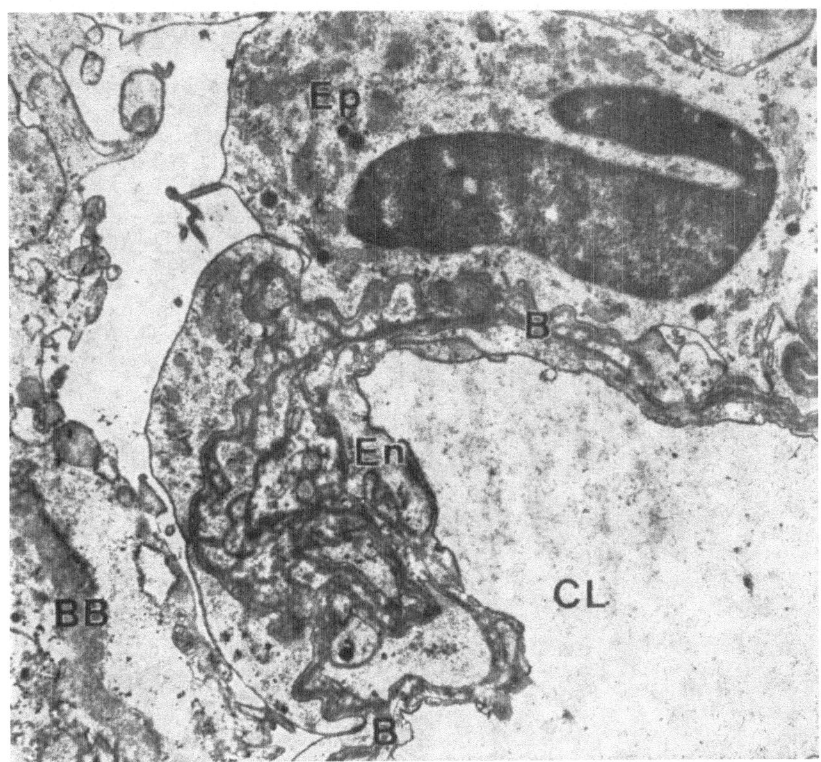

Abb. 3. Material wie Abb. 2. Basalmembranschnitt (B) mit multiplen, korallen-stockartigen Aufsplitterungen. Veränderungen der Begleitzellen siehe Text. Ep = Epithelzelle, En = endotheliales Cytpolasma (umgewandelte Lamina fene-strata), CL = Capillarlumen, BB = Basalmembran der Bowmanschen Kapsel. Präparation wie in Abb. 2; 10 600×

Wir hoffen, daß eine weitere Analyse der biochemischen und morpho-logischen Parameter uns erlauben wird, auch dieses interessante Teil-problem allmählich besser zu verstehen.

Literatur

1. ABRAHAMS, C., C. L. PIRANI, and V. E. POLLAK: Ultrastructure of the Kidney in a Patient with Multiple Myeloma. J. Path. Bact. **92**, 220 (1966).
2. COLEMAN, R. F., C. H. LUPTON, and J. F. A. McMANUS: Renal Lesions in Inbred Mice with Plasma-cell Tumors. Arch. Path. **74**, 6 (1962).

3. Fisher, E. R., E. Perez-Stable, and Z. A. Zawadzki: Ultrastructural Renal Changes in Multiple Myeloma with Comments Relative to the Mechanism of Proteinuria. Lab. Invest. **13**, 1561 (1964).
4. Harrison, J. F., J. D. Blainey, J. Hardwicke, D. S. Rowe, and J. F. Soothill: Proteinuria in Multiple Myeloma. Clin. Sci. **31**, 95 (1966).
5. McIntyre, K. R., and M. Potter: Studies of Thirty Different Bence-Jones Protein-producing Plasma Cell Neoplasms in an Inbred Strain of Mouse. J. nat. Cancer Inst. **33**, 631 (1964).
6. Mohr, U. u. W. Dontenwill: Organ- und Blutveränderungen beim KG-13-Plasmocytom des Goldhamsters. Z. Krebsforsch. **66**, 29 (1964).
7. Zollinger, H. U.: Niere und ableitende Harnwege. In: Doerr, W. u. E. Uehlinger (Hrsg.): Spezielle pathologische Anatomie, Bd. 3. Berlin-Heidelberg-New York: Springer 1966.

Untersuchungen an einem Plasmocytom des Goldhamsters
c) Cytogenetische Besonderheiten dieses Tumors

Von

O. WIESER

Es ist bekannt, daß mit zunehmender Entdifferenzierung einer Transplantationsgeschwulst die Hetero-Transplantation möglich wird. Der Versuch, das KG-13-Plasmocytom des syrischen Goldhamsters auf andere erwachsene, nicht konditionierte Nager zu transplantieren, gelang bisher nicht. Daher stellte sich die Frage, ob das Chromosomenkomplement dieses stabilen Tumors im Vergleich zum unstabilen Zajdela-Hepatom der Ratte Unterschiede zeigt.

Material und Methode

Untersucht wurden das KG-13-Plasmocytom des syrischen Goldhamsters und das Zajdela-Hepatom der Ratte in Ascitesform. Mit Desacethyl-Methylcolchicin wurden in vivo die Mitosen arretiert, danach der Ascites abpunktiert, die Zellen in Hankscher Salzlösung gewaschen, in 0,9% Natrium-citricum-Lösung gequollen und in Eisessig-Alkohol fixiert. Die Zellsuspension wurde im Spreading-Verfahren auf eingefrorene Objektträger aufgebracht, getrocknet und mit Aceto-Orcein gefärbt. Gut ausgebreitete Metaphaseplatten wurden mit dem Orthomaten (Leitz) fotografiert. Auswertung der Positive bei einer Vergrößerung von ca. 1:3000.

Ergebnisse und Diskussion

Das KG-13-Plasmocytom des syrischen Goldhamsters ist ein pseudotetraploider Tumor mit ausgeprägter Stammlinie von $S = 88$. Bei einer ersten Auszählung von 952 Metaphaseplatten fanden sich 40% Stammzellen, 36% Plus- und 24% Minusvarianten. Die letzten Zählungen von 712 Metaphaseplatten zeigten eine Stammlinie mit 41%; die Plusvarianten betrugen dabei 17, die Minusvarianten 42%.

Durch den Verlust einzelner Chromosomen bei der Präparation sollen sich nach RUTISHAUSER [2] unter den Minusvarianten zahlreiche Stammzellen verbergen.

O. Wieser

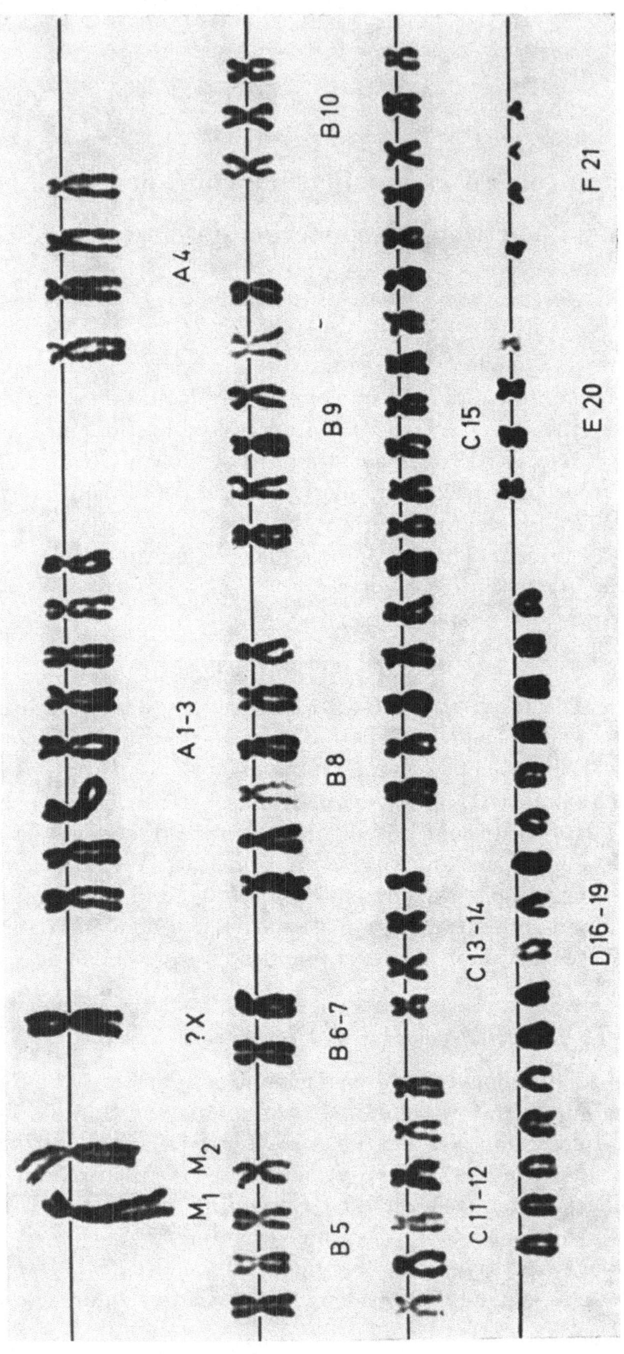

Abb. 1. Karyogramm einer Plasmocytomzelle

Die Histogramme zeigten eine Stabilität des Stammlinienkonzeptes über längere Zeit. Ähnlich war auch das Ergebnis der Chromosomenanalysen, wobei die Einordnung der Chromosomen nach dem Schema von ISHIHARA u. Mitarb. [1] erfolgte. Bei dem pseudotetraploiden KG-13-Plasmocytom ist von Platte zu Platte die Anzahl der Chromosomen in einzelnen Gruppen unterschiedlich. Dennoch zeigten die früheren und auch die letzten 90 Analysen eine Konstanz der Chromosomen in den

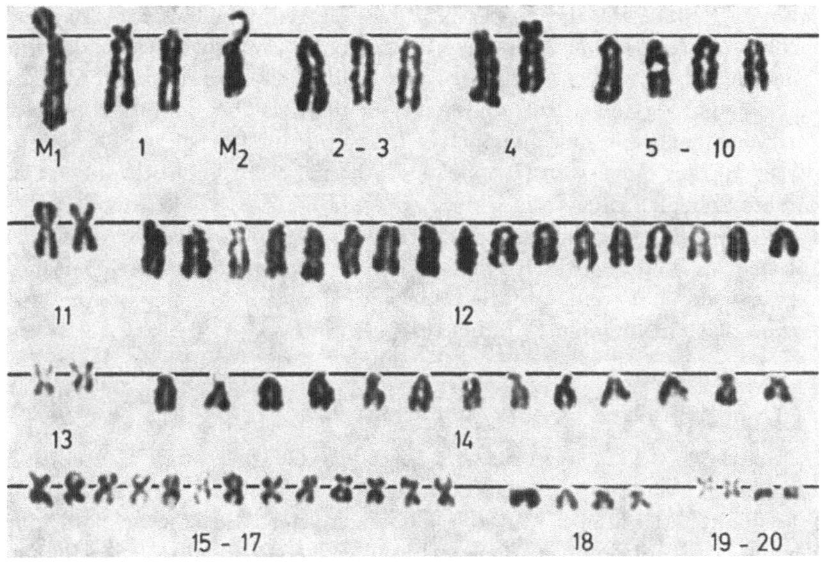

Abb. 2. Karyogramm einer Hepatomzelle

Gruppen D 16–19 mit 16 und in den Gruppen E 20 und F 21 mit je 4 Chromosomen. Auch die zwei größten meta- bis submetazentrischen Chromosomen fanden sich in der Hälfte aller Platten (Abb. 1).

Im Gegensatz dazu stehen die Ergebnisse des heterotransplantablen Zajdela-Hepatoms. Hierbei wurde das Chromosomenkomplement zwischen der 150. und 282. Passage 3mal untersucht. Bei der ersten Auswertung ließ sich keine klare Stammlinie abgrenzen. Es fand sich ein breitbasiges Histogramm mit 67 Chromosomen in 12%. Bei der zweiten Untersuchung wurde, offenbar durch Selektionsprozesse begünstigt, eine Stammlinie von 68 Chromosomen erkannt. Bei der letzten Auswertung (Passage 282) war diese Stammlinie nur mehr bei 25% der untersuchten Zellen nachweisbar.

Jetzt gelang auch die Transplantation auf andere nicht konditionierte Nager (Mäuse, syrische und chinesische Hamster). Dabei änderte sich das Histogramm erneut im Sinne einer Entdifferenzierung. Die Stammlinie zeigte 67 Chromosomen inmitten eines breitbasigen Histogramms. Das Rattenkomplement war jedoch trotz Heterotransplantation erkennbar geblieben.

Die zahlreichen Passagen des Tumors auf der Ratte führten zu erheblichen morphologischen, lichtmikroskopisch sichtbaren Chromosomen-Veränderung. Bei der ersten Untersuchung des Komplements wurde nur ein Markerchromosom, ein submetazentrisches Chromosom der ersten Gruppe mit negativ heterochromatischen kürzeren Chromatiden, gefunden. 132 Passagen später zeigten sich 4 unterscheidbare Markerchromosomen (Abb. 2). In keiner Platte fehlte der Marker M 1, der um etwa ein Drittel größer als das größte der übrigen Chromosomen war. In ca. 80% der Platten wurde ein Marker beobachtet, bei dem die kürzeren Chromatidenanteile miteinander verdrillt und um 180° eingerollt waren. Dieser Marker der ersten Gruppe zeigte häufig auch heterochromatische kürzere Schenkel mit Kernfärbung an den Enden.

Gelegentlich fand sich ein telozentrisches Chromosom der Gruppe 5–10 mit negativ heterochromatischer Bande in Chromatidenmitte. Seltener war in Gruppe 14 ein weiteres Markerchromosom mit negativ heterochromatischen kürzeren Chromatiden.

Zusammenfassung

Das KG-13-Plasmocytom des syrischen Goldhamsters zeigte über Jahre ein konstantes Chromosomenkomplement. Bei einem anderen Transplantationstumor (Zajdela-Hepatom der Ratte) erfolgte im gleichen Zeitraum eine Entdifferenzierung der Geschwulst. Die Heterotransplantation wurde möglich. Dabei änderte sich das Chromosomenkomplement hinsichtlich Morphologie und Stammlinie.

Literatur

1. ISHIHARA, T., G. E. MOORE, and A. A. SANDBERG: Chromosome Constitution of two Tumors of the Golden Hamster. J. nat. Cancer Inst. **29**, 161 (1962).
2. RUTISHAUSER, A.: Cytogenetik transplantabler tierischer und menschlicher Tumoren. Neujahrsblatt 1963.

Untersuchungen an einem Plasmocytom des Goldhamsters
d) Immunreaktionen an Gewebekulturen des KG-13-Plasmocytoms in vitro*

Von

V. KINZEL und H. J. SEIDEL

Die Ähnlichkeit des KG-13-Plasmocytoms (GARCIA, BARONI and RAPPAPORT [2]) beim Goldhamster mit Plasmocytomen des Menschen (MOHR u. DONTENWILL [*12*]) veranlaßte uns, diese Geschwulst für verschiedene Untersuchungen in vitro zu kultivieren. Neben der Morphologie und dem Verhalten des Tumors in vitro (KINZEL, SEIDEL u. MOHR [*8*]) erschien der Ablauf von Immunreaktionen an den Zellen von Interesse.

Material und Methode

Zellen des KG-13-Plasmocytoms lassen sich aus der soliden Form der Geschwulst im sogenannten hängenden Tropfen aus Hühnerplasma und Hühnerembryonalextrakt bei 37 °C kultivieren. Nach 5–6 Tagen können die Präparate unter Zusatz von Salzlösung nach Hanks in Durchströmungskammern (KINZEL [*7*]) übertragen werden. Bei den Versuchen wurde ein Medium aus gleichen Teilen Salzlösung (nach Hanks), inaktiviertem Kaninchen-Serum und 10fach verdünntem Meerschweinchen-Komplement verwandt. Beobachtung und mikrokinematographische Registrierung erfolgten im Phasenkontrastmikroskop unter dem Hüllthermostaten bei 37 °C. Zur Anwendung kam: 1. Serum normaler, unvorbehandelter Kaninchen, 2. Serum von Kaninchen, die mit Homogenat aus Milzen normaler Hamster und 3. Serum von Kaninchen, die mit Homogenat aus solidem KG-13-Plasmocytom behandelt worden waren. Zur Herstellung der Antiseren erhielten ausgewachsene Kaninchen 3mal wöchentlich für 4 Wochen 0,5 ml frisches Homogenat und 0,5 ml Freunds Adjuvans subcutan.

Ergebnisse und Besprechung

Seren normaler, unvorbehandelter Kaninchen können den Zellen des KG-13-Plasmocytoms in vitro zugesetzt werden, ohne daß eine Zellreaktion sichtbar wird. Einige Normalseren bewirken jedoch eine Um-

---

* Mit Mikrofilmdemonstration.

gestaltung der kompakten Plasmocytomzellen in lang ausgezogene, fibro-blastenartige Zellen.

Serum von Kaninchen, die mit Homogenat aus Milzen normaler Hamster immunisiert worden waren, bewirkt an Zellen des KG-13-Plasmocytoms in vitro unmittelbar nach Zugabe beginnende reversible Veränderungen – Steigerung der Eigenbeweglichkeit mit nachfolgender Zellabrundung –, die als antikörper-bedingte anabole Reaktionsformen aufzufassen sind (LETTERER [10]). Ähnliche Veränderungen sind an der Walker-Carcinomzelle in vitro in einem vergleichbaren System zu finden (KINZEL [7]).

Serum von Kaninchen, die mit Homogenat aus solidem KG-13-Plasmocytom immunisiert worden waren, führt bei Zellen dieses Tumors in vitro zu irreversiblen Veränderungen. Bis zum Beginn der sichtbaren Immunreaktion erfolgt nach Serumzugabe eine etwa 10 min dauernde Latenzzeit, in der Pinocytose und Bewegungsvorgänge normal oder etwas verstärkt ablaufen (s. auch GOLDBERG and GREEN [3]). Der Beginn der Reaktion wird durch die zunehmende Agglutination von Cytoplasma-Granula, die ihre gerichtete Bewegung anfangs noch beibehalten, und eine Bewegungsunruhe der Zellmembran angezeigt. Später wird die Agglutination vollständig, wobei sich der sichtbare Zelldurchmesser zunächst verkleinert. Die Zelle scheint für kurze Zeit wie fixiert, löst sich dann aber aus der Starre. Die Cytoplasma-Granula zeigen die sogenannte Brownsche Bewegung im kontrastlosen Cytoplasma. Die sichtbare Immunreaktion beginnt somit ähnlich wie an Zellen des Walker-Carci-noms auch bei der Plasmocytomzelle in vitro im gesamten Cytoplasma-Bereich gleichzeitig, was auf die während der Latenzzeit abgelaufene Pinocytose zurückzuführen ist (LETTERER [10]). Gerinnungsähnliche Veränderungen finden am Cytoplasma nicht statt, und die Zellmembran bleibt bei der Plasmocytomzelle in ihrer Kontinuität erhalten (Abb. 1) (s. auch KAISER u. SPRINGER [6]). Das Phänomen der Potocytose ist bei der Plasmocytomzelle nach der sichtbaren Immunreaktion im Gegensatz zur Walker-Zelle (Abb. 2) nur schwach ausgeprägt. Das Golgi-Feld zeigt außer einer Kontraststeigerung keine im Phasenkontrastmikroskop faß-baren Veränderungen.

Der Zellkern wird während der letzten Phase der Cytoplasmareaktion (s. auch LATTA [9]) zunehmend kleiner und dunkler – anscheinend dich-ter. Seine Bestandteile lassen sich nicht mehr deutlich differenzieren. Gleichzeitig mit der Pyknose werden ein oder mehrere direkt am Kern entstehende Bläschen beobachtet, die diesen zu halbmondförmiger Gestalt zu imprimieren scheinen (Abb. 1). Ihr Kontrast ist heller als der des umgebenden entmischten Cytoplasmas, aber dunkler als der Kontrast der etwa zuvor durch Pinocytose aufgenommenen Tröpfchen. Im Mikro-film mutet dieser Vorgang in Zeitraffung wie ein Auspressen von Kern-

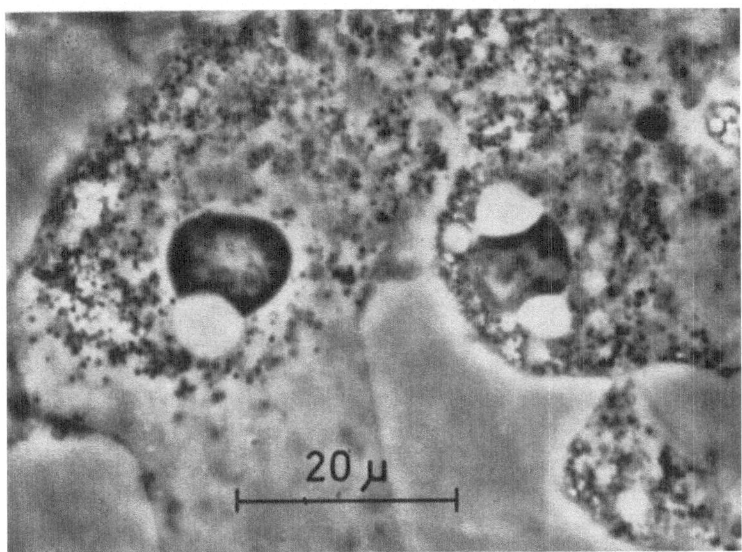

Abb. 1. Zwei Plasmocytomzellen nach Immuncytolyse. Pyknose der Zellkerne mit anliegenden Bläschen

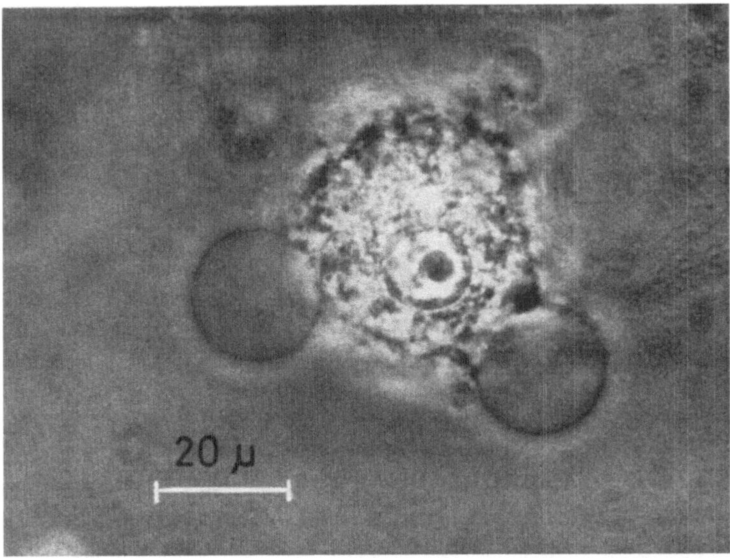

Abb. 2. Walker-Carcinom-Zelle nach Immuncytolyse. „Glänzender" Kern, Poto-cytose

flüssigkeit in diese Bläschen an, doch ist der Mechanismus unklar. Pyknose und Bläschenbildung geschehen also gleichzeitig, nicht wie an anderen Systemen nacheinander (Latta [9]). Diese Form des Kernsubstanzverlustes scheint zwischen dem morphologisch nicht faßbaren Ausströmen von Kernflüssigkeit (Lumsden [11]) und dem Reißen der Kernmembran (Letterer [10]) zu stehen.

An elektronenoptischen Präparationen wurden bei Zellen nach Immuncytolysen Auftreibungen der Doppelmembran des Kernes – der paranukleären Zisternen – festgestellt (Latta [9]; Green and Goldberg [4]; Kaiser u. Springer [6]). Inwieweit diese Veränderungen am Zellkern mit den Expulsionsvacuolen nach hypoxydotischer Herzmuskel-Schädigung bzw. denen nach akuter Hemmung der zellulären Oxydation (Grundmann [5]; Doerr u. Becker [1]) vergleichbar sind, läßt sich nicht sagen.

Während sonst nach Immuncytolyse – auch an der Walker-Carcinom-Zelle (Abb. 2) (Kinzel [7]) – der Zellkern im Phasenkontrastmikroskop das Bild des glänzenden Kernes (Zollinger [13]) zeigt, was wohl auf eine Akkumulation von Nukleoplasma an der Innenseite der inneren Kernmembran (Latta [9]) zurückzuführen ist, reagiert die Plasmocytomzelle in vitro auf Zusatz von Antiserum und Komplement mit einer akut verlaufenden phasenoptisch darstellbaren Kernpyknose. Ob diese für das System des Plasmocytoms charakteristisch ist, bleibt Gegenstand weiterer Untersuchungen. Die beschriebenen Veränderungen sind irreversibel.

Zusammenfassung

Kulturzellen des transplantablen KG-13-Plasmocytoms vom Goldhamster reagieren in vitro auf Zusatz heterologen Antiserums und Komplement mit charakteristischen, phasenkontrastmikroskopisch beobachtbaren Veränderungen:

1. Nach einer dem Immunserumzusatz folgenden Latenzzeit verfallen alle Plasmocytomzellen einer sehr schnell ablaufenden Cytolyse.

2. Der Zellkern zeigt nicht wie sonst nach Immuncytolyse das Bild des „glänzenden" Kernes, sondern eine bereits im Phasenkontrastmikroskop erkennbare Pyknose.

3. Während der Pyknose entstehen ein oder mehrere dem Kern anliegende, große Bläschen, deren Genese im Zusammenhang mit sogenannten Expulsionsvakuolen diskutiert wird.

Literatur

1. Doerr, W. u. V. Becker: Das morphologische Äquivalentbild der Niere nach experimenteller Vergiftung mit Cyankalium und Malonsäure. Verh. Dtsch. Ges. Path. **35**, 222 (1951).

2. GARCIA, H., C. BARONI, and H. RAPPAPORT: Transplantable Tumors of the Syrian Golden Hamster. J. nat. Cancer Inst. **27**, 1323 (1961).
3. GOLDBERG, B. and H. GREEN: The Cytotoxic Action of Immune Gamma Globulin and Complement. on Krebs Ascites Tumorcells. J. exper. Med. **109**, 505 (1959).
4. GREEN, H. and B. GOLDBERG: The Action of Antibody and Complement on Mammalian Cells. Ann. N.Y. Acad. Sci. **87**, 352 (1960).
5. GRUNDMANN, E.: Histologische Untersuchungen über die Wirkungen experimentellen Sauerstoffmangels auf das Katzenherz. Beitr. path. Anat. **111**, 36 (1950).
6. KAISER, E. u. K. SPRINGER: Elektronenoptische und biochemische Untersuchungen über cytotoxische Wirkung heterologer Antisera gegen Tumorzellen. Wien. klin. Wschr. **75**, 312 (1963).
7. KINZEL, V.: Über die Cytolyse von Tumorzellen in vitro durch Antiserum. Z. Krebsforsch. **68**, 209 (1966).
8. —, H. J. SEIDEL u. U. MOHR: Lebendbeobachtungen zur Struktur des Golgi-Feldes bei Zellen eines transplantablen Plasmocytoms in vitro. Z. Zellforsch. **77**, 435 (1967).
9. LATTA, H.: A cellular reaction to antibody in tissue culture studied with electron microscopy. J. biophys. biochem. Cytol. **5**, 405 (1959).
10. LETTERER, E.: Morphische Folgen der Antigen-Antikörper-Reaktion. Verh. Dtsch. Ges. Path. **46**, 83 (1962).
11. LUMSDEN, C. E.: Effects of antibodies on cells in tissue culture. In: GRABAR-MIESCHER (Hrsg.) Immunopathology Bd. I, 1. Internat. Symposium in Basel/Seelisberg 1958, p. 262. Basel: Schwabe & Co. 1959.
12. MOHR, U. u. W. DONTENWILL: Organ- und Blutveränderungen beim KG-13-Plasmocytom des Goldhamsters. Z. Krebsforsch. **66**, 29 (1964).
13. ZOLLINGER, H. U.: Phasenmikroskopische Beobachtungen über Zelltod. Schweiz. Z. Path. **11**, 276 (1948).

B.

2. wissenschaftliche Sitzung am Dienstag, den 26. 9. 1967

Vorsitz: W. Doerr

Über die „Mutationstheorie der Geschwulstentstehung" und deren Fortentwicklung

Von

K. H. BAUER

Einleitung

Eine Krebsforschung im wissenschaftlichen Sinne gibt es erst seit VIRCHOWS „Cellularpathologie" (1858). Für sie ist „die Zelle wirklich das letzte Form-Element aller lebendigen Erscheinung, sowohl im Gesunden als im Kranken".

Speziell für die Krebskrankheiten gilt seit BORST (1924) der Satz: „Alle Geschwülste nehmen ihren Ausgang von den Zellen unseres Körpers" und setzen sich „in all ihren Teilen aus körpereigenen Zellen zusammen".

Bis heute kennt man, je nach Lokalisation, an die *150 Krebsarten*, ihrerseits mit vielen Varianten und mit überaus wechselvollen Verlaufsformen. Bildlich gesprochen: Krebs kleidet sich in vielerlei Gewänder.

Aber so variabel wie die Krebsformen, so variabel sind auch die *Krebs-Ursachen*. Ihr Katalog umfaßt heute an die 500 krebserzeugende, sogenannte carcinogene Stoffe und krebsauslösende Strahlungen.

Ganz von selbst drängt sich da die Frage auf: Welches ist denn nun angesichts dieser vielhundertfältigen kausalen Genese *der formalgenetisch einheitliche Grundvorgang*, der eine Körperzelle in eine Krebszelle verwandelt? Oder anders ausgedrückt: Welches ist das intrazelluläre Primärereignis, dem wir die Krebsumwandlung, die *Cancerisierung von Körperzellen*, zuzuordnen haben?

Der Grundvorgang der Cancerisierung historisch gesehen

Natürlich war man sich immer schon bewußt, daß der Cancerisierung, wie BORST [*10*] es ausdrückte, „eine tiefgreifende Änderung des Zellcharakters" entsprechen muß. v. HANSEMANN sprach von „Anaplasie", BENEKE von „Kataplasie" und BORST selbst, ein Wort HAUSERS variierend, von einer „neuen Zellrasse".

Herrn Prof. HANS v. SEEMEN zum 70. Geburtstag.

Was es aber natürlich an Stelle der bloßen Wortprägungen braucht, das sind objektive Tatbestände zunächst der *Geschwulstmorphologie*. Gerne hält man sich natürlich an die beim Krebs so besonders häufig pathologischen Kernteilungsfiguren. Kein Wunder, daß diese *Kernverwilderung* schon 1914 zum Ausgangspunkt einer Theorie der Geschwulstentstehung gemacht wurde. Der Zoologe BOVERI [*11*] experimentierte an Seeigeleiern, die er doppelt befruchtete. Natürlich erhielt er

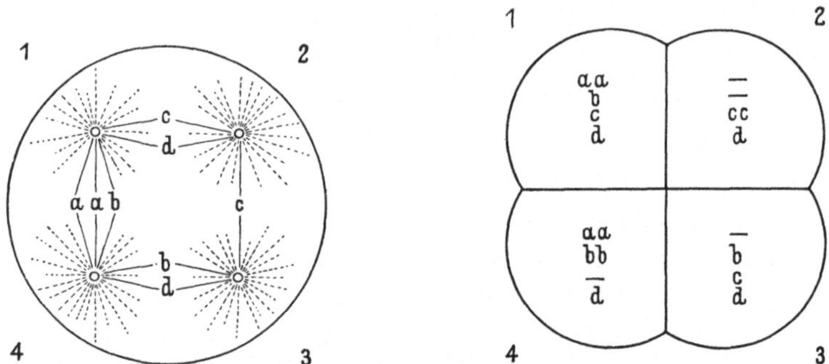

Abb. 1. Verteilungsmöglichkeiten der Chromosomen in doppelt befruchteten Seeigeleiern bei einer 4- (statt 2-)poligen Zellteilung. Effekt: Abnorme Chromosomenzahlen in den 4 Tochterzellen (BOVERI, 1914)

in diesen meist dreikernigen Eiern häufig pluri- bzw. tetrapolare Zellteilungen (Abb. 1), notwendigerweise mit „fehlerhaften Chromosomenkombinationen". Mit dem Primärgeschehen der Krebsentstehung haben aber die BOVERIschen pathologischen Mitosen nichts zu tun, denn die BOVERIschen „fehlerhaften Chromosomenkombinationen" waren ja lediglich die Folge einer bei der Krebsentstehung nie vorkommenden, (durch die Doppelbefruchtung) künstlich hervorgerufenen Chromosomenzahlerhöhung. Außerdem waren ja die entstandenen Zellen keine Krebszellen. Die BOVERIsche Versuchsanordnung begründet also keine Theorie der Geschwulstentstehung, sondern bedeutet nur einen Beitrag zur Erzeugung abnormer Mitosen.

Auch gibt es ja Chromosomenabnormitäten in nichtkrebsigen Geweben, so z. B. bei der Regeneration und Hyperplasie. Und wenn schon in Krebszellen im Vergleich mit ihren Mutterzellen abnorm hohe Chromosomenzahlen häufig genug vorkommen, so stets nur als Folge der bereits stattgehabten Cancerisierung, aber nicht als deren Ursache.

Was aber ist denn nun *krebsspezifisch?* Es ist dies

1. die Potenz eines beschleunigten Zellteilungsrhythmus durch einen Defekt in dessen Regulation. Hinzu kommt

2. ein Defekt in der Gewebsgebundenheit der Zellen.

Während normalerweise die Körperzellen allesamt an die Ordnung des Zellverbandes gebunden bleiben, können sich Krebszellen aus dem Gewebsverband ablösen und lokal in die Nachbargewebe einwachsen, oder sie können in ferne Gewebe oder Organe abgesiedelt – „metastasiert" – werden. Beide, der Regulationsdefekt der Zellteilung mit der Folge des schrankenlos expansiven Wachstums und der Defekt der Gewebsgebundenheit mit der Folge des infiltrierenden Wachstums machen zusammen das aus, was allgemein als Attribut der Malignität gilt: Die *autonom-destruktive Wucherung*. Soweit die Lehrmeinung Mitte der 20er Jahre.

Erbbiologische Voraussetzungen für eine genetisch-entwicklungs-physiologische Krebstheorie

Lassen Sie mich nun bitte den eigenen Weg hin zum Krebsproblem rekapitulieren, nicht etwa dergestalt, daß ich ex post rückwärtsspekuliere, sondern lassen Sie mich bitte nach dem ex-ante-Prinzip meine eigenen damaligen Formulierungen verwenden.

Ende November 1918 ging es vom Rückmarsch aus Frankreich weg nach Freiburg zu dem Pathologen LUDWIG ASCHOFF. Gleich der erste Tag war schicksalsentscheidend. ASCHOFF übergab dem homo novus eine Fehlgeburt mit angeborener Knochenbrüchigkeit (Osteogenesis imperfecta). Es bestanden Hunderte von Frakturen. Es ließ sich zeigen (K. H. BAUER, 1920) [3] – wörtlich! –: „daß die . . . Veränderungen *nicht nur auf das Knochensystem* beschränkt, sondern daß *auch zahlreiche andere Gewebe*, wie das Zahnsystem, die verschiedenen Arten von Knorpel, alle Sorten von Bindegewebe, die Blutgefäße, das lymphatische, das blutbildende Gewebe usw. gleichzeitig *mitbetroffen* waren." . . . „Es war also alles mesenchymale Gewebe erkrankt, alles ekto- und endodermale Gewebe verschont." . . . Morphogenetische Elektivität: „Störung der Grundsubstanzproduktion, Grad der Störung abhängig vom phylogenetischen Alter: Die erste angeborene *Mesenchymkrankheit* war morphologisch als solche ausgewiesen."

In der Chirurgie in Göttingen kamen ab 1919 weitere Fälle hinzu. Von der Morphologie ging es zur Erbbiologie: Die Osteogenesis imperfecta war vererbbar. Bald folgten 7 weitere chirurgische Systemerkrankungen (K. H. BAUER, 1923) [5], alle gleichfalls vererbbar. Die für damals neue Frage lautete: „Was bedeutet das im Lichte des Mendelismus . . .?"

Die Antwort lautete – wörtlich! –: „Aus der Tatsache, daß sich alle Beispiele nach dem Einfaktor-Schema einfach dominant vererben, läßt sich ‚mit Sicherheit ableiten', daß *der bunten Fülle ihrer klinischen Erscheinungen ein, und zwar nur ein einziger pathologischer Erbfaktor zugrunde liegt.*"

Sofort heißt es weiter: „In der Genetik nennt man nun einen solchen pathologischen Erbfaktor ..., der in einer bislang völlig gesunden Generationsfolge plötzlich auftritt, dann aber sich streng gesetzmäßig weitervererbt, und der seine Existenz einer dem Wesen nach noch unbekannten pathologischen Abänderung eines normalen Erbfaktors, einem scheinbar spontanen Erbumschlag verdankt, eine Mutation." Nun, die Früchte reiften schnell. „Erbkonstitutionelle Systemerkrankungen und Mesenchym" lautete der Habilitationsvortrag.

Die damals berüchtigtste chirurgische Erbkrankheit war die Bluterkrankheit, die Hämophilie. Ein Vortrag im März 1922 in Leipzig auf der Naturforscher-Tagung (anläßlich der 100-Jahrfeier ihrer Gründung) galt der „Bluter-Regel" „nur Männer erkranken, vererben aber nicht, nur Frauen vererben, sind selbst aber gesund" und deren Interpretation als geschlechtsgebunden-rezessive Vererbung eines Semiletalfaktors. Der Vortrag brachte eine Einladung nach Brünn zur Feier von GREGOR MENDELS 100. Geburtstag. Malen Sie sich selbst bitte die Gefühle aus, die den jungen Privatdozenten im Klostergärtlein in Brünn am Ort der Kreuzungsversuche MENDELS bewegten!

Der anschließende Vortrag [4] in Wien auf dem 1. Deutschen Vererbungskongreß trug den Titel „Über die Erbbiologie der Hämophilie und deren Bedeutung für unsere Vorstellungen von der Natur der Gene" (K. H. BAUER, 1923) [4]. Der Kernsatz schlug die Brücke von der Mutationstheorie zur Biochemie. Er lautete: „Das Gen Hämophilie und der ihr zugrunde liegende chemisch-fermentative Defekt – der Mangel an Thrombokinase – muß in allen Zellen des Organismus gesucht werden."

Damit war eindeutig zum Ausdruck gebracht, daß ein Gen-Defekt einer Keimzelle allen Körperzellen zuerteilt wird; auch war die spätere „*Ein-Gen – ein-Enzym-Hypothese*" für den speziellen Fall der Hämophilie klar ausgesprochen worden.

Auch war damals schon an Hand klinischer Beispiele von Erbkrankheiten der Tatsacheninhalt der Mutationstheorie von DE VRIES aus dem Jahre 1901 bereits erfaßt. Es war klar: Ein Gen verrät sich als distinkte Erbeinheit erst durch die Auswirkungen seiner Mutation. Mutationen sind eben in ihrer großen Mehrzahl Defektmutationen. Sie bedingen nicht nur Erbkrankheiten und Mißbildungen, sondern auch biochemische Defekte. Ein Gen kann, wenn es erst mutiert ist, weder entbehrt, noch durch andere ersetzt, noch geheilt werden. Alle klinischen Beispiele lehrten: Der Vorgang ist irreversibel.

Das Selbstvertrauen des jungen Privatdozenten war offenbar groß: Im Wintersemester 1924 hielt er bereits eine erbbiologische Vorlesung für Hörer aller Fakultäten. Man kannte um diese Zeit die Anwendung der Mendelschen Gesetze auf die Humanpathologie, die Lokalisation der Erbfaktoren in den Chromosomen, dort deren lineäre Anordnung und die

Erbfaktorenkombination der befruchteten Eizelle als genetische Grundlage der Individualität. Man wußte aber nichts, rein gar nichts, über die Mutationsverursachung.

Die Mutationstheorie der Geschwulstentstehung in ihrer ersten Form

In diese Situation platzte 1928 die Nachricht hinein, daß es MULLER [22] an Drosophila gelungen war, die spontane Mutationsquote in Keimzellen durch Röntgenbestrahlung der Keimdrüsen bis auf das 150fache zu steigern.

Sogleich stellte sich der furor combinatorius die Frage: „Wenn schon Röntgenstrahlen in Keimzellen Mutationen erzeugen, und wenn schon die gleichen Röntgenstrahlen in Körperzellen Krebs erzeugen, ist dann nicht vielleicht der Primärakt der Cancerisierung auch ein Mutationsvorgang, nur nicht an Genen in Keimzellen, sondern an Genen in Körperzellen?"

Wie schon vor 2 Jahren an gleicher Stelle berichtet, schlug die Ideenassoziation „Krebs als Folge einer Mutation im Zellerbgut somatischer Zellen" ein auf einer Bahnfahrt mit der BORSTschen „Allgemeinen Pathologie der malignen Geschwülste" als Reiselektüre und der Entdeckung von MULLER als wissenschaftlichem Novum.

Voraussetzung für die Richtigkeit einer solchen Vorstellung war natürlich, daß die Somazellen auch wirklich alle Gene der Keimzellen übertragen erhalten. Man war sich aber bereits damals darin einig: Sämtliche Körperzellen erhalten von ihrer Stammutter, der befruchteten Eizelle, deren sämtliche Chromosomen und deren sämtliche Gene übertragen.

Wohl werden bei der Ontogenese, vor allem bei der Differenzierung der Gewebe und Organe nicht alle Genwirkungen realisiert – weil sie ja nicht überall gebraucht werden –; daß sie aber in allen Zellen des Organismus vorhanden sind, läßt sich cytologisch in jeder sich teilenden Körperzelle nachweisen, werden ja doch jeder Tochterzelle alle Chromosomen neu zugeteilt. Anders ausgedrückt: Die befruchtete Eizelle gibt allen Tochterzellen, schließlich denen des gesamten Organismus, das gesamte Befehlsbuch mit, dessen Befehle die Somazellen, wenn dies notwendig wird, überall auszuführen in der Lage sind.

Wenn nun aber alle Körperzellen die gleichen Gene wie die befruchtete Eizelle besitzen, warum sollen die Körperzell-Gene bei adäquater Einwirkung nicht in gleicher Weise mutieren können wie die Keimzell-Gene?

MULLER stimmte der Konzeption sofort zu. Drei Monate später erschien die „*Mutationstheorie der Geschwulstentstehung*" [6], die die Cancerisierung als „Übergang von Körperzellen in Geschwulstzellen durch Gen-Änderung" nach allen Richtungen des damaligen Wissens durchdiskutierte.

Natürlich war es klar: Ein Analogieschluß – hier von Keimzellen auf Somazellen – ist natürlich noch kein allein zureichender Beweisgrund. Weitere Indizienbeweise waren notwendig. Was sofort faszinierte, war die *Parallelität zwischen Mutationsauslösung und Krebsauslösung*:

Beide entstehen plötzlich.
Beide sind durch gleiche Mittel exogen induzierbar.
Bei beiden entstehen neue Eigenschaften bei Erhaltung der meisten alten.
Bei beiden handelt es sich um einen Defekt, einmal in den Genen der Keimzellen, das andere Mal um den geschilderten Regulationsdefekt gegenüber den Körperzellen.
Beide sind irreversibel.

Das zweite Argument ist die weitgehende *Parallelität keimzell-mutagener und körperzell-carcinogener Wirkung* gleicher chemischer Agentien.

Inzwischen waren ja – als ein wahrer Triumph der damaligen Krebsforschung – den Klinikern schon lange geläufige stofflich-komplexe Krebsursachen, wie Rauch, Ruß, Teer, Pech etc., durch das Prisma der chemischen Analyse in ein großes Spektrum chemisch strukturell genau definierbarer Stoffe zerlegt und aufgeklärt worden. Aus den an die 500 chemischen und physikalischen krebsauslösenden Faktoren sei hier lediglich an die Fülle der Krebsnoxen, die inhaliert Bronchialkrebs auszulösen vermögen, erinnert.

Ferner hat die Chemogenetik schon von 1930 an gezeigt, daß es mit einer ganzen Reihe chemischer Carcinogene möglich ist, in Keimzellen Mutationen auszulösen, so z. B. mit Senfgas und Lostderivaten, mit Urethan, Arsen, mit carcinogenen Kohlenwasserstoffen wie Benzpyren, Methylcholantren, 1,2,5,6-Dibenzanthracen und vielen anderen Stoffen mehr. Die Mutationsauslösung durch Schädigungen aus unserer technisierten Umwelt mit der drohenden Erbgutverschlechterung des Menschen ist heute ein weltweites Forschungsgebiet geworden. Neben den Arbeiten von MULLER, OEHLKERS, CH. AUERBACH sei vor allem auf MARQUARDT [*19, 21*] sowie auf VOGEL und seine Schule [*34, 35*] verwiesen.

Nun hat man gefordert, die Kongruenz keimzell – mutativ/körperzell – carcinogen müsse eine 100%ige sein, sonst sei die ganze Gen-Mutationstheorie widerlegt. Tatsächlich sind nicht alle chemischen Mutagene zugleich carcinogen und umgekehrt. Aber HECKER [*15*] hat bereits darauf hingewiesen, daß die Prüfung auf mutagene Wirkung fast ausschließlich an Bakterien, Pilzen und Bakteriophagen vorgenommen wird, also an Objekten, die vom (für die Carcinogenität verwendeten) Wirbeltier phylogenetisch sehr weit entfernt sind.

Sodann gibt es sogenannte resorptiv, d. h. nicht am Ort der Applikation, sondern fernab wirksame Carcinogene, die wie z. B. das Dimethyl-
amino-azobenzol (Buttergelb) oder das Betanaphthylamin nur durch ihre
Umwandlungsprodukte und dann „organotrop", nur in bestimmten
Organen carcinogen sind, in anderen Organen jedoch nicht. Wie sollen
solche Körperzell-Carcinogene auf Keimzellen mutagen wirken, wenn
diese Carcinogene die Keimzellen selber ja überhaupt nicht erreichen
können?

Die 100%ige Mutagen-Carcinogen-Übereinstimmung ist jedoch dort
gewährleistet, wo strahlende Energien Körpergewebe und Keimzellen in
gleicher Weise durchfluten. Hier sind alle Strahlenenergien mit Wellenlängen kürzer als das sichtbare Licht samt und sonders zugleich mutagen
und zugleich carcinogen. Es kann dies um so weniger Zufall sein, als auch
die Gegenprobe nicht fehlt: Strahlen mit größeren Wellenlängen, wie
z. B. die Strahlen des sichtbaren Lichtes oder die Radiowellen, erzeugen
keinen Krebs, sie erzeugen auch keine Mutation.

So wird gerade die *Parallelität gleicher mutationsauslösender und
gleicher krebsinduzierender Strahlen* zugleich *das stärkste Argument* für die
Schlüssigkeit der Mutationstheorie der Krebsentstehung.

Nun haben natürlich – und mit Recht – Skeptiker Einwände zur
Hand. Der wichtigste Einwand lautet: Es fehlt der experimentelle Beweis.
Es ist richtig, der experimentelle Beweis fehlt. Er wird aber immer
fehlen, weil wir wohl den Effekt der experimentellen Krebserzeugung –
nämlich den Krebs – nachweisen können, niemals jedoch die Gen-
Veränderung am Gen-Ort selbst; erfolgt ja diese Gen-Änderung im
molekularen Bereich und ist daher auch durch 100000fache Vergrößerung
im Elektronenmikroskop nicht faßbar, sondern nur erschließbar.

Nun gibt es aber nicht bloß Laborexperimente, sondern auch Natur-
experimente, und diese sind dann beweisschlüssig, wenn die theoretische
Forderung praktisch voll erfüllt ist.

Schon 1937 hat der damals führende Theoretiker der Genetik TIMO-
FÉEFF-RESSOVSKY folgendes postuliert (Abb. 2): Tritt eine Erbgut-
änderung nicht in Keimzellen, sondern erst nach der Befruchtung der
Eizelle, also als *somatische Mutation* ein, so muß sie im Falle a – Mutation
einer Zelle im Zweizellenstadium – die eine Körperhälfte befallen, die
andere verschonen. Bei späterem Eintritt im Falle b muß sie einen ganzen Körperabschnitt, im Falle c bei noch späterer Auslösung nur eine
beschränkte Körperpartie betreffen. Dazu 4 Fälle:

1. Eine streng *halbseitige Chondromatose* des Knochensystems
(Abb. 3),

2. eine sogenannte *Melorheostose* als eine über eine ganze Gliedmaße
sich erstreckende, expansiv wachsende Geschwulstbildung (Osteomatose),

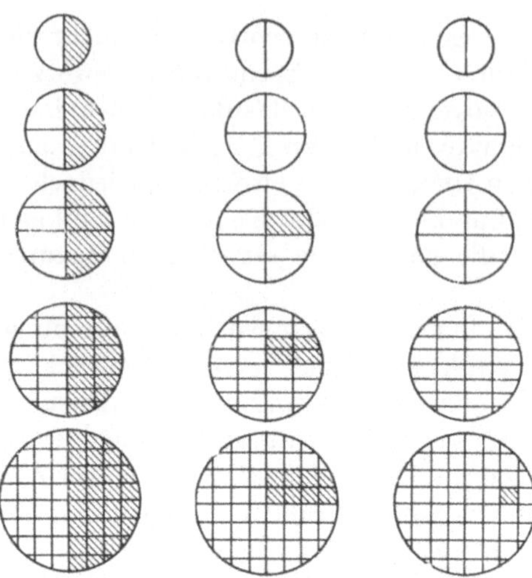

Abb. 2. Die Auswirkungen somatischer Mutationen in ihrer Verschiedenheit je nach dem Zeitpunkt ihres Auftretens (n. TIMOFÉEFF-RESSOVSKY, 1937)

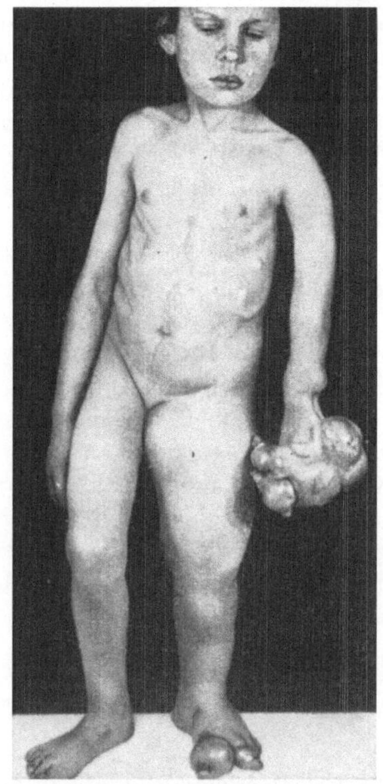

Abb. 3. Rein halbseitige Chondromatose des Knochensystems

3. eine ausschließlich periphere, beiderseits identisch-symmetrische *Chondromatose* beider Hände*,

4. ein isoliertes *Chondrom* nur einer Phalange**.

Die aufgeführten Beispiele lassen die theoretische Forderung des Genetikers durch die praktische Erfahrung im experimentum naturae an einer solchen blastogenetischen Reihe als voll erfüllt erscheinen.

Ganz von selbst erhebt sich nunmehr die Frage: Entsteht Krebs durch die gleiche Mutation zahlreicher, z. B. Hunderter somatischer Zellen, oder ist Krebs durch die somatische Mutation nur eines einzigen Gens einer Zelle bedingt?

Man erinnere sich bei dieser Frage der Hämophilie. Sie zeigt, daß, wenn unter den Tausenden von Genen eines Menschen nur dieses eine Gen, welches das entscheidende Enzym für die spontane Blutgerinnung determiniert, fehlt oder defekt ist, dann auch die Tausende noch vorhandenen Gene das Fehlen des einen mutierten Gens nicht zu kompensieren vermögen, weil jedem einzelnen Gen eine einmalige, streng spezifische und unersetzbare Bedeutung, in diesem Falle für das Enzymgeschehen, zukommt.

Das ausschlaggebende Argument liefern die *monohybrid*, d. h. nach dem Einfaktorschema *vererbbaren menschlichen Krebskrankheiten*. Sie können *nur durch die Mutation eines einzigen Gens* der Keimzellen ausgelöst sein.

Ich nenne als Beispiele nur die nach dem Mendelschen Grundgesetz vererbbare *Polyposis intestini*, die meist schon früh zu oft multiplen Dickdarmcarcinomen, und das *maligne Retinoblastom*, welches gleichfalls fast immer zum Tode führt.

Wenn es sich bei einer erblichen und dann generalisierten Polyposis dem Erbgang nach mit Sicherheit um die Mutation nur eines Gens in den Keimzellen eines Elters handelt, warum soll es sich dann bei dem primär solitären, aber morphologisch identischen Einzelpolypen nicht um die gleiche, diesmal somatische Mutation des gleichen Gens handeln?

Man könnte einwenden, daß gegen die Ein-Gen-Annahme die Tatsache spräche, daß wenigstens bei einer malignen Erkrankung, nämlich bei bestimmten Formen myeloischer Leukämie im sogenannten Philadelphia-Chromosom eine chromosomale Änderung am Genom der Leukämiezellen nachgewiesen ist. Es ist dies unzweifelhaft richtig – nebenbei auch in Heidelberg soeben ein als konstant aberrierendes Chromosom bei 2 Kindern mit akuter myeloischer Leukämie bestätigt (SCHLEIERMACHER, 1967) –; doch ist diese chromosomale Abweichung – gerade wegen der

---

* Vgl. Abb. 148, S. 536 in K. H. BAUER, Das Krebsproblem. 2. Aufl. 1963.
** Vgl. Abb. 149, S. 537, ibid.

Einzigartigkeit ihrer Konstanz – doch sehr viel wahrscheinlicher nur die Folge einer mutagenen Störung an einem Gen der Mitose-Regulation.

Dies war 1948 der Stand der Dinge, der es erlaubte, in dem Buch „Das Krebsproblem" das damalige Wissen um das Krebsgeschehen in der Sprache und dem Vorstellungsgehalt der Mutationstheorie der Geschwulstentstehung einheitlich darzustellen; galt es ja alsbald als ebenso sicher wie selbstverständlich: *Die Cancerisierung einer Körperzelle beginnt mit einer von nun an irreversiblen Änderung jener Erbstruktur, die die Regulation des Zellwachstums determiniert.*

Was aber inzwischen seit damals neu hinzugekommen ist, das ist die Fortentwicklung der sogenannten klassischen Genetik zur molekularen Genetik.

Die Fortentwicklung der Mutationstheorie

Hatte auch die klassische Genetik mit dem Mendelismus, der Genanalyse bestimmter Lebewesen, vor allem der Drosophila, der linearen Anordnung der Gene in den Chromosomen, gipfelnd in den „Chromosomenkarten" MORGANS Großartiges geleistet, so war andererseits die *biochemische Natur der Gene* unbekannt geblieben. Nehmen wir das Endergebnis gleich vorweg: Als Erbsubstanz aller Lebewesen gilt heute die hochmolekulare Desoxyribonukleinsäure (abgekürzt DNS) als erwiesen. Ihre Ausgangssubstanz war schon 1869 von MIESCHER entdeckt worden. Aber erst 1943 wurde von AVERY nachgewiesen, daß die DNS die in den Genen der Keimzellen niedergelegte, wie wir heute sagen, genetische Information speichert und beim Aufbau jedes neuen Organismus auf alle Körperzellen überträgt.

Die DNS stellt ein einziges langfädiges Makromolekül dar, welches – genetisch betrachtet – aus einer fortgesetzten Kette von Genen besteht. Dem Einzel-Gen ist jeweils – Beispiel Hämophilie! – eine ganz bestimmte, aber nur diese Aufgabe zuerteilt.

Vom Thema her interessiert natürlich am meisten die Frage, ob sich die *Mutationsauslösung und die Krebsauslösung an der DNS durch gleiche chemische Stoffe* durch gleiche molekular-genetische Veränderungen befriedigend erklären lassen.

Dazu ist es erforderlich, zunächst kurz auf die *Struktur der DNS* einzugehen. Diese ist unter Zugrundelegung der Arbeiten von WATSON u. CRICK, sowie von WILKINS u. a. in letzter Zeit häufig dargestellt worden. Wir beziehen uns auf BRESCH (1964) [12] und auf HECKER (1967) [15] (Abb. 4 und 5). Für unseren Zusammenhang genügt es, an einem Teilstück der DNS auf das für die chemische Reaktion mit Carcinogenen entscheidende Prinzip der Basenpaarung, und zwar auf die Partner Guanin und Cytosin bzw. Adenin und Thymin hinzuweisen.

Wie einer Abbildung HECKERS [15] zu entnehmen ist, vermag hier die Base Guanin der DNS (Abb. 5) mit dem Carcinogen Dimethylnitrosamin in Reaktion zu treten, mit dem Effekt einer ganz bestimmten chemischen Abänderung.

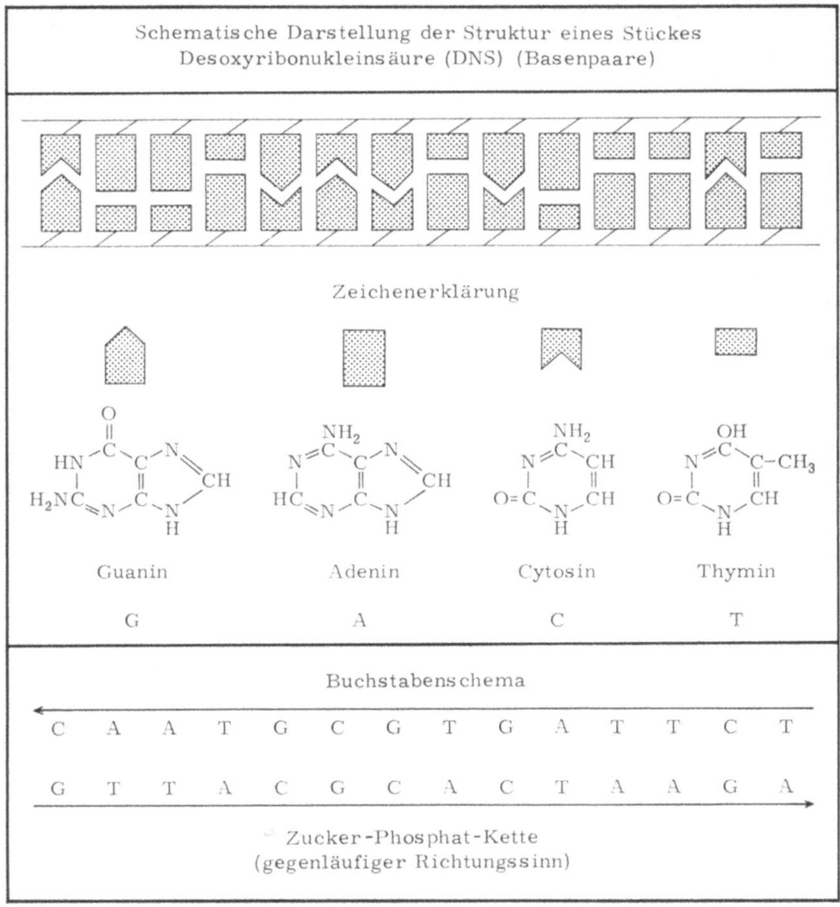

Abb. 4. Ein Teilstück der Desoxyribonukleinsäure schematisch. Oben Basenpaare, darunter Strukturformeln, unten Buchstabenschema der Basenpaare (Schema kombiniert aus mehreren Abbildungen bei BRESCH [12])

Vergleichbares gilt für die Abänderung der Basen Thymin und Guanin, einmal durch Röntgen-, sodann durch Ultraviolettstrahlen (Abb. 6), welche beide ja zugleich mutagen und carcinogen sind.

Damit ist zunächst etwas grundsätzlich Wichtiges ausgesagt: Carcinogene Stoffe und Strahlungen gelangen wirklich an die DNS heran, sie reagieren mit ihr und vermögen biochemisch wichtige Strukturelemente des DNS, nämlich Basen derselben, chemisch abzuändern.

Es ist aber andererseits damit natürlich noch nicht ausgesagt, daß gerade diese oder jene molekular-genetische Abänderung die Cancerisierung selbst dokumentieren würde. Die chemische Basenänderung zeigt jedoch eindeutig an, daß Teilstücke der Desoxyribonukleinsäure, auf denen die Gene hintereinander aufgereiht sind, chemisch abgeändert zu werden vermögen.

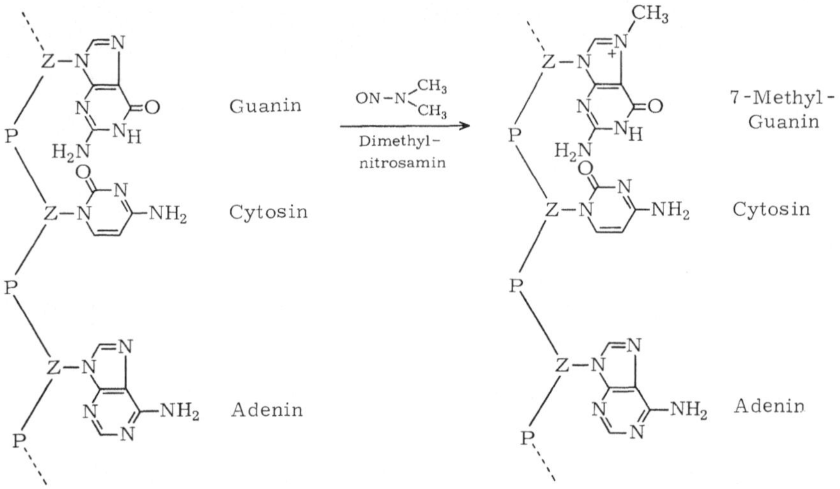

Abb. 5. Veränderungen der Desoxyribonukleinsäure durch Reaktion mit Dimethylnitrosamin (nach E. HECKER, 1967)

Aber noch eindrucksvoller ist *der strahlenphysikalische Indizienbeweis*. Seit langem ist es bekannt, daß beim „Lichtkrebs" der Seeleute und Ackerbauern die Krebsentstehung durch die jahrelange Einwirkung ultravioletter Strahlen des Lichtes ausgelöst wird. Nun weiß man seit langem, daß sich die Mutabilität der Gene durch *Ultraviolettstrahlung* ebenso steigern läßt, wie durch Röntgenstrahlen. Was aber hier entscheidend erscheint: Das Wirkungsspektrum der Ultraviolettstrahlung und das Absorptionsspektrum der DNS stimmen genau überein. Das bedeutet: „Licht der Wellenlänge um 260 mμ, das gerade von der DNS stark absorbiert wird, hat zugleich die stärkste mutagene Wirkung" (KARLSON, 1961). Da auch der carcinogene Effekt im gleichen Wellenbereich gelegen ist, so ist das ein ungemein eindrucksvoller Beweis dafür, daß die Wirkung die gleiche ist, gleichviel, ob es sich um die Absorption der DNS selbst oder um die Mutations- bzw. um die Krebsauslösung handelt.

Es würde zu viel Zeit beanspruchen, wollte ich versuchen, die Bedeutung der DNS als biochemisches Substrat der Erbsubstanz ausführlicher zu bringen. Nur so viel: Es besteht heute Einigkeit darüber, daß die Auswahl und die Reihenfolge der Basen in der DNS den sogenannten

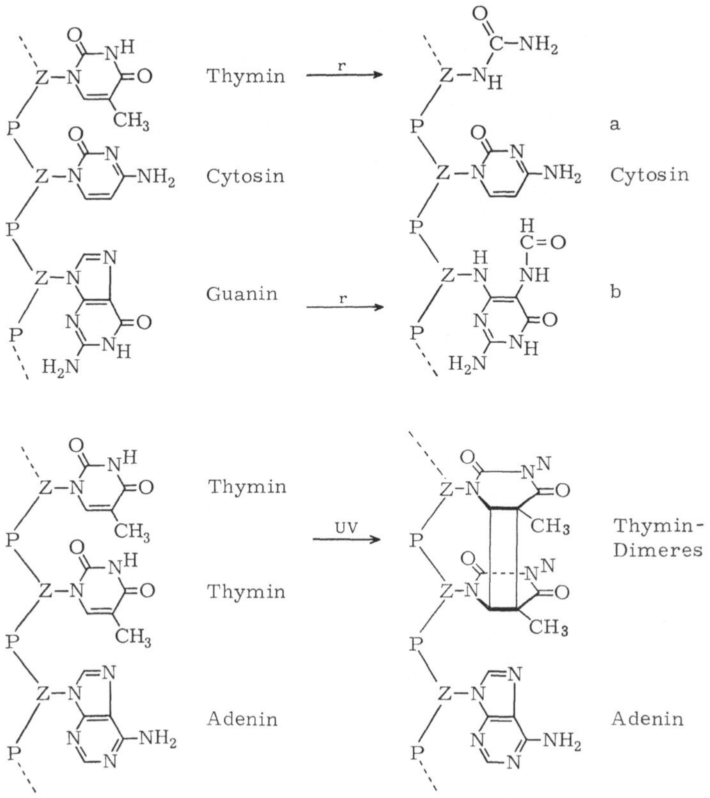

Abb. 6. Veränderungen der Desoxyribonukleinsäure durch Röntgen- (oben), bzw. UV-Strahlen (unten) (nach E. HECKER, 1967)

genetischen Code darstellt, der im ganzen Organismenbereich die gleichen 4 Basen der DNS benutzt, um durch die Übertragung dieses Codes auf die Proteine mit 20 Aminosäuren zu arbeiten (vgl. A. KÜHN, 1965) [17].

Das Entscheidende für die Mutationstheorie der Geschwulstentstehung ist die Tatsache, daß die DNS-Basen auf chemische Stoffe und Strahlen reagieren, die experimentell zugleich als mutagen und zugleich als carcinogen erwiesen sind.

Nun schien es eine Zeit lang, als ob die seit dem Roussarkom des Huhnes (1906) bereits bekannten *Virustumoren* mit der Mutationstheorie absolut unvereinbar seien. Daß es sich um Geschwulstkrankheiten

handelt, ist unbestreitbar. Ebenso unbestreitbar ist aber, daß sich Virustumoren von allen geläufigen menschlichen Organkrebsen und durch so
gut wie alle Krankheitserscheinungen unterscheiden. Worauf es entscheidend ankommt, ist die Frage, ob die Mutationstheorie auch die
Virustumoren befriedigend zu interpretieren in der Lage ist.

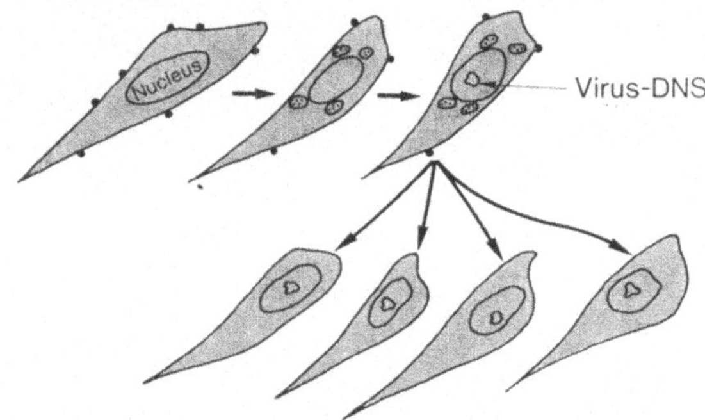

Abb. 7. „Neoplastische Transformation" von Hamsterembryozellen durch Infektion
mit Virus-DNS (nach R. DULBECCO, 1967)

Das ist nun tatsächlich der Fall, seit sich gezeigt hat, daß die Viren
vorwiegend aus Eiweiß und Nukleinsäuren bestehen, die sich nur in
lebenden Zellen zu vermehren vermögen, und daß sie in die DNS-
Synthese der Zelle eingreifen.

Vielleicht zeigt eine schematische Zeichnung eines führenden Viro-
logen – DULBECCO, San Diego [13] –, wie er sie kürzlich in unserem
Heidelberger Krebskolloquium demonstrierte, am einfachsten, worum es
dabei geht. Das Bild (Abb. 7) zeigt: Viruspartikel dringen in die Mäuse-
embryo-Zelle ein und lagern sich dem Zellkern an; die in den Zellkern
eindringende Virus-DNS bewirkt die „maligne Transformation", die
sich dann gleichartig auf die Zellnachkommen überträgt. Diese Nach-
kommenzellen weisen ihrerseits ihre neoplastische Transformation dadurch aus, daß sie a) ihre Steuerungsfähigkeit verloren haben (kenntlich
daran, daß ihre Gewebekulturen dank ihres raschen Wachstums dichter
wachsen) und b) dadurch, daß ihre zellulären Nachbarbeziehungen abgeändert sind; sie wachsen unregelmäßig, besonders deutlich daran
erkennbar, daß sie einander zum Teil „überlappen" (Abb. 8).

So besteht heute, nachdem es gesichert ist, daß diese onkogenen Viren
in die DNS-Synthese eingreifen, kein Gegensatz mehr zwischen der
sogenannten Virus- und der Mutationstheorie. Im Gegenteil: Die Vor-

gänge bei der viralen Tumorgenese haben den Vorteil, daß man an diesen onkogenen Viren, wie MUNK (1967) [23] es ausdrückte, „den Vorgang der neoplastischen Transformation, d. h. die Umwandlung einer normalen Zelle in eine Tumorzelle, bis in molekular-biologische Dimensionen hinein verfolgen kann."

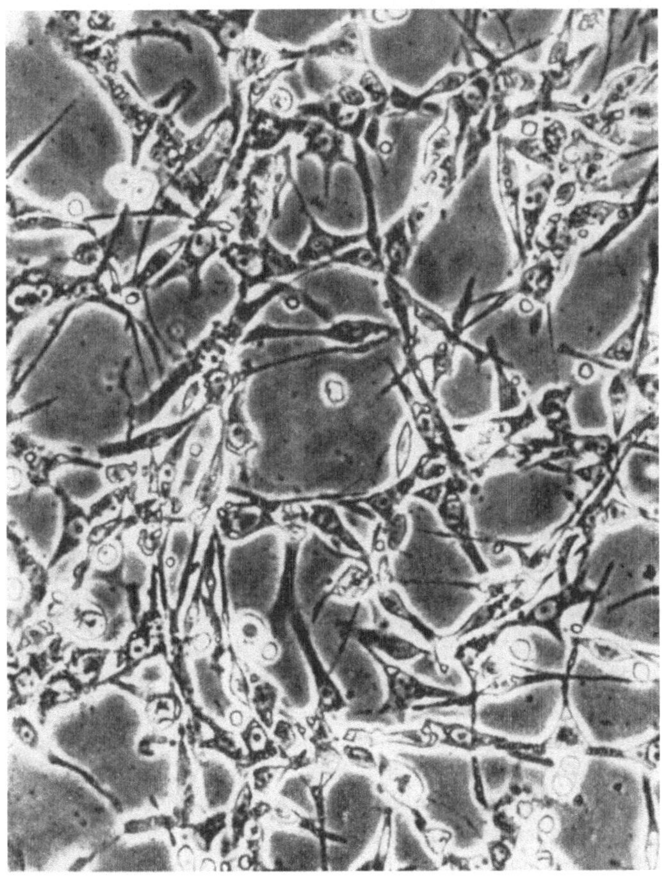

Abb. 8. Durch Virus-DNS neoplastisch transformierte Hamsterembryozellen in der Gewebekultur (nach R. DULBECCO, 1967)

Mutations- und Virus-Theorie schließen sich also nicht nur nicht gegenseitig aus, vielmehr bedeutet der Sonderfall „maligne Transformation durch Viren" nur eine weitere Bestätigung der molekular-biologischen Mutationstheorie.

So ist abschließend zu sagen, daß auch die großen neuen Fortschritte der molekularen Genetik – und hier besonders der Nachweis der Desoxyribonukleinsäure als universelles Substrat für die Vielzahl der Gene –, und speziell der Nachweis, daß onkogene Viren mit der Desoxyribonukleinsäure der befallenen Zellen in Reaktion treten, eine Fortentwicklung und Neufundierung der Mutationstheorie mit sich gebracht haben.

Neue Fragestellungen und Ausblicke in die Zukunft

Der Hauptprüfstein einer Theorie ist jedoch, daß sie auch zu neuen Fragestellungen Anlaß gibt. Lassen Sie mich zunächst bitte auf eine eigene Überlegung zurückgreifen, über die ich vor 2 Jahren in meinem Vortrag über die Anfänge einer zusätzlichen Krebstherapie kurz vortrug. Ich sagte mir:

Röntgenstrahlen, auf *Keimzellen* appliziert, erzeugen Mutationen,

Röntgenstrahlen, auf *Körperzellen* appliziert, erzeugen Krebs,

Röntgenstrahlen, auf *Krebszellen* appliziert, erzeugen Krebsheilung.

Was geschieht nun, so habe ich mich gefragt, wenn man statt der carcinogenen Röntgenstrahlen das zugleich keimzell-mutative und krebserzeugende Benzpyren auf Krebszellen selbst appliziert?

Nun, es hat sich an den dem direkten Kontakt zugänglichen Hautcarcinomen gezeigt, daß die Krebszellen eine erneute mutative Abänderung ihres schon defekten Zellerbgutes nicht vertragen und, genau wie durch Röntgenstrahlen, durch Carcinogene auch chemisch geheilt zu werden vermögen. Ich zeige nur kurz rekapitulierend zwei solcher Fälle, die jenen Grundversuch und sein Ergebnis dokumentieren*.

Selbstverständlich sollte dies von allem Anfang an keine „neue Krebstherapie" darstellen, sind ja solche Hautcarcinome operativ und strahlentherapeutisch einfacher und zugleich sicherer zu heilen. Worum es ging, das war der Grundversuch!

Inzwischen gibt es eine Unzahl von Chemotherapeutika gegen den Krebs, unter diesen auch solche, die sich als Lost-Derivate von Kampfstoffen des 1. Weltkrieges ableiten. Solche Lost-Derivate sind es auch gewesen, mit denen CHARLOTTE AUERBACH zum erstenmal in der Geschichte der Mutationsforschung Mutationen in Keimzellen chemisch ausgelöst hat.

Zu solchen Lost-Derivaten stehen auch die heute am meisten verwendeten Krebsheilmittel *Endoxan* und *Trenimon* in Beziehung. Vom Trenimon ist die mutagene Wirkung von RÖHRBORN (1967) nachgewiesen

---

* Die Original-Diapositive wurden erstmals auf dem Deutschen Chirurgenkongreß 1937 demonstriert und in 3 Abbildungsreihen im Kongreßbericht (s. Lit.-Verz.) veröffentlicht. Weitere Wiedergaben finden sich in beiden Auflagen des Buches „Das Krebsproblem" und im Heidelberger Symposionbericht über „Aktuelle Probleme aus dem Gebiet der Cancerologie" (1966) veröffentlicht.

worden. SCHMÄHL (1967) hat inzwischen im Tierexperiment gezeigt, daß diese beiden Krebs-Heilmittel

a) ausgesprochen *lebensverkürzend* wirken und

b) schon in therapeutisch üblichen Dosen selbst als *krebserzeugend* angesehen werden müssen.

Nur in Parenthese: So bestürzend es erscheint, daß die geläufigsten Krebsheilmittel auf lange Sicht selbst krebserzeugend sind, so gering ist die praktische Gefahr; erhalten ja jene Mittel fast ausschließlich aussichtslos krebskranke Menschen mit nur noch kurzer Lebenserwartung. Andererseits wird man natürlich diese Mittel bei denjenigen Krebskranken nicht mehr verwenden, die aller ärztlichen Voraussicht nach geheilt sind, und demzufolge, besonders als Jugendliche, noch eine lange Lebenserwartung vor sich haben.

Eine zweite Fragestellung: In den 30er Jahren erfreute sich das Röntgenkontrastmittel *Thorotrast*, weil es ganz ausgezeichnete Röntgenbilder lieferte, großer Beliebtheit. Da das Kontrastmittel Thoriumdioxyd enthält, macht es jedoch die betreffenden Kranken wegen der Beta- und Gammastrahlung, wenn auch nur schwach, so aber fürs ganze Leben radioaktiv. Nach der Mutationstheorie wirken entsprechend den Ergebnissen der Strahlenphysik sämtliche Strahlen mit Wellenlängen kürzer als das sichtbare Licht – bei entsprechender Dosis und Zeit – carcinogen. So warnte ich denn 1943 vor dem Gebrauch des Thorotrastes und wagte die Vorhersage, daß 12–18 Jahre nach der Applikation maligne Thorotrasttumoren zu erwarten seien. Es wurden damit Krebsgeschwülste beim Menschen vorausgesagt, die es bis dahin nicht gab. Tatsächlich kam alsbald genau 12 Jahre nach der Thorotrastapplikation das erste Hämangiosarkom der Leber zur Publikation. Seitdem sind über 100 Fälle von malignen „Thorotrastomen" der verschiedensten Lokalisation beschrieben worden. Wie viele werden nicht beschrieben sein, da man oft nichts von der Thorotrast-Applikation weiß oder weil nicht daran gedacht wird! Die Militärbehörden waren einsichtig genug, auf meine Vorstellungen hin das Thorotrast zu verbieten. Wieviele Tausende damaliger Soldaten mögen vor schweren Thorotrastschäden, vor allem der Leber, und wieviele vor thorotrastinduzierten malignen Tumoren bewahrt geblieben sein! Der Kliniker kennt viele Beispiele, bei denen bei der Krebsentstehung – leicht ausweisbar – eine Vielheit von Schädigungen, sei es gleichzeitig oder nacheinander, sei es carcinogener oder nur sonst schädigender Art bei der Krebsentstehung zusammengewirkt haben. Ich prägte dafür 1948 den Ausdruck *Syncarcinogenese*. SCHMÄHL hat inzwischen durch geistreiche Variation der Versuchsbedingungen mit Hilfe verschiedener Carcinogene und nichtcarcinogener sonstiger Schädigungen die heuristische Bedeutung des Begriffs „Syncarcinogenese" experimentell unterbaut und damit auch für die Krebsverhütung wichtige Unterlagen geschaffen.

SCHMÄHL [*29–31*] zeigte in einer Serie von Arbeiten (Zusammenfassung 1966), daß eine Syncarcinogenese dann vorliegt, wenn carcinogene Substanzen mit gleicher Organ- oder Gewebsbezogenheit gleichzeitig oder nacheinander einwirken oder wenn Hormongaben die Voraussetzung für die Wirkung eines Carcinogens in dem hormonabhängigen Organ schaffen. Es fehlt auch nicht der Gegenbeweis: Carcinogene mit verschiedener Organbezogenheit sind ohne syncarcinogenetische Wirkung. Umgekehrt wiederum verstärkt ein nicht carcinogenes Organgift die krebserzeugende Wirkung eines auf dieses Organ wirkenden Carcinogens.

Das therapeutische Gegenstück zur Syncarcinogenese ist die *Syncarcinokolyse*, d. h. die Krebsbehandlung mit Carcinostatika zellulär verschiedener Angriffspunkte.

Zwei Beispiele*: Fall 1: eine 39jährige Frau wurde nach einem Brustkrebs, bei ausgedehnten Ovarial-, Hilus- und riesigen Lungenmetastasen bis 10 cm Durchmesser wie folgt behandelt: Ovariektomie, Testoviron, Arsen, Cholchizin, Urethan, Stickstoff-Lost und Chinin. Die riesigen Lungenmetastasen gingen von Kontrolle zu Kontrolle so weit zurück, daß sie zum Schluß röntgenologisch nicht mehr ausweisbar waren. Dreijährige Überlebensdauer.

Fall 2: Bei einem 40jährigen Mann großzelliges Carcinom im Halsbereich, ausgedehnte Hautmetastasen mit stets übler Prognose, Halsumfang 64 cm. Nach einer 1. Serie mit Stickstoff-Lost, Arsen, Cholchizin und Urethan Rückgang des Halsumfanges um 12 cm, Gewichtszunahme, aber noch Hautmetastasen. Auf eine 2. gleiche Kur Rückbildung auch dieser. Klinisch das Bild völliger Heilung. Wiederaufnahme der Arbeit als Heizungs-Ingenieur. Über 1 Jahr später plötzlicher Tod nach Querschnittslähmung infolge Halswirbelmetastase.

Die kombinierte Chemotherapie nach dem Prinzip der Syncarcinokolyse wird heute in den verschiedensten Kombinationen durchgeführt.

Ausblick in die Zukunft

Der Krebs ist mit dem Fortschritt aufs Engste gekoppelt, und zwar bereits seit Urbeginn des technischen Fortschrittes, seit Prometheus und seiner Feuererzeugung und Feuerbewahrung. Mit der Feuererzeugung vermochte der Mensch zum ersten Male seine naturgegebene Umwelt zu seinen Gunsten künstlich umzugestalten. Gleichzeitig zogen jedoch mit

---

* Die vorgezeigten Bilder entsprechen den Abb. 204 und 205 (Fall 1) und der Abb. 203a und b in K. H. BAUER: Das Krebsproblem. 2. Aufl. S. 811–813, 1963.

dem Rauch, Ruß und den Abgasen der unvollkommenen Verbrennung die ersten Carcinogene in die vom Menschen nunmehr ständig manipulierte Umwelt ein.

Seitdem ist der technische Fortschritt mit allem, was er sonst noch gebracht hat, die letzte Ursache der Krebszunahme, und zwar gleich auf doppelte Weise: Auf der einen Seite haben alle großen Erfindungen, nicht zuletzt die 600000 neu synthetisierten Stoffe, darunter die Vitamine, Hormone, Enzyme, hochwirksame Medikamente usw., es dahin gebracht, daß sich die Lebenserwartung im letzten Jahrhundert im Durchschnitt mehr als verdoppelt hat, so daß der heute Neugeborene die reelle Chance hat, das biblische Alter von 75 Lebensjahren zu erreichen.

Mit der Erreichung hoher Altersstufen erreichen jedoch die Menschen zugleich das Ende der Latenzzeit des Krebses, das sie früher nicht erlebten. Das Alter erzeugt zwar nicht den Krebs, aber es ermöglicht und begünstigt ihn.

Die Kehrseite des segensreichen Fortschritts, den uns die erwähnten 600000 neuen Stoffe beschert haben, besteht darin, daß in der ungefähren Größenordnung von 1 : 1000 gewissermaßen als Neben- und Abfallprodukte an die 500 Carcinogene in unsere Umwelt eingeschleust worden sind.

So wird Krebs weiterhin zunehmen,

a) weil die durchschnittliche Lebensdauer ansteigt, und

b) weil die Ursachen, die den Krebs bedingen, selbst noch weiterhin zunehmen.

Wie sehr die Zunahme der Carcinogene abhängt von der Produktion ihrer Rohstoffe, dafür nur einen Beleg:

Eine Tabelle* zeigt ab 1900 die Zunahme der Produktion, z. B. von Kohle, Teer, Briketts, Asphalt, Asbest, Arsen, Chrom und anderen Chemikalien; alles zugleich die Zunahme chemischer Carcinogene industrieller Provenienz.

Die Konsequenzen sind dreifacher Art:

1. Es braucht ein erschöpfendes Register aller Carcinogene.
2. Es braucht eine spezielle Krebsforschung, die die Summe neuer Stoffe schon vor ihrem Gebrauch auf Carcinogenität prüft.
3. Es braucht gesundheitspolitisch eine aktive Krebsverhütung durch größtmögliche Ausschaltung der Carcinogene unserer Umwelt.

Daß eine solche aktive Krebsverhütung viel vermag, beweist der *Magenkrebs.* Er ist vor allem dank der gesetzgeberischen Ausschaltung der chemischen Fremdbeimischungen zu den Lebensmitteln in den

---

* Im Vortrag vorgezeigt, im Original publiziert im „Krebsproblem" [2] als Abb. 213 S. 884.

letzten 30 Jahren fast auf die Hälfte zurückgegangen und geht weiter zurück.

Umgekehrt steigt der *Bronchialkrebs* an. Beim Manne macht er heute mit 25,06% genau ein Viertel aller Krebs-Todesfälle aus. Jeder 4. Mann, der an Krebs verstirbt, stirbt an Bronchialkrebs. Den Magenkrebs hat er 1965 bereits um 11% überholt.

Das Diagramm* dokumentiert einerseits unsere Hauptsorge um die weitere Krebs-Zukunft, sie dokumentiert andererseits am Beispiel Magenkrebs: *Rein gesetzgeberisch hat die Antikrebs-Zukunft bereits begonnen.* Im Kampf gegen den Krebs bleibt jedoch immer noch sehr viel mehr zu leisten, als bereits geleistet worden ist.

Was aber im Rahmen unseres Themas besonders irritiert, ist – wieder aus der Sicht der Mutationstheorie – die Tatsache, daß die gleichen Noxen, die in Körperzellen Krebs verursachen, in Keimzellen Mutationen und damit eine *Erbgutverschlechterung* der Kulturvölker auslösen.

Stimmt es nicht nachdenklich, daß der Entdecker der Röntgen-Mutationen, MULLER-Texas, in großer Sorge darüber starb, daß die Erbgutverschlechterung bereits nicht mehr aufzuhalten sei. Und auch die Entdeckerin der chemisch induzierten Mutationen CHARLOTTE AUERBACH äußert sich besorgt und pessimistisch. Aber es ist wohl immer so, daß große Entdecker die Welt vornehmlich durch das Prisma ihrer eigenen Entdeckung und damit einseitig verzerrt sehen.

Nicht, als ob die Gefahr verkleinert werden soll, aber die Selbsthilfe der Natur in Gestalt der Ausmerze ist eben doch beachtlich. An die 50% der Mutationen verlaufen letal, d. h. sie führen zum Absterben der Keimzellen oder der Früchte. Von den restierenden 50% bedingt ein Teil Sterilität und damit Selbstausschaltung. Von dem Rest gehen neun Zehntel mit einer Minderung der Vitalität einher und damit mit einer Minderung der Fortpflanzungschance. Auf lange Sicht bleibt jedoch – bedingt durch die carcinogene Verseuchung unserer Umwelt – unleugbar eine genetische Gefahr.

So setzen wir denn unsere Haupthoffnung auf die Wissenschaft. Die Geschichte der Medizin lehrt: Noch immer ist in der Krankheitsbekämpfung der Ursachen-Aufklärung die Ursachen-Verhütung alsbald nachgefolgt.

Würden Sie mich fragen, was ich selbst als größtes wissenschaftliches Erlebnis meines Lebens ansehe, so würde ich sagen: es ist das Miterleben der Dynamik des Fortschrittes seit 1900.

Der Fortschritt wächst eben exponentiell. Warum? Natürlich gibt es mehr Forscher, sie haben mehr Hilfskräfte, beide zusammen mehr Hilfsmittel, eine umfassende und schnelle Information und heute eine viel-

---

* publiziert in G. WAGNER (Hrsg.): Krebs – Dokumentation und Statistik maligner Tumoren, Abb. 7, S. 144. (F. K. Schattauer Verlag, Stuttgart 1966).

fache Automatisierung der Forschungsgeräte. Übertrieben ausgedrückt könnte man sagen: Zum Teil forscht der Forscher heute weiter, auch wenn er schläft. Entscheidend fällt mit ins Gewicht die Gruppenarbeit. Je mehr wir wissen, um so weniger weiß der Einzelne Alles. Das „Alles Wissen" ist eben heute an die Vielzahl der Spezialisten gebunden.

Aber dies ist vielleicht doch nur das Äußere: Das Großartige am Fortschritt ist die Tatsache, daß der Fortschritt selber die Folge des Fortschritts und gleichzeitig die Ursache weiteren Fortschritts ist. Der Fortschritt fließt, fließt wie die Zeit. Die Zeit ist ja selbst seine nährende Mutter. Der Fortschritt ist ein eigengesetzliches Phänomen moderner Naturwissenschaft und Technik geworden.

Speziell in der Krebsforschung liegen die größten Möglichkeiten in der molekularen Genetik. Stellt man sich im Sinne der Mutationstheorie die exogen ausgelöste Cancerisierung vor als „specific injury to the genome of a cell causing a false genetic code" – wie es HUGGINS [16] hier an dieser Stelle vor 2 Jahren ausdrückte –, so erscheint es eben heute weitgehend sicher, daß der in der DNS niedergelegte Code zu entziffern sein wird. Eines Tages wird es möglich sein, das große Gesetzbuch der Natur, niedergelegt in den langfädigen Molekülen der Desoxyribonukleinsäure, ähnlich zu lesen, wie man heute die Keilschrift oder die Hieroglyphen zu lesen vermag.

Dann wird wohl auch der Tag kommen, an dem die Chiffre „Krebs" als Mutation somatischer Zellen im Bereich eines Regulator- oder Operator-Gens für uns lesbar geworden sein wird.

Wann und wo? Wir wissen es nicht! Wir wissen es *noch* nicht!! Aber wir *werden* es wissen.

Literatur

1. BAUER, K. H.: Mutationstheorie der Geschwulstentstehung. Übergang von Körperzellen in Geschwulstzellen durch Gen-Änderung. Berlin: Springer 1928.
2. — Das Krebsproblem. Einführung in die Allgemeine Geschwulstlehre. Für Studierende, Ärzte und Naturwissenschaftler. Berlin-Heidelberg: Springer 1949. 2. Aufl. 1963.
3. — Über Osteogenesis imperfecta. (Zugleich ein Beitrag zur Frage einer allgemeinen Erkrankung sämtlicher Stützgewebe). Dtsch. Zschr. Chir. **154**, 166 (1920).
4. — Über die Erbbiologie der Hämophilie und deren Bedeutung für unsere Vorstellungen von der Natur der Gene. Z. indukt. Abstamm. Vererb.lehre **30**, 314 (1923).
5. — Erbkonstitutionelle „Systemerkrankungen" und Mesenchym. Klin. Wschr. **2**, 624 (1923).
6. — Die Mutationstheorie der Geschwulstentstehung. In: Neuere Ergebn. a. d. Geb. d. Krebskrkh. Leipzig: Hirzel 1937.
7. — Die Mutationstheorie der Krebsentstehung im Lichte ihrer physikalischen und chemischen Beweismittel. Münch. med. Wschr. **90**, 681 (1943).

8. BAUER, K. H.: Über Syn- und Anticarcinogenese. Klin. Wschr. **27**, 118 (1949).
9. — Über „Krebstheorien" im Wandel der Zeit. SRW-Nachrichten, H. **29**, I–X (1966).
10. BORST, M.: Allgemeine Pathologie der malignen Geschwülste. Leipzig: Hirzel 1924.
11. BOVERI, TH.: Zur Frage der Entstehung maligner Tumoren. Jena: Fischer 1914.
12. BRESCH, C.: Klassische und molekulare Genetik. Berlin: Springer 1964.
13. DULBECCO, R.: Krebsentstehung durch Viren. Umschau **67**, 548 (1967).
14. GIERER, A.: Über die Funktion der Desoxyribonukleinsäure und die Theorie der Regulation der Genwirkung. Naturwissenschaften **54**, 389 (1967).
15. HECKER, E.: Neue biochemische Gesichtspunkte bei der Cancerisierung. Krebsforsch. Krebsbekämpf. **6**, 77 (1967).
16. HUGGINS, CH.: Function of the Cancer Cell. Z. Krebsforsch. **67**, 106 (1965).
17. KÜHN, A.: Entwicklungsphysiologie. 2. Aufl. München: Bergmann 1965.
18. LETTRÉ, H. u. R. LETTRÉ: Biochemische Eigenschaften von Krebszellen und Mutationstheorie. Langenbecks Arch. klin. Chir. **294**, 473 (1960).
19. MARQUARDT, H.: Neuere experimentelle Ergebnisse zur Mutationshypothese der chemisch induzierten krebsigen Entartung. Dtsch. med. Wschr. **90**, 398 (1965).
20. — Neuere Ergebnisse der somatischen Genetik. Naturwissenschaften **54**, 217 (1967).
21. — Mutationsauslösung und Krebsauslösung. Umschau **67**, 59 (1967).
22. MULLER, H. J.: Artificial Transmission of the Gene, Science **66**, 84 (1927).
23. MUNK, K.: Grundzüge der Virusätiologie von Tumoren nach neueren Ergebnissen. Ergebn. Mikrobiol. **38**, 224 (1964).
24. — Molekularbiologische Vorgänge bei der viralen Tumorgenese. Krebsforsch. Krebsbekämpfg. **6**, 35 (1967).
25. ORTH, J.: Geschwülste des Nebennierenmarks nebst Bemerkungen über die Nomenklatur der Geschwülste. Z. Krebsforsch. **10**, 42 (1911).
26. RÖHRBORN, G.: Die mutagene Wirkung von Trenimon bei der männlichen Maus. Humangenetik **1**, 576 (1965).
27. — Über einen Geschlechtsunterschied in der mutagenen Wirkung bei der Maus. Humangenetik **2**, 81 (1966).
28. SCHLEIERMACHER, E., W. KROLL, M. HERTL und N. REINHARDT: A constant chromosome aberration in two children with acute myeloic leukaemia. Humangenetik **5**, 80 (1967).
29. SCHMÄHL, D.: Entstehung, Wachstum und Chemotherapie maligner Tumoren. Aulendorf: Editio Cantor 1963.
30. — Die experimentelle Syncarcinogenese. In DOERR-LINDER-WAGNER (Hrsg.): Aktuelle Probleme aus dem Gebiet der Cancerologie, S. 81 ff. Berlin-Heidelberg-New York: Springer 1966.
31. — Syncarcinogenese. Dtsch. med. Wschr. **91**, 1799 (1966).
32. — Carcinogene Wirkung von Cyclophosphamid und Triazichon bei Ratten. Dtsch. med. Wschr. **92**, 1150 (1967).
33. VIRCHOW, R.: Die Cellularpathologie. 2. Aufl. Berlin: Hirschwald 1859. 4. Aufl. 1871.
34. VOGEL, F.: Genetic Prognosis in Retinoblastoma. Mod. Trends Ophthal. Vol. IV, p. 34. London: Butterworth 1967.
35. — u. Mitarb.: Mutationen durch chemische Einwirkung bei Säuger und Mensch. Dtsch. med. Wschr. **92**, 2249, 2315, 2343, 2382 (1967).

Die Bedeutung eines Kernreaktors für die experimentelle und klinische Krebsforschung

Von

K. E. SCHEER

Ein Kernreaktor ist ein Gerät, in dem eine Kernspaltungsreaktion kontrolliert und gesteuert abläuft. Man kann ihn dazu verwenden, die umgesetzte Wärmeenergie auszunutzen, wie dies bei einem Kraftwerksreaktor der Fall ist. Man kann die Wärme in mechanische Energie verwandeln; man macht dies bei Schiffsreaktoren, um das Schiff anzutreiben. Oder aber man legt auf die Wärmebildung keinen Wert und will nur die Neutronen, die bei der Kettenreaktion frei werden, ausnutzen, um mit ihnen wieder Kernreaktionen auszulösen. Das ist die Aufgabe eines Forschungsreaktors. Ein solcher Reaktor steht dem Deutschen Krebsforschungszentrum zur Verfügung.

Am 29. August 1966 wurde der Reaktor zum ersten Mal kritisch und am 24. Oktober wurde er von der Gutehoffnungshütte, die ihn als Lizenznehmerin der Fa. General Atomic gebaut hatte, dem Deutschen Krebsforschungszentrum übergeben. Danach verging ein halbes Jahr mit dem Probebetrieb, Leistungsmessungen, Strahlenschutzmessungen und Erfüllung der zahlreichen Auflagen, die von der Genehmigungsbehörde gemacht worden waren. Seit nunmehr fünf Monaten kann der Reaktor für die praktische Forschungsarbeit eingesetzt werden.

Der Reaktor ist so konstruiert, daß man mit einem möglichst geringen thermischen Energieumsatz einen möglichst hohen Fluß von Neutronen erhält. Es handelt sich um einen Schwimmbadreaktor, bei dem der eigentliche Kern auf dem Boden eines Tanks angeordnet ist, der mit einer 5,5 m hohen Wasserschicht bedeckt ist. Das Wasser ist entmineralisiert und dient sowohl zum Moderieren der Neutronen als auch zum Wärmetransport und zur Abschirmung der Strahlung nach oben zum Reaktorraum hin. Alle Proben müssen durch die Wasserschicht nach unten in den Kern gebracht werden, der mehrere Einrichtungen für die Probenaufnahme enthält.

Der höchste Neutronenfluß mit 10^{13} n cm^{-2} sec^{-1} an thermischen Neutronen besteht im Zentrum des Kerns, in das das zentrale Bestrahlungsrohr führt. Hier können zwei Probekapseln eingeführt werden. An der Peripherie des Kerns liegt eine Rohrpoststation, die eine Probe aufnehmen kann. Hier beträgt der Fluß $5 \cdot 10^{12}$ n cm^{-2} sec^{-1} an thermischen Neutronen. Die Rohrpost gestattet es, Proben in kürzester Zeit bei laufendem Reaktor in die Bestrahlungsposition einzubringen und wieder herauszuführen.

Außerhalb des Kerns befindet sich das Bestrahlungskarussell, das 80 Proben aufzunehmen gestattet und einen Neutronenfluß von $2 \cdot 10^{12}\, n$ $cm^{-2}\, sec^{-1}$ an thermischen Neutronen aufweist. Das Karussell kann während der Bestrahlung in Drehbewegung gehalten werden, so daß die Proben unabhängig von etwaigen Feldinhomogenitäten gleichmäßig bestrahlt werden. Das ist vor allem für die Neutronenaktivierung von Bedeutung, bei der die Meßwerte auf einen mitbestrahlten Standard bezogen werden.

Der hohe Neutronenfluß auf kleinem Raum bei einer verhältnismäßig kleinen Energieumsetzung (maximal 250 kW) ist nur durch Verwendung von ^{235}U angereichertem Uran zu erzielen. Bei einem Anreicherungsgrad von 20% beträgt die Gesamtmenge ^{235}U, die zum Betrieb erforderlich ist, 2,3 kg. Dieser Brennstoff ist in 59 Brennelementen in einer Matrix aus Zirkonhydrid untergebracht. Das Zirkonhydridbrennelement ist durch seinen negativen Temperaturkoeffizienten charakterisiert. Daraus ergibt sich eine sehr hohe Betriebssicherheit des Reaktors, so daß die Bauausführung sehr einfach gehalten werden konnte. Nur dank des negativen Temperaturkoeffizienten war es möglich, den Reaktor unmittelbar in unserem Institutsgebäude unterzubringen und so kürzeste Wege zwischen den Isotopenlaboratorien, den Meßräumen und dem Reaktor zu erhalten.

Wir haben diesen Reaktor bisher sowohl für die Neutronenaktivierungsanalyse als auch zur Herstellung kurzlebiger Radionuklide verwendet. Für beides möchte ich einige Beispiele anführen.

Im Rahmen eines größeren Untersuchungsprogramms über die Auswirkungen des radioaktiven Kontrastmittels Thorotrast, das in den 30er und 40er Jahren verwendet wurde, stellte sich die Aufgabe, in Blut- und Gewebsproben von Patienten Thorium-Bestimmungen vorzunehmen. Bei der außerordentlich kleinen zu erwartenden Thoriummenge bot von vornherein nur die Neutronenaktivierungsanalyse eine Aussicht auf Erfolg. Bereits die ersten Versuche an unserem Reaktor zeigten, daß mit einer einfachen Methodik eine hohe Empfindlichkeit zu erzielen war. Es liegt dabei eine (n, γ)-Reaktion zugrunde, bei der ein thermisches Neutron von dem nachzuweisenden Kern eingefangen und ein γ-Quant abgegeben wird. Die Reaktion hat den folgenden Ablauf:

$$^{232}Th\ (n,\ \gamma)\ ^{233}Th\ \xrightarrow[22,4\ \text{min}]{\beta^-}\ ^{233}Pa\ \xrightarrow[27\ \text{d}]{\beta^-}\ ^{233}U$$

Es kann nun entweder das zunächst erzeugte ^{233}Th oder das aus diesem durch radioaktiven Zerfall frei werdende, ebenfalls radioaktive ^{233}Pa bestimmt werden.

Da ^{233}Thorium eine Halbwertzeit von 22,4 min hat, wird es zwar in höherer Aktivität gebildet als das ^{233}Protaktinium mit 27 Tagen Halbwertzeit, doch klingt die Aktivität des ersteren auch rasch ab, so daß Störaktivitäten aus ^{38}Cl und ^{24}Na vorhanden sind, deren Abklingen nicht abgewartet werden kann. Dieser Nachweis gibt zwar die höchste Empfindlichkeit, doch dann ist eine chemische Aufarbeitung der aktivierten Probe notwendig, um Chlor und Natrium zu entfernen.

Trotz der geringeren erzeugten Aktivität erwies es sich daher als günstiger, den Thorium-Nachweis über die Strahlung des aus dem Zerfall von ^{233}Th gebildeten ^{233}Pa durchzuführen. Infolge der langen Halbwertzeit dieses Nuklids kann das Abklingen von ^{24}Na und ^{38}Cl abgewartet werden. Es sind keine chemischen Arbeiten an der aktivierten Probe notwendig. Am günstigsten ist es, 400 Std nach der Bestrahlung zu warten und dann die Aktivität zu messen, die jetzt nur noch aus ^{233}Pa besteht.

Versuche mit verschiedenen Gewebsarten haben gezeigt, daß bei einer 4-stündigen Bestrahlungszeit im Karussell des Reaktors bei einem Neutronenfluß von $2 \cdot 10^{12}$ n cm^{-2} sec^{-1} eine Thorium-Menge von 0,02 μg in 1 g Gewebe noch gut bestimmt werden kann. Mit Hilfe dieser sehr einfachen Methodik, die in kurzer Zeit am Institut für Nuklearmedizin des DKFZ entwickelt werden konnte, ist es möglich, den Thorium-Blutspiegel bei Patienten zu bestimmen, die vor mehr als 20 Jahren eine Thorotrast-Injektion erhalten haben.

Unter den kurzlebigen Radionukliden, die wir bisher mit diesem Reaktor erzeugen konnten, hat uns besonders ^{128}J und ^{18}F interessiert. Jod ist eines der wichtigsten Elemente für die radioaktive Indikatortechnik, da sich dieses Element wegen seiner Reaktionsfreudigkeit in zahlreiche organische Verbindungen einbauen läßt. Für die klinische Geschwulstdiagnostik haben radiojodmarkierte Verbindungen in den letzten Jahren eine besondere Bedeutung erlangt. Da bisher fast nur das Isotop ^{131}J zur Verfügung stand, das eine Halbwertzeit von 8 Tagen hat, sind die Mengen an Aktivität, die einem Patienten verabreicht werden können, begrenzt. Das Isotop ^{128}J hat eine Halbwertzeit von nur 25 min, so daß bei gleicher Strahlenbelastung eine rund 1000fach höhere Aktivität verabreicht werden kann. Es entsteht durch Bestrahlung des inaktiven ^{127}J im Reaktor durch eine (n, γ)-Reaktion mit thermischen Neutronen.

Da bei (n, γ)-Reaktionen das entstehende Radionuklid ein Isotop des inaktiven Ausgangsnuklids ist, können mit dieser Reaktion allein keine hohen spezifischen Aktivitäten erzielt werden, da sich das erzeugte radioaktive Isotop vom stabilen Isotop mit chemischen Methoden nicht trennen läßt. Eine solche Trennung ist aber während der Kernreaktion möglich mit Hilfe der Szilard-Chalmers-Reaktion. Dabei wird das inaktive Jod in Form von Acetyljodid bestrahlt. Bei der Kernreaktion werden die umgewandelten Jodkerne wegen ihrer hohen Rückstoßenergie aus dem Molekülverband herausgeschlagen, so daß man nach Ausschütteln des Methyljodids in einem wäßrigen Medium überwiegend aktivierte Jodkerne in der wäßrigen Phase enthält.

Ein anderes Isotop, das sich vor allem für die Früherkennung von Knochenmetastasen als besonders günstig erwiesen hat, ist das radioaktive Fluor ^{18}F. Es handelt sich hierbei um einen Positronenstrahler mit einem Neutronenmangel gegenüber dem inaktiven Fluor ^{19}F. Im Reaktor läßt es sich nur über einen doppelten Kernprozeß erzeugen und zwar nach der Reaktion

$$^6\text{Li (n, t) }^4\text{He}; \quad ^{16}\text{O (t, n) }^{18}\text{F}.$$

Bestrahlt man Lithiumcarbonat im Reaktor, so kommt es am stabilen Isotop ^{6}Li zu einem Neutroneneinfang mit Emission eines Tritium- und eines Heliumkerns. Der energiereiche Tritiumkern reagiert seinerseits mit dem stabilen Sauerstoffkern im Carbonat und führt zum Isotop ^{18}F,

Tabelle 1. *Im TRIGA Mark I-Reaktor erzeugte Radioisotope und deren Anwendung*

Nuklid	$T_{1/2}$	γ-Strahlung MeV	%	Targetmaterial	Anwendung
^{18}F	1,7 h	0,511	2 · 100	Li_2CO_3	Knochenscintigraphie
^{87m}Sr	2,8 h	0,388	79	^{86}Sr (angereichert)	Knochenstoffwechsel
^{24}Na	15,4 h	1,37	100		
		2,75	100	Na_2CO_3	Physiologische
^{42}K	12,5 h	1,53	18	K_2CO_3	Untersuchungen
^{64}Cu	12,8 h	0,511	38	Cu- ⎱ Phtalocyanin	Hirn- ⎱ Scintigraphie
^{69m}Zn	13,9 h	0,438	94	Zn- ⎰	Pool- ⎰
^{72}Ga	14,1 h	0,830	75	$Ga(OH)_3$	Nieren- { Scintigraphie
		0,630	24		{ Autoradiographie
^{128}J	25 m	0,450	18	Acetyljodid	Schilddrüsenscintigraphie
^{198}Au	2,7 d	0,411	96	Au-Draht	Hypophyse (Therapie)
				Au-Plättchen	Auge
				Au-Kolloid	Ergüsse, abdom. Metastas.

das eine Halbwertzeit von 1,7 Std hat. Das Bestrahlungsprodukt enthält neben dem erzeugten ^{18}F noch eine größere Menge von Tritium. Es muß daher eine vorsichtige Destillation vorgenommen werden, die dann zu einem Produkt von radioaktivem Fluor führt, das nur noch in vertretbarer Menge mit Tritium verunreinigt ist.

Intravenös injiziertes ^{18}F tauscht sehr schnell gegen die Hydroxylgruppe des Apathits im Knochen aus, und der Grad seines Einbaus ist ein Maß für die Größe des Knochenstoffwechsels. Einige erste klinische Untersuchungen geben Hinweise dafür, daß eine beginnende Knochenmetastasierung, die mit Röntgenmethoden noch nicht nachweisbar ist, sich bereits durch eine vermehrte ^{18}F-Einlagerung bemerkbar macht.

Die Tabelle gibt eine Übersicht über diejenigen kurzlebigen Radionuklide, die wir bisher mit dem Reaktor erzeugt haben, und einen Hinweis für deren klinisches Anwendungsgebiet (Tab. 1).

Nach fünf Monaten praktischer Arbeit mit dem TRIGA Mark I-Forschungsreaktor des Deutschen Krebsforschungszentrums läßt sich sagen, daß sich dieser Reaktor als ein sehr leicht zu bedienendes und betriebssicheres Gerät erwiesen hat. Sowohl Neutronenaktivierungsanalysen als auch die Erzeugung kurzlebiger Radioisotope lassen sich gut durchführen, und die Erwartungen, die in diesen ersten deutschen Forschungsreaktor für medizinisch-biologische Aufgaben gesetzt wurden, haben sich bisher voll erfüllt.

Die Computerscintigraphie in der Tumordiagnostik*

Von

W. E. Adam und W. J. Lorenz

Tumordarstellungen durch nuklearmedizinische Methoden basieren auf zwei unterschiedlichen Verfahren:

Eine positive Darstellung durch vermehrte Akkumulation von Aktivität, als sogenannter *warmer Bereich*, gelingt immer dann, wenn eine radioaktiv markierte Verbindung eine selektive Affinität zu entsprechendem Tumorgewebe hat oder wenn die Tumorkapsel eine große Permeabilität aufweist. Dazu gehören Absiedlungen mancher bösartiger Schilddrüsentumoren, die selektiv radioaktives Jod, Hirntumoren, die bestimmte Quecksilberverbindungen, und Knochenmetastasen, die ^{18}F speichern.

Der infiltrierende oder metastatische Tumor in seiner Eigenschaft als „raumfordernder Prozeß" läßt sich als *kalter Bereich* darstellen, wenn man eine radioaktive Substanz appliziert, die in den Organen selbst gespeichert wird. Das läßt sich bei infiltrierenden Tumoren der Schilddrüse mit Jod, bei der Leber mit Radiogold, bei den Nieren und bei der Milz mit Quecksilberverbindungen durchführen.

Die Messung der Radioaktivitätsverteilung erfolgt von außen entweder mit einer Meß-Sonde, die schrittweise oder kontinuierlich den Untersuchungsbereich abfährt, oder mit Hilfe eines sogenannten stehenden Detektors, der simultan die Aktivitätsverteilung registriert. Der Umfang der dabei gewonnenen Informationen hängt unter anderem von der Güte des Detektorsystems ab. Fortschritte der *Datengewinnung* sind zu erwarten durch Erhöhung der Empfindlichkeit der Detektoren und durch Kollimatoren mit größerem Auflösungsvermögen.

Demgegenüber verfolgen wir als Ziel eine Verbesserung der Darstellung der gewonnenen Informationen mit Hilfe der *Datenverarbeitung* [1–4]. Wenn der Tumor die Aktivität selektiv speichert, bereitet es keine Schwierigkeit, ihn bei der Bildbetrachtung zu entdecken. Das gleiche gilt für Aktivitätsaussparungen in parenchymatösen Organen, die durch infiltrierendes oder metastasierendes Wachstum bedingt sind. Im Falle einer geringen Aktivitätsanreicherung wird die Beurteilung jedoch

* Mit Unterstützung der Deutschen Forschungsgemeinschaft.

schwierig oder unmöglich, da die Strahlenemission in zufälliger Verteilung erfolgt. Die gleiche Schwierigkeit bereiten kleine Gewebsdefekte, die durch die Strahlung benachbarter Parenchymbereiche überlagert und verwischt werden, oder auch größere tiefliegende Geschwülste, wenn sie von gesundem Organgewebe überlagert sind.

Diese von der Klinik her bekannten, der nuklearmedizinischen Methodik angelasteten falsch negativen Ergebnisse sind in vielen Fällen Versager sinnesphysiologischer Informationsverarbeitung.

Nach WINKLER [5] werden Unterschiede der Impulsdichte im Scintigramm erst dann visuell erkennbar, wenn sie größer als etwa die vierfache Streubreite der Impulsdifferenz werden. Das gilt für Areale bis zu 5 cm Durchmesser, wie sie üblicherweise in der Tumordiagnostik in Frage kommen. Das bedeutet in der Tat, daß bei der visuellen Auswertung scintigraphischer Bilder ein Teil der Information verloren geht. Üblicherweise sucht man dieser Gefahr durch eine Kontrastverstärkung zu begegnen. Dabei können geringste Impulsdifferenzen deutlich sichtbar gemacht werden. Es besteht jedoch die Gefahr, daß es sich bei den kontrastreich hervorgehobenen Bezirken um Zufallsdifferenzen handelt, die durch statistische Schwankungen bedingt sind. Die digitale Darstellung in einem Kernspeicher gestattet demgegenüber, die Prüfung auf eine statistische Signifikanz der Differenzen zweier benachbarter Areale durchzuführen.

Als Computer verwenden wir einen PDP-8 der Firma Digital Equipment Corporation mit 8 K Speicherplätzen. Die Primärinformation nehmen wir von der Scintillationskamera auf einem Analogband auf und spielen sie über zwei Analog-Digital-Converter in unseren Computer ein. Jedem Areal des Detektors wird ein Speicherplatz eindeutig zugeordnet. Vor der Analyse des scintigraphischen Bildes erfolgt eine Korrektur der Primärinformationen, da das gesamte System auf der Aufnahmeseite Inhomogenitäten aufweist, die bei ungünstiger Justierung der Photomultiplier zu Schwankungen der Empfindlichkeit von $\pm$ 20% um den Mittelwert führen. Abb. 1 zeigt die Inhomogenität der Registrierempfindlichkeit des Kristalls (linke Bildseite) im Vergleich zum korrigierten Bild desselben homogenen Phantoms (rechte Bildseite). Die Abbildung gibt gleichzeitig ein Beispiel für die sogenannte isometrische, also perspektivisch-dreidimensionale Darstellung der Aktivitätsverteilung unseres homogenen Modells. Abb. 2 zeigt ein Beispiel für eine Bildanalyse durch Querschnitte. Das Primärbild der Anger-Kamera (Mitte) ergibt außer einer relativ homogenen Aktivitätsverteilung keine Auffälligkeiten; erst die Horizontalschnitte mit auseinandergezogener Matrix lassen einen Bereich verminderter Aktivität im Zentrum des Phantoms erkennen. Ihm entspricht ein bandförmiger kalter Bereich von 1,0 cm Durchmesser.

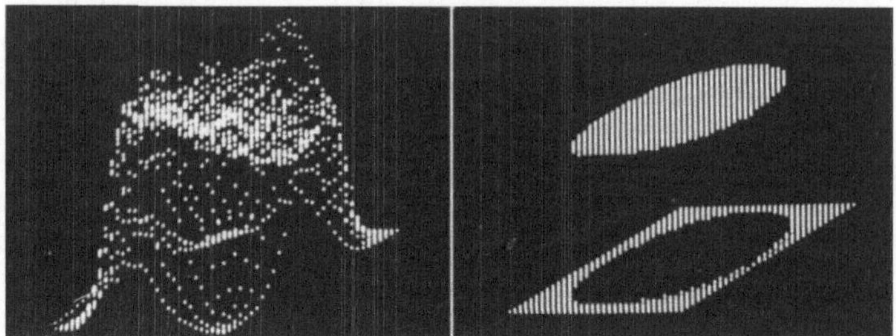

Abb. 1. Isometrische Darstellung eines homogenen Phantoms vor (links) und nach (rechts) Computerkorrektur

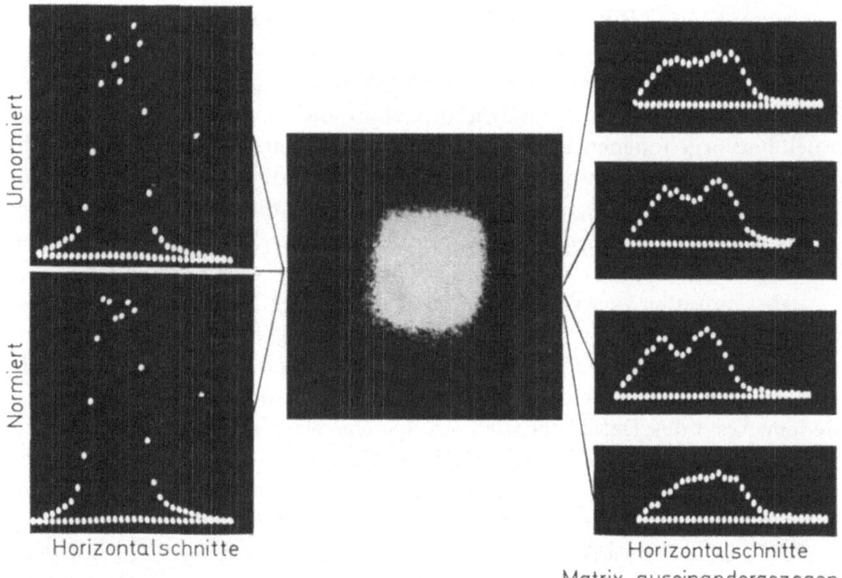

Abb. 2. Homogenes Kastenphantom mit einem vertikal verlaufenden kalten Bereich von 1,0 cm Durchmesser. Der kalte Bereich ist im Angerkamerabild nur undeutlich zu erkennen, deutliche Darstellung auf den Schnittbildern, insbesondere bei auseinandergezogener Matrix

Beispiele für eine Konturdarstellung gibt Abb. 3. Es handelt sich um das Rezidiv eines linksseitigen Schädeltumors, der auf der AP-Aufnahme der Scintillationskamera zur Darstellung kommt. Bei der Konturdarstellung wird die untere Schwelle schrittweise angehoben. Dabei läßt sich deutlich eine Asymmetrie der Speicherung im Bereich des Hirn-

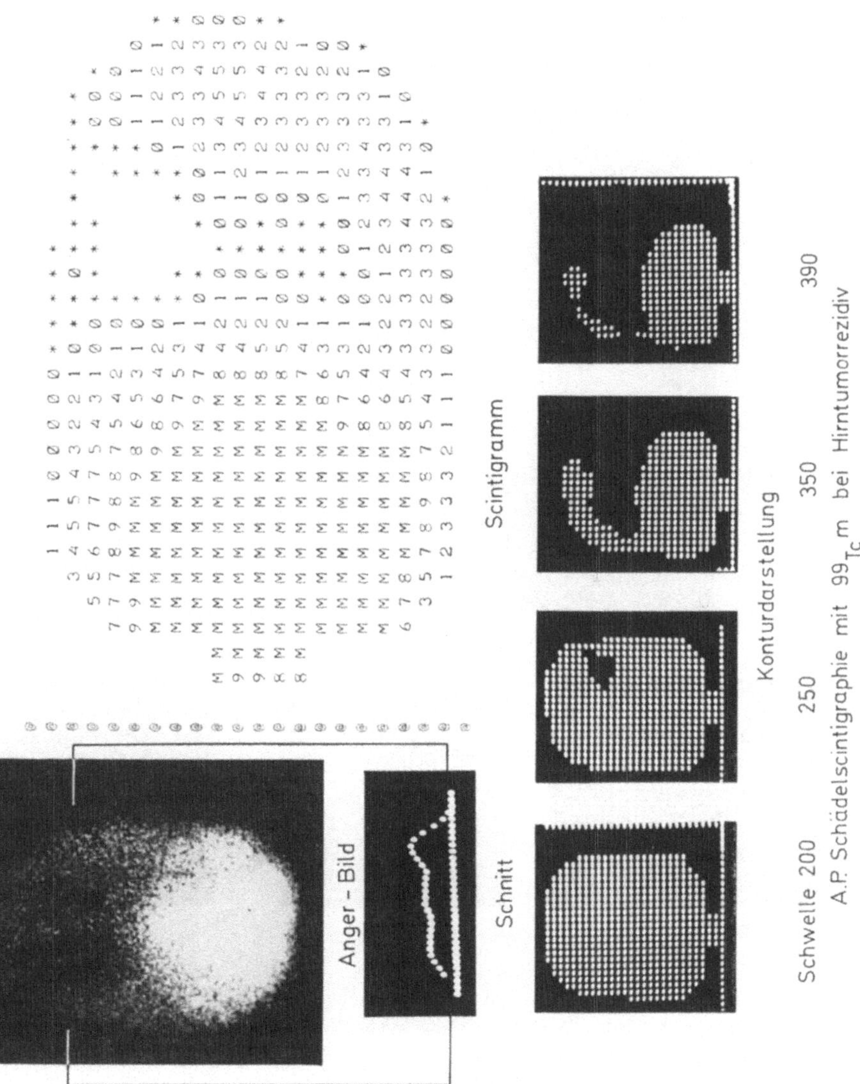

Abb. 3. Die vermehrte Aktivitätsakkumulation im Bereich des Hirntumorrezidivs links kommt sowohl auf dem Horizontalschnitt als auch bei der Konturdarstellung (seitenverkehrt) zur Darstellung

schädels nachweisen, es bleibt schließlich ein dem Tumor entsprechender isolierter Aktivitätsbezirk zurück. Ein Horizontalschnitt durch den Hirnschädel weist ein entsprechendes Maximum linksparietal auf.

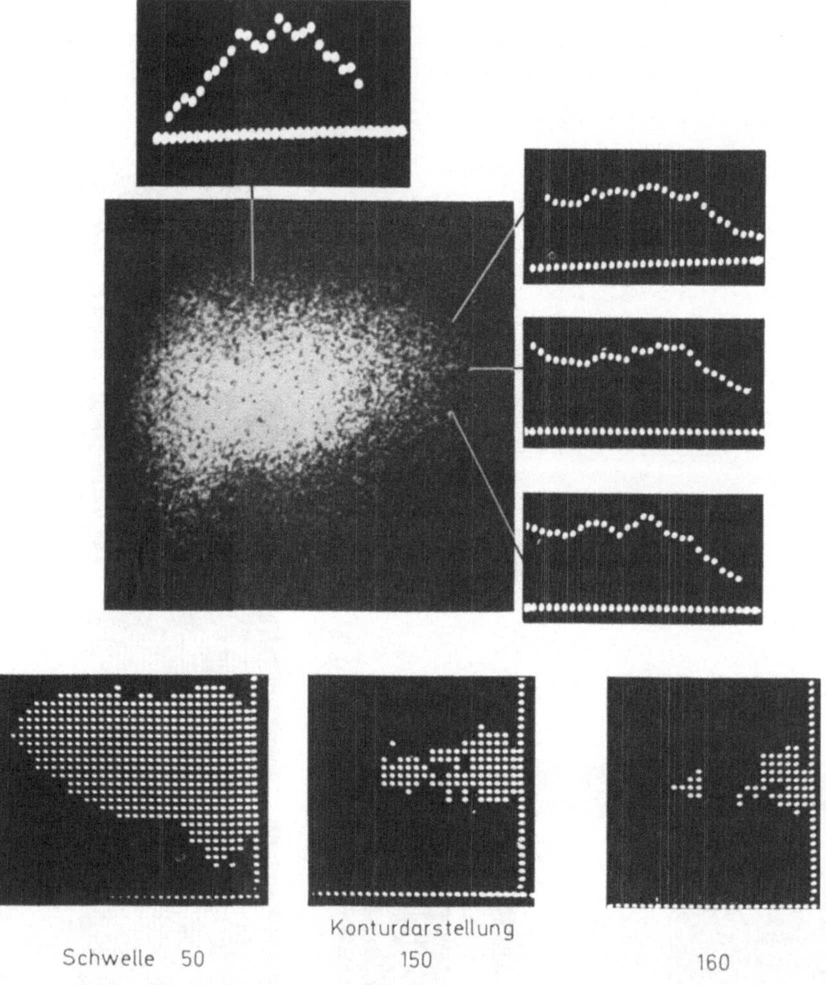

Abb. 4. Leber eines Patienten mit einem Bronchialcarcinom. Unauffälliges Leberszintigramm mit homogen erscheinender Aktivitätsverteilung. Im Sagittalschnitt unregelmäßige Kontur mit Einsenkungen, ebenso in einem Horizontalschnitt, Metastasen entsprechend

Infiltrativ wachsende, raumfordernde Prozesse sind scintigraphisch häufig schwierig zu entdecken, da Randstrahlen aus benachbarten Geweben und Strahlen aus normalem darüberliegendem Gewebe kalte

Bereiche überdecken können. Der Informationsgewinn durch die Computerscintigraphie soll im folgenden dargestellt werden.

Die normale Leber speichert die Aktivität homogen, d. h. das Zentrum zeigt im scintigraphischen Bild die stärkste Schwärzung; sie nimmt zur Peripherie hin gleichmäßig ab. Das läßt sich sowohl an Hand der Schnitte

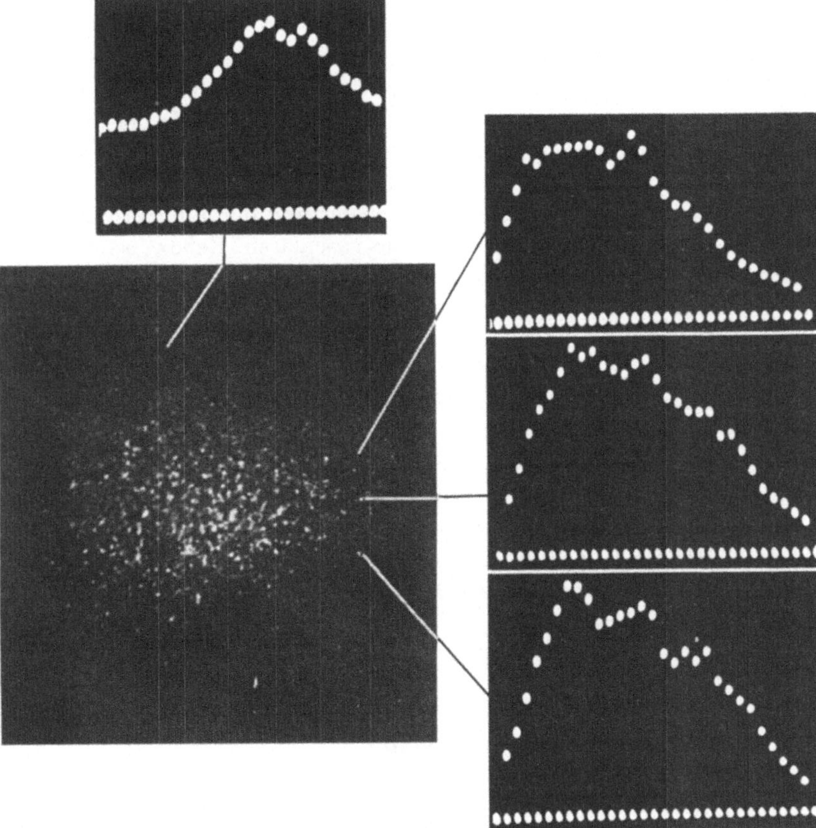

Abb. 5. Leber eines Patienten mit einem Magenkarzinom. Klinisch Metastasen der Leber nicht nachweisbar. Originalaufnahme der Scintillationskamera unauffällig. Die Horizontalschnitte zeigen Stufen und Einsenkungen ihrer Kontur, Metastasen entsprechend

als auch auf Grund der Konturdarstellung mit schrittweiser Erhöhung der Subtraktionsrate nachweisen. Abb. 4 zeigt eine Metastasenleber. Die Originalaufnahme mit der Scintillationskamera läßt keine Besonderheiten gegenüber der Aufnahme einer normalen Leber erkennen. Dagegen stellen sich auf zahlreichen Schnitten muldenförmige Einsenkungen dar, die Metastasen entsprechen.

Die Analyse einer Leberscintigraphie bei einem Patienten mit einem Magenkarzinom stellt Abb. 5 dar. Weder röntgenologisch noch scintigraphisch konnten Metastasen nachgewiesen werden. Erst die Computeranalyse ergab signifikante Aktivitätsverminderungen im Leberparenchym. Es handelte sich also um Metastasen, die bildlich als Einsenkungen in den Horizontalschnitten und im Vertikalschnitt der Leber zum Ausdruck kommen.

Mit der Analyse stehender scintigraphischer Bilder sind jedoch die Möglichkeiten der Computerscintigraphie nicht erschöpft. In der Form der sogenannten quantitativen Funktionsscintigraphie lassen sich schnelle kinetische Vorgänge gleichzeitig morphologisch und in Form von Funktionskurven erfassen. Die Durchblutungsdrosselung einer Lunge, wie wir sie als Modellfall einer Minderbelüftung der Lungen durch ein Bronchialcarcinom über einen alveolo-vasculären Reflex beim Hund experimentell erzeugt haben, läßt sich schließlich quantitativ darstellen. Die Durchblutung eines Tumors sowie die Anreicherung markierter Substanzen im Tumorgewebe lassen sich von außen ohne Eingriff und ohne Katheterisierung in weitaus exakterer Weise bestimmen, als das bisher bei Radioisotopenuntersuchungen mit einem blind aufgesetzten Detektor möglich war.

Die Computerscintigraphie kann in der Klinik Erhebliches zur Diagnose und frühzeitigen Erkennung von Tumoren leisten. In ihrer Form als „quantitative Funktionsscintigraphie" ist sie darüber hinaus durch die glückliche Kombination einer Darstellung morphologischer und funktioneller Größen geradezu prädestiniert zum Einsatz in der experimentellen Krebsforschung.

Literatur

1. ADAM, W. E., W. J. LORENZ u. K. E. SCHEER: Quantitative Untersuchungen mit der Szintillationskamera. In HOFFMANN-SCHEER (Hrsg.): „Radioisotope in der Lokalisationsdiagnostik". Stuttgart: F. K. Schattauer 1967.
2. BROWN, D. W.: Digital Computer Analysis and Display of the Radionuclide Scan. J. nucl. Med. 7, 740 (1966).
3. PIZER, S. M. and H. G. VETTER: The Problem of Display in the Visualisation of Radioisotope Distributions. J. nucl. Med. 7, 773 (1966).
4. SCHEPERS, H. and G. WINKLER: An Automatic Scanning System, using a Tape Perforator and Computer Techniques. Medical Radioisotope Scanning, Vol. I. IAEA, Vienna 1964.
5. WINKLER, C.: Szintigraphischer Nachweis minimaler Aktivitätsdifferenzen infolge von Parenchymdefekten in Schilddrüse, Leber, Nieren und Pankreas. In J. BECKER (Hrsg.): Bericht über die 45. Tagung der Deutschen Röntgengesellschaft vom 9.–13. April 1964 in Wiesbaden, S. 59. Stuttgart: Georg Thieme 1965.

Comparative Incidence of Cancer in Three Regions in Texas*

By

E. J. MACDONALD and P. F. WOLF

The Texas cancer program began in 1944 as a new venture to be molded by experience and evaluated by results. Essentially, it embodies the stimulation and dissemination of conscious knowledge of the disease and its implications among the profession and the populace, and the supplementation of existing diagnostic and therapeutic resources. It has been tempered to a degree of sensitivity to existing needs, and has maintained its pliability for the accommodation of progressive change. The incorporation of corrections and the omission of proved inadequacies as determined by analysis of continuing studies have been the tools in the tempering process.

The agencies in the state concerned with cancer set up a representative advisory group. Duplication of effort and unanimity of purpose is subscribed to through this voluntary sharing of plans. The University of Texas M. D. Anderson Hospital and Tumor Institute at Houston with its unequalled facility for basic and clinical research lies at the heart of the state program. Through its department of epidemiology, surveys and clinical trials are conducted of different population segments. Differences are found between the same ethnic groups living under the different environments existing in Texas.

Most of Texas' 254 counties cover 1,000 or more square miles; seven are as large as Connecticut. This huge land mass of 267,339 square miles divides naturally into 21 hospital regions around major population and treatment centers. Around these regions are miles of lightly populated areas, often deserts. The regions have varied environments – subtropical and temperate climate, high and low altitude, high and low humidity,

* Grateful acknowledgement is made to MARCO FIORENTINO, MARY S. JOHNSON, SUE A. ALLEN, and the staff of epidemiology of The University of Texas M. D. Anderson Hospital and Tumor Institute at Houston, to the Common Research Computer Facility, and to USPHS Grant FR-00254 and NCI Grant CS-9299 for assistance in compiling this report.

varied industries, and most forms of agriculture. Oil is produced in nearly every county. Although cowboys and ranchers are the trademark of Texas, the state's largest business is cotton.

The three regions included in this report are El Paso County, Travis County, and Taylor-Jones Counties (Abilene) combined. A comparison

Table 1. *Population and Geographical Characteristics*

	Abilene	Travis	El Paso
Population 1950	85,517	160,980	194,968
Population 1960	120,377	212,136	314,070
Average rainfall (inches)	23.35	32.58	7.89
Percent possible sunshine hours	70	63	82
Altitude	1600–2400	400–1400	3500–7100
Density/square mile, 1960	64.6	209.0	298.0
Median age, 1960	25.9	25.3	22.6
Median income, 1960	4,706	5,058	5,157
Area in square miles	1,863	1,015	1,054
Average temperature F.	64	67	62
Humidity			
6 a.m.	75%	85%	53%
6 p.m.	45%	55%	28%
Economic index	844	1.108	1.763
No. of farms	2,213	1,406	482
No. of employed, 1960	41,534	77,451	86,946
Percent net change population	+ 40.76	+ 31.8	+ 61.1

with European proportions may elucidate the distances involved. If El Paso County were placed over Paris, Travis County would cover Berlin, and Taylor-Jones Counties would fall between Hamburg and the border of Denmark. The physical and other characteristics of the three regions are shown in Table 1.

From 1944 through 1958 inclusive, an intensive survey was made to determine the incidence rates of cancer by site in these widely-separated counties. When real differences were noted in El Paso County between Latin Americans and Anglo-Americans in sites of cancer, comparisons were sought between the Anglo-Americans in two additional counties to see if there were real differences in the same ethnic group in different environments. Significant differences were found, and the epidemiologist is now studying environmental factors in depth to try to explain the reasons for these differences.

Anglo-Americans in the three geographical areas differed significantly in incidence of head and neck cancer excluding skin, stomach cancer and rectal, urinary tract, and male genital tract cancers. Latin American men had a significantly higher incidence of stomach, liver and reticulo-endothelial system cancer and lower incidence of intestinal and lip cancer than their Anglo-American neighbors.

Table 2. *Average Annual Age-Adjusted* Cancer Incidence Rates per 100,000 Males 1949–1953*

	Abilene (*Taylor-Jones*)	Travis	El Paso *Anglo*	El Paso *Latin*
All sites	177.72	461.13	489.94	189.15
All sites except skin	169.03	214.08	223.79	163.97
Lip	7.04	14.94	25.54	0.92
Upper respiratory except lip	6.41	13.13	20.34	8.90
Stomach	15.81	14.82	18.03	22.25
Intestines except rectum	15.08	19.21	18.02	4.14
Rectum	1.99	7.15	7.67	3.61
Liver	6.70	4.18	4.27	9.13
Pancreas	9.95	9.11	9.28	7.81
Lung	15.70	16.11	27.01	10.04
Breast	1.07	0.00	0.47	0.00
Male genital tract	28.42	—	—	—
Prostate	26.89	31.54	22.23	26.26
Kidney	4.00	5.02	3.81	5.28
Urinary tract	10.57	10.39	14.38	9.74
Melanoma	1.48	5.88	3.28	2.31
Skin except melanoma	8.69	247.05	266.15	25.18
Skin of the exposed areas	8.15	220.50	241.61	17.57
Brain	1.88	2.67	2.19	0.77
Thyroid gland	1.62	3.19	0.28	0.00
Bone	1.47	1.04	0.95	0.00
Soft parts	2.44	3.84	4.36	5.87
No primary discovered	14.33	23.52	16.81	22.64
Reticuloendothelial system	18.08	19.56	19.35	15.12
Lymphoma	7.38	10.39	6.86	7.11
Leukemia	9.28	6.96	10.58	7.48

* Adjusted to 1950 United States population.

Anglo-American women in the three areas differed significantly in incidence of cancers of the head and neck, lung, breast, thyroid, pancreas, reticuloendothelial system and female genital tract. Latin American women had a significantly higher incidence of cancer of the stomach, liver, lung, and cervix than the Anglo-American women and a signi-ficantly lower incidence of cancer of the breast, intestines, rectum and urinary tract.

     E. J. Macdonald and P. F. Wolf

The highest incidence rates of skin cancer were in Travis County, which has less direct sun light, but higher humidity and temperature readings than the other two areas. Even disregarding skin cancer, total

Table 3. *Average Annual Age-Adjusted* Cancer Incidence Rates per 100,000 Females 1949–1953*

	Abilene (Taylor-Jones)	Travis	El Paso Anglo	El Paso Latin
All sites	176.27	382.69	412.69	285.12
All sites except skin	172.98	228.53	285.88	256.83
Lip	0.46	1.08	2.39	0.86
Upper respiratory except lip	5.14	3.46	8.16	8.93
Stomach	3.27	7.44	12.12	12.56
Intestines except rectum	21.90	19.16	23.28	7.11
Rectum	6.09	5.60	8.74	3.89
Liver	3.68	5.07	5.76	14.92
Pancreas	2.91	5.31	3.90	6.38
Lung	4.18	2.98	5.89	11.95
Breast	31.90	56.37	67.35	32.88
Female genital tract	46.21	61.12	82.96	80.44
Cervix uteri	19.79	34.68	44.06	46.80
Corpus uteri	16.06	14.47	23.72	18.72
Ovary, fallopian tube and broad ligament	10.37	11.97	15.17	14.93
Kidney	1.42	2.90	3.30	2.18
Urinary tract	4.28	3.73	6.14	2.77
Melanoma	4.64	7.31	6.06	2.18
Skin except melanoma	3.29	154.16	126.82	28.29
Skin of the exposed areas	2.88	137.76	113.52	21.55
Brain	2.71	4.30	2.08	2.75
Thyroid gland	2.82	5.55	4.67	5.27
Bone	0.50	1.90	0.49	2.52
Soft parts	1.92	5.60	6.59	2.44
No primary discovered	12.62	13.86	16.25	37.86
Reticuloendothelial system	11.18	9.00	11.52	10.62
Lymphoma	3.76	4.59	3.74	6.31
Leukemia	7.41	3.61	7.79	3.25

* Adjusted to 1950 United States population

cancer incidence was higher in Travis County than elsewhere. Travis County is more comparable to the District of Columbia in structure, with education, government, and recreational facilities its main occupations. The main University of Texas and the state capitol are at Austin. In a state-by-state and District of Columbia mortality study, the latter followed no regional pattern as did each state. Travis County may represent the same situation in a state milieu. Tables 2 and 3 give 5-year average age-adjusted incidence rates by site of cancer.

The age-adjusted incidence rates for total cancer incidence show different regional patterns in Texas. Regression lines with slopes representing average yearly changes were fitted to yearly age-adjusted incidence for each region for the entire period. Fig. 1 shows the differences

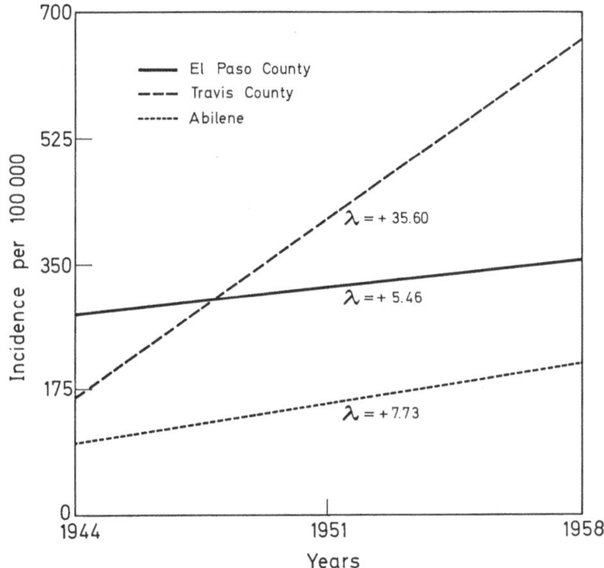

Fig. 1. Cancer of all sites. Age-adjusted incidence trends, total population 1944–1958

with the annual increments of change. Fig. 2 shows the age-adjusted total cancer incidence rates for Latin and other Americans in El Paso County. In Figs. 3 and 4, the percentage distribution by sex and ethnic group is shown by cancer site excluding skin. El Paso Anglo-Americans, under the heading of Other El Paso, and El Paso Latin Americans show the differences in the one community. Taylor-Jones Counties are shown under the name of the regional medical center, Abilene.

The regression lines for the age-adjusted mortality rates from 1949 through 1961 are shown in Fig. 5. The rates were declining for El Paso County, where there has been an active medically sponsored follow-up program since 1950. The trend was beginning to fall in Taylor-Jones (Abilene) Counties, and rising in Travis County.

Because of the environmental and ethnic differences observed in the three regions, it should be of great interest to have sufficient data for a comprehensive analysis of comparative cancer incidence in Texas. The

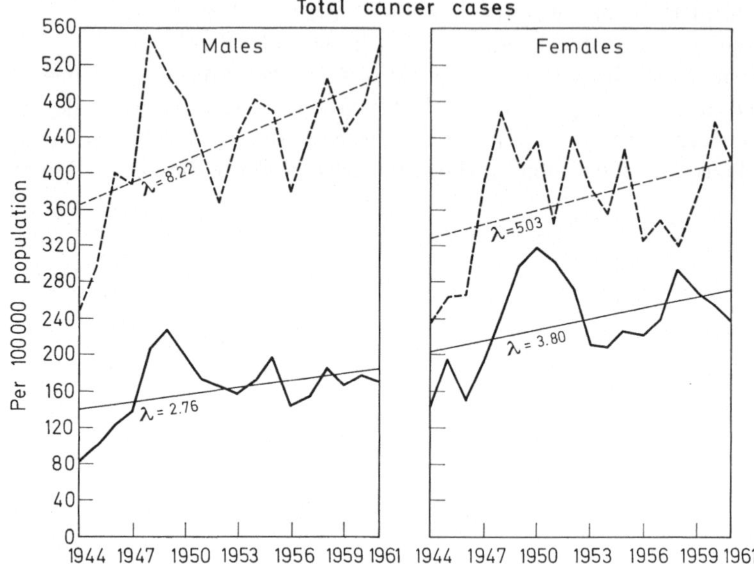

Fig. 2. El Paso County. Age-adjusted cancer incidence rates per 100,000 population, by sex and ethnic group 1944–1961

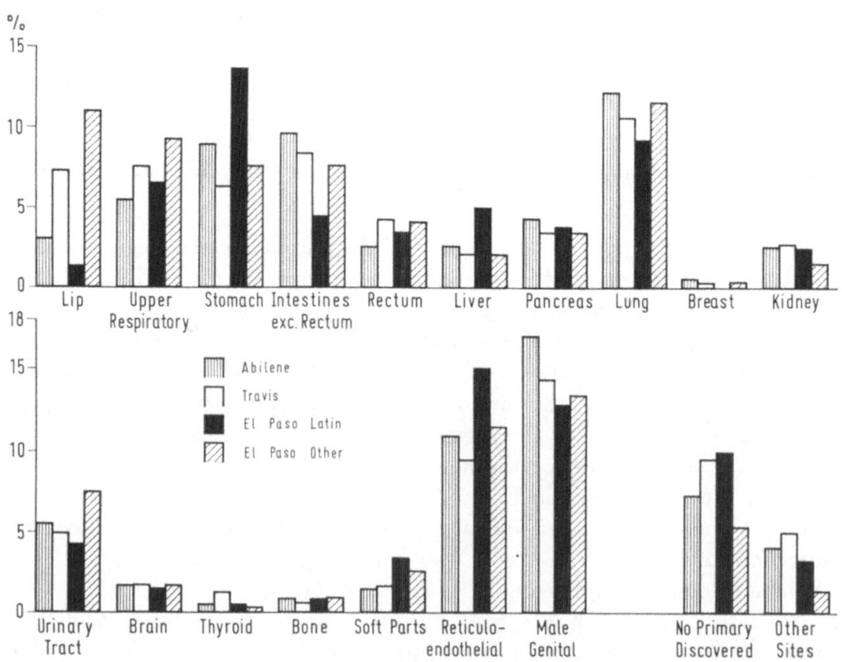

Fig. 3. Cancer of all sites minus skin, percentage distribution (males)

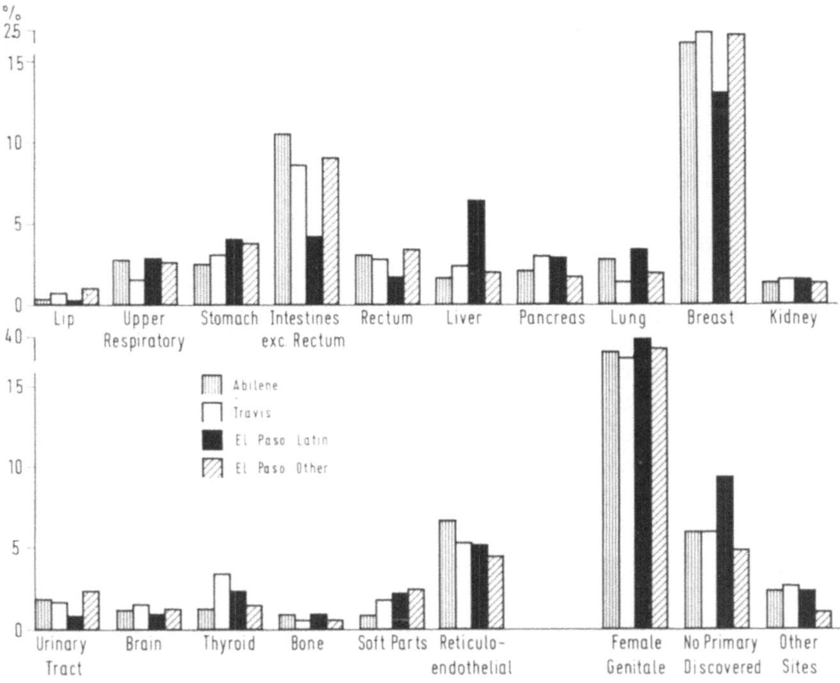

Fig. 4. Cancer of all sites minus skin, percentage distribution (females)

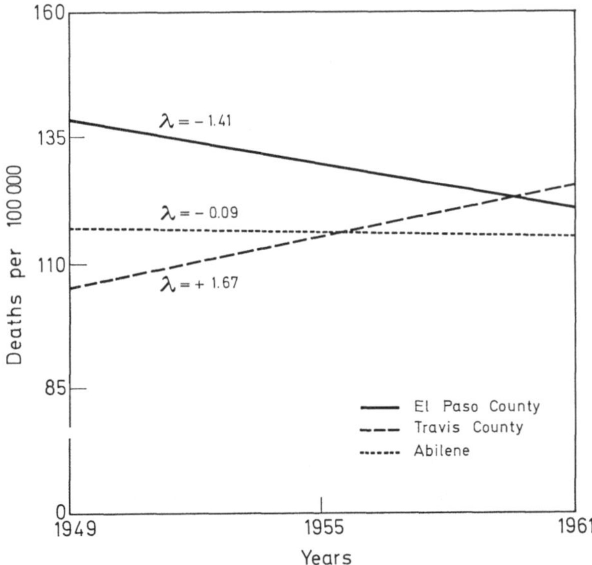

Fig. 5. Cancer of all sites. Age-adjusted mortality trends, total population 1949–1961

necessity for cancer registries often is not understood. However, true incidence rates can be obtained only if all cases are accounted for and each individual is counted only once – not once from each hospital attended.

Most large hospitals in the state have sent abstracts to the Anderson Hospital central registry since 1944 for varying periods of years up to 1958, 1960, or to the present. It was decided to make this information current and to add abstracts from each hospital, laboratory, dermatology office, and other source of cancer patient information. Funds for this purpose recently became available and plans were made to complete one large region at a time.

The population of Texas in 1967 is estimated as about 11,000,000 of which three quarters are urban dwellers and one quarter rural dwellers. For the first time in history, there are more women than men in the population. There is a faster increase for Caucasians than for Negroes. Negroes constitute 12.3 per cent or one and a quarter million persons of the total population, and individuals with Latin American surnames constitute 15 per cent or just over one and one half million persons of the total.

A survey is underway which eventually will include all 510 general hospitals and other information sources from 1944 through 1967. Since fall, 1966, three regions including about 30 counties have been completed and are being coded. Approximately 200,000 of the potential 600,000 accessions are registered. This will increase our population coverage when completed to 11 million and will give the cancer incidence among Negroes. This is one component of the population not covered in the 1944–1958 study. Negroes in Texas represent an economic cross section just as do the other ethnic groups. There are 17 millionaire Negroes in Houston. They have an arts and sciences state supported university in Houston with a 1964 enrollment of 4,220 and at summer school of 5,333. A state sponsored agricultural and mechanical college is at Prairie View with a 1964 enrollment of 3,548. In addition, Texas has eight privately supported Negro colleges with a 1964 enrollment of 3,535. Thus, one of every 100 Negroes in the state attended college in 1964, assuming all students attending were Negroes. Negroes are admitted to all area hospitals but also have two private hospitals in Houston, one with a cancer program accredited by the American College of Surgeons.

Concurrently with this collection of data, an intensive study of environmental conditions in each county and each metropolitan area is in progress. When differences such as those observed in the 1944–1958 survey are noted in cancer types occurring in the same ethnic groups in different areas of the same state, environmental factors must be evaluated for relationships. When, as in El Paso County, cervical cancer has a different prognosis in women of one ethnic group, even when matched by stage of disease at time of treatment, both environmental and genetic factors must be explored to find the reason, and, if possible, to remove or alter the factors responsible.

It is anticipated that with more than 20 years' coverage in this vast state of 21 regions with its three ethnic groups and different environments, and with data analysis centrally and consistently performed, the effect of exogenous factors may be measured in a specific way. The data could not have been analyzed without a giant computer and adequate programmers to process data in such quantities. Corrective measures to alter these factors for the advantage of the cancer patient will then have a scientific foundation. The cooperation of different disciplines in interpreting this information and effecting the application of scientific knowledge as it develops in the laboratory should enable interruption of the sequence of cancer development and eventually prevent some, if not all, of its manifestations.

Über Modelle zur Carcinogenese

Von

G. Wagner und W. J. Bühler

Die expansive Entwicklung der Wissenschaften in den letzten Jahrzehnten hat nicht nur zu einer erheblichen Verbreiterung der klassischen Wissenschaftsbereiche geführt, sondern auch ganz neue Wissenschaftszweige entstehen lassen. Das Eindringen mathematisch-statistischer Gedankengänge und Methoden in den Bereich der biologischen Wissenschaften hat zu einer enormen Entwicklung der Biometrie geführt; daneben ist eine Wissenschaft im Entstehen, die man als „mathematische Biologie" bezeichnen kann, ein Begriff, unter dem alle die Bestrebungen zusammengefaßt werden können, die versuchen, biologische Vorgänge und Sachverhalte in Modellvorstellungen zu beschreiben.

Die Möglichkeit, theoretisch-mathematische Modelle zur Aufklärung biologischer Phänomene heranzuziehen, beruht auf dem Konzept der Isomorphie. Zwei Systeme bezeichnet man als isomorph, wenn ihre Faktoren oder Elemente und die Beziehungen bzw. Wirkungen zwischen diesen Elementen einander entsprechen. Das Ziel jeder mathematischen Modellanalyse ist es, eine möglichst optimale Isomorphie zwischen biologischem System und mathematischem Modell zu finden. Aussagen, die das Modell gestattet, können dann analog auf das biologische System übertragen werden.

In praxi geht man dabei von einigen wichtigen empirischen Tatsachen aus, wobei man weniger wichtig erscheinende Details zunächst außer Betracht läßt. Die daraus abgeleiteten Grundannahmen müssen in einem mathematischen Formalismus ausgedrückt werden, der das primäre Gerüst für alle weiteren Deduktionen darstellt. Es ist also keineswegs erforderlich – und in praxi auch gar nicht möglich – a priori *alle* Elemente des biologischen Systems im Modell zu berücksichtigen; man wird sich zunächst auf die wesentlichsten Einflußfaktoren beschränken müssen und versuchen, das Modell schrittweise zu erweitern. Modellanalyse und Experiment bzw. Beobachtung können sich dabei gegenseitig befruchten, indem die Ergebnisse der Modellanalyse die Aufmerksamkeit des Beobachters oder Experimentators gezielter auf bisher nicht oder wenig beachtete Faktoren lenken und dadurch neue Beobachtungsdetails bekannt werden, die ihrerseits wiederum zu einer Verbesserung der Modellvorstellungen führen können. Der Fortschritt der Erkenntnis vollzieht sich dabei stufenweise und ist charakterisiert durch ein wechselseitiges Geben und Nehmen zwischen Theorie und Praxis.

Jede Aufstellung eines mathematischen Modells ist ein Akt der Formalisierung der Natur, der notwendigerweise um so schwieriger ist, je verwickelter die empirischen Phänomene sind. Ohne bestimmte A-priori-Vorstellung über einen empirischen Sachverhalt ist die Konstruktion eines Modells nicht möglich. Nicht selten tritt aber der Fall ein, daß die aus dem primären Modell zu ziehenden Schlußfolgerungen der beobachtbaren Wirklichkeit wenig entsprechen. Die dem Modell zugrunde liegenden Annahmen erweisen sich damit als unrichtig bzw. unvollständig und müssen dann modifiziert oder ergänzt werden.

Die größte Schwierigkeit jeglichen Bemühens auf diesem relativ neuen Forschungsgebiet beruht somit darin, eine adäquate Adaption des Modells an die Wirklichkeit zu erreichen. Die Gegenstände und Verhaltensweisen alles Lebendigen sind äußerst komplex und kompliziert; im Vergleich dazu sind die mathematischen Modellvorstellungen elementar und notgedrungen fragmentarisch. Ein allzu vereinfachtes Modell hat jedoch wenig Erkenntniswert, auch dann, wenn es mit den beobachteten Fakten gut in Einklang zu bringen ist. Andererseits besteht aber auch keine Gewähr dafür, daß komplizierte mathematische Modelle der Wirklichkeit näherkommen als einfachere. Theoretisch gibt es nämlich keinen absoluten Beweis für die Richtigkeit eines Modells. Die einzig vollständige Repräsentation eines biologischen Systems oder Geschehens ist das System oder Geschehen selbst – ein Modell ist immer nur eine mehr oder weniger zutreffende Beschreibung in Symbolform, die die Wirklichkeit niemals 100%ig erreichen kann. Der große Vorzug mathematischer Modellvorstellungen besteht jedoch darin, daß dabei alle in die Rechnung eingehenden Parameter bekannt sind und beliebig variiert werden können, während das Experiment der Natur oder des Menschen in der Regel nur ein Gesamtresultat erkennen läßt.

Wir stehen heute noch ganz im Anfang einer solchen mathematischen Biologie, von der sich noch nicht vorhersagen läßt, ob sie jemals die gleiche Bedeutung wie die experimentelle Biologie erlangen kann, die aber – darüber besteht wohl schon heute kein Zweifel mehr – letztere sicher fruchtbringend beeinflussen wird.

Einer der frühesten Meilensteine auf dem Gebiete der mathematischen Modellvorstellungen biologischer Phänomene waren die Studien von VOLTERRA in den 20er Jahren unseres Jahrhunderts. VOLTERRA versuchte beispielsweise, mit Papier und Bleistift herauszubekommen, was passiert, wenn sich zwei Tierarten eine nur in begrenztem Maße zur Verfügung stehende Nahrung gegenseitig streitig machen. Dabei ging er von der Überlegung aus, daß ein Anwachsen der Individuenzahl notwendigerweise zu einer Verknappung der Nahrung führen muß, das darauf eintretende Verhungern von Individuen aber den Nahrungsvorrat wieder ansteigen läßt. Die natürliche Proportionalität jeder Spezies zwischen Geburt und Todesfällen erfährt also eine Störung bzw. Veränderung durch das jeweils zur Verfügung stehende Nahrungsangebot. Das ganze Geschehen stellt eine Art Regelungsvorgang dar, der in einen biologischen Gleichgewichtszustand einmündet und sich durch eine Koppelung von Differentialgleichungen mathematisch beschreiben läßt.

Die Modelle von VOLTERRA waren noch rein deterministisch; sie setzten ein unveränderliches Milieu und ein absolut gleichartiges Verhalten aller Individuen voraus und ließen das Spiel des Zufalls völlig außer acht. Erst die weitere Entwicklung der Wahrscheinlichkeitstheorie hat es möglich gemacht, Modelle zu entwickeln, in denen auch die Rolle des Zufalls berücksichtigt ist. Solche Modelle nennt man indeterministisch oder stochastisch. Die meisten dieser Modelle gehen davon aus, daß zukünftige Entwicklungen vom gegenwärtigen Zustand abhängig sind, nicht aber davon, wie es zu diesem gegenwärtigen Zustand gekommen ist. Die entsprechenden Zufallsprozesse sind dann Markoffsche Prozesse.

Es versteht sich von selbst, daß derartige, den Zufall berücksichtigende Modellvorstellungen einen sehr viel größeren Rechenaufwand beanspruchen als die wesentlich einfacheren deterministischen Modelle. Ihre Behandlung und Weiterentwicklung ist überhaupt erst durch den Einsatz von elektronischen Datenverarbeitungsanlagen möglich geworden, die uns heute in die Lage versetzen, auch Modelle, die einen großen Rechenaufwand beanspruchen, unter beliebiger Veränderung der einzelnen Parameter durchzuspielen und dabei zu verfolgen, in welcher Weise die dabei ermittelten Resultate sich den Ergebnissen der Experimente bzw. Beobachtungsreihen anpassen.

Im Rahmen dieser mathematisch-biologischen Forschung spielen die *stochastischen Krebsmodelle* eine zunehmend wichtige Rolle, da man hofft, vielleicht auch auf diesem Wege dem Rätsel der Krebsentstehung einen Schritt näher zu kommen.

Diese Modelle der Carcinogenese gehen fast ausnahmslos von der Mutationstheorie der Krebsentstehung aus, d. h. davon, daß sprunghafte, bei der Zellteilung vererbliche Veränderungen der Zellen erfolgen, die dann zum Wachstum von Tumoren führen. Je nachdem, wieviele solche Veränderungen als nötig postuliert werden, unterscheidet man Ein-, Zwei- und Mehrstufen-Modelle. Oft wird angenommen, daß die Zellveränderungen durch die Einwirkung eines Carcinogens, z. B. durch Treffer von energiereicher Strahlung, erfolgen. Jeder Stufe entspricht dann ein Treffer und man spricht von Ein-Treffer- bzw. Mehr-Treffer-Theorien.

Tab. 1 soll einen Überblick über die bisher vorliegenden Modelle vermitteln. Das Modell von IVERSEN und ARLEY [14] wurde 1950 als erstes stochastisches Modell der Krebsentstehung vorgeschlagen. In ihrem Modell setzen die Autoren einen Treffer durch das Carcinogen voraus, dem eine variable Induktionszeit bis zur Manifestation eines

Tabelle 1. *Modelle der Krebsentstehung*

Übersicht – Stochastische Modelle

Autoren		Beschreibung des Modells
ARLEY, S. IVERSEN	1950	Ein Treffer, dann Induktionszeit
NEYMAN	1958	Ein Treffer, spontane Zweitmutation
STOCKS	1953	C Stufen, dann Latenzzeit, $C = 5$
NORDLING	1953	$C = 6$, Poisson – Prozeß
ARMITAGE, DOLL	1954	verschiedene Raten für versch. Stufen
ARMITAGE, DOLL	1957	Erster Treffer: exponentielles Wachstum Zweiter Treffer: Krebsentstehung
H. G. TUCKER	1961	Erster Treffer: Hyperplasie, diese kann durch zweiten Treffer maligne werden
D. G. KENDALL	1960	Zwei-Treffer-Modell, Geburts- und
WAUGH	1961	Todes-Prozesse für Erst- bzw. Zweit-
NEYMAN, E. L. SCOTT	1961	mutanten
PREHN	1964	Carcinogen wirkt selektiv toxisch
KREYBERG	1965	Kritische Dosis des Carcinogens
O. H. IVERSEN, BJERKNES	1963	Feedback-Modell der normalen Haut

Tumors folgt. Unter gewissen Annahmen über die Trefferrate (proportional zur verabreichten Dosis) und die Wahrscheinlichkeitsverteilung der Induktionszeit leiteten die Autoren Aussagen ab über die zu erwartende Zeit zwischen der Verabreichung der Dosis und dem Auftreten von Tumoren und über die Anzahl der zu erwartenden Tumoren. Diese Aussagen wurden mit experimentellen Ergebnissen verglichen. Die Übereinstimmung war überraschend gut, bis ARLEY und IVERSEN versuchten [5], ihr Modell auf Versuche von H. BLUM [9] anzuwenden, der außer der Gesamtdosis auch den Zeitplan ihrer Verabreichung in Teildosen variiert hatte.

Ähnlich liegen die Dinge bei dem Modell von NEYMAN [19], der annahm, das Carcinogen löse eine erste Mutation aus und die Nachkommen der mutierten Zelle(n) unterlägen dem Risiko einer (spontanen) Zweitmutation. Hinzu kommen Annahmen über die Art der Vermehrung der mutierten Zelle. Da nach dem ersten Treffer der Prozeß nicht mehr vom Einfluß des Carcinogens abhängig ist, kann man insgesamt NEYMANS Modell als eine Variante des ARLEY-IVERSENschen Modells bezeichnen.

Die Modelle von STOCKS [23, 24], NORDLING [21] und ARMITAGE und DOLL [6] setzen mehrere (5 oder 6) Treffer voraus und wurden im wesentlichen zur Erklärung epidemiologischer Daten konstruiert. Wir werden auf das STOCKSsche Modell noch näher eingehen. ARMITAGE und DOLL zeigen später [7], daß zur Erklärung dieser Daten auch ein Zwei-Treffer-Modell ausreicht, bei dem der erste Treffer den Nachkommen der mutierten Zelle einen selektiven Vorteil verschafft. Diese Nachkommen sind dann dem Risiko einer Zweitmutation unterworfen. In TUCKERS [25] Modell sind ebenfalls zwei Treffer erforderlich; der erste erzeugt eine Hyperplasie, aus der bei einem zweiten Treffer ein Tumor entsteht. Die Modelle von KENDALL [16], WAUGH [26], NEYMAN und SCOTT [20] verlangen ebenfalls zwei Treffer; getroffene Zellen vermehren sich nach einem Geburts- und Todesprozeß, der für die Erstmutanten subkritisch verläuft, d. h. im Endeffekt zu ihrem Aussterben führt, für die Zweitmutanten (Tumorzellen) jedoch superkritisch verläuft. Genauer gesagt, wenn $f(t)$ die Dosisfunktion zur Zeit t ist (Intensität von Strahlung, Konzentration einer chemischen Substanz), so soll in der NEYMAN-SCOTTschen Version dieses Modells in der Zeit von t bis $t + \mathrm{d}t$ die Wahrscheinlichkeit für das Auftreten eines Erstmutanten $f(t)\mathrm{d}t$ sein. Jeder Erstmutant bzw. Nachkomme eines solchen soll mit der Wahrscheinlichkeit

$\lambda\,\mathrm{d}t$ sich in zwei Zellen gleicher Art teilen,

$\mu\,\mathrm{d}t$ sterben oder

$[\nu_0 + \nu_1 f(t)]\mathrm{d}t$ in eine Tumorzelle mutieren.

Jede Tumorzelle soll mit der Wahrscheinlichkeit $\Lambda\,\mathrm{d}t$ sich vermehren, mit $M\,\mathrm{d}t$ sterben.

PREHN [22] schlägt ein Modell vor, in dem mehrere Mutationen zur Cancerisierung führen. Diese Mutationen erfolgen spontan; die Einwirkung eines Carcinogens besteht in seiner Toxizität, die selektiv wirkt zugunsten der Zellen, die schon einige Schritte auf dem Wege zum Krebs fortgeschritten sind. Das Modell ist mathematisch nicht ausgearbeitet. KREYBERG [18] möchte mit seinem Modell insbesondere die Entstehung von Bronchialkrebs beim Raucher beschreiben.

Das Modell von O. H. IVERSEN und BJERKNES [13] bezieht sich zunächst nur auf normale Mäusehaut; an eine Erweiterung zum Krebsmodell ist gedacht. Die Simulation des Modells auf einem Analog- bzw. Digitalrechner ergab gute Übereinstimmung mit dem Verhalten normaler Mäusehaut.

Die meisten dieser Modelle sind konstruiert worden, um gewisse empirische Daten zu erklären. Da in jedem Modell einige Parameter vorkommen, deren Werte a priori unbekannt sind, ist es nicht allzu erstaunlich, wenn die Parameterwerte so angepaßt werden können, daß das Modell den vorliegenden Daten gut entspricht. Der Versuch, das Modell auf Daten mit einer anderen Struktur anzuwenden, kann dann u. U. zeigen, daß das Modell doch von der Wirklichkeit zu weit entfernt ist. Ein Beispiel wurde schon erwähnt, der Mißerfolg des ARLEY-IVERSEN-Modells bei der Anwendung auf Versuche mit fraktionierten Bestrahlungsdosen. Ähnlich war NEYMANS Ein-Treffer-Zwei-Stufen-Modell unzureichend zur Erklärung der Lungentumorausbeute bei Mäusen bei fraktionierter Injektion von Urethan.

Dieses Scheitern des Modells veranlaßte NEYMAN [20] und andere [16, 26], das Modell zu modifizieren und zu erweitern zu dem schon beschriebenen Zwei-Treffer-Modell. Dieses Modell enthält nun sechs unbekannte Parameter und eine unbekannte Funktion $f(t)$, die in der NEYMAN-SCOTT-Version durch zwei weitere Parameter beschrieben wird. Dadurch ist das Modell so komplex geworden, daß man in die Gefahr gerät, durch geeignete Manipulation mit den Parametern eine gute Adaption an alle möglichen Daten zu erhalten, selbst dann, wenn zwischen Modell und Wirklichkeit keine enge Beziehung bestehen sollte. Um dieser Gefahr auszuweichen, muß man zweierlei tun:

1. muß man versuchen, aus dem Modell weitere Aussagen abzuleiten über Größen, die bisher nicht betrachtet wurden, und diese dann mit den Ergebnissen neuer Versuche vergleichen. Hierbei treten große mathematische Schwierigkeiten auf; aber selbst wenn diese überwunden werden können, auch Schwierigkeiten experimenteller Natur. So hat beispielsweise KLONECKI [17] Aussagen über die gemeinsame Verteilung der Anzahl der Erstmutanten und der Gruppen von Zweitmutanten im NEYMAN-SCOTT-Modell gewonnen; wegen der Schwierigkeiten beim Auszählen der vermuteten Erstmutanten konnten seine Ergebnisse aber nicht experimentellen Daten gegenübergestellt werden.

2. muß man versuchen, Werte für wenigstens einige der Parameter zu bestimmen, evtl. auch in Versuchen, die unabhängig sein können von den Experimenten zur Tumorerzeugung, um so den Spielraum für Manipulationen mit den Parametern des Modells einzuengen. Experimente dieser Art sind in Berkeley im Gange.

Aber auch mathematisch weniger komplizierte Modelle unterliegen der Gefahr der Manipulierbarkeit. Dies soll an dem Beispiel des STOCKS-schen Modells [23] gezeigt werden. STOCKS führte sein Modell 1953 zur Erklärung der Sterberaten an Magenkrebs in England und Wales ein und wendete es 1966 auch auf den Lungenkrebs an [24]. STOCKS setzt voraus, zur Entstehung eines Krebses seien mehrere (C) Schritte erforderlich. „Der Einfachheit halber" – wie er wörtlich schreibt – nimmt er an, in einem Jahr könne höchstens ein Schritt erfolgen. Die Wahrscheinlichkeit, mit der der Prozeß der Cancerisierung in einem gegebenen Jahr um einen Schritt weiter führt, soll für jeden Schritt gleich q sein. Nach Erreichen der Stufe C soll dann eine weitere Zeit L vergehen, nach der der Tod eintritt.

Unter diesen Annahmen werden Todesfälle an der betrachteten Krebsart nicht vor dem Alter von $C + L$ Jahren zu erwarten sein. Nach $C + L$ Jahren wird der Anteil der Bevölkerung sterben, der im Alter von C Jahren auf der Stufe C angelangt war, also der Anteil q^C. Entsprechend wird die Sterberate im Alter $C + L + X$ bestimmt sein durch die Wahrscheinlichkeit, nach $C + X$ Jahren die Stufe C zu erreichen, also durch

$$q^C (1 - q)^X \; \frac{(C + X - 1)(C + X - 2) \ldots (C + 1)\, C}{1 \cdot 2 \ldots \cdot X} \tag{1}$$

gegeben sein.

STOCKS verglich nun die Kurve der Raten (1) mit der Kurve der Sterberaten an Lungenkrebs bei Männern in England und Wales und fand, daß „keine Übereinstimmung möglich war außer für $C = 5$", und daß die Anpassung für $q = 0{,}043$ und $L = 20$ am besten war. Das hieße mit anderen Worten: Lungenkrebs benötigt für seine Entstehung 5 Schritte (also mindestens 5 Jahre); in jedem gegebenen Jahr gehen 4,3% der Bevölkerung einen Schritt weiter ins Krebsrisiko und nach Erreichen der Stufe C vergehen noch 20 Jahre, bis der Krebs zum Tode führt.

Die im Modell vorkommenden Größen C und L wurden von STOCKS nicht in Beziehung gesetzt mit (wenigstens im Prinzip) beobachtbaren biologischen Größen. Eine Isomorphie zwischen Modell und Wirklichkeit in dem eingangs erwähnten Sinn wurde also nicht hergestellt. Mit den drei unbekannten Parametern C, q, L ist das Modell schon so flexibel, daß eine gute Anpassung der Raten (1) an die beobachteten Streberaten nicht überraschend erscheint. Um diese Anpassung weiter zu verbessern, nahm STOCKS ohne genauere biologische Begründung noch eine Altersabhängigkeit von L mit in sein Modell auf. Weiterhin erscheint die Annahme, jeder Schritt benötige gerade ein Jahr, nicht zwingend.

Aus allen diesen Gründen haben wir die STOCKSschen Ergebnisse nicht unbesehen hingenommen, sondern nochmals die durch das STOCKSsche Modell vorhergesagten Raten nach (1) für verschiedene Parameterwerte errechnet und mit den von STOCKS publizierten Sterberaten verglichen.

Eine einigermaßen vollständige Übersicht über die durch das Modell gegebenen Möglichkeiten zur Anpassung an die Sterberaten hätte mehrere hundert Stunden Rechenaufwand auf Tischrechenmaschinen erfordert. Das Problem wurde daher mit Hilfe der elektronischen Datenverarbeitungsanlage (IBM 360/30) am Institut für Dokumentation, Information und Statistik des Deutschen Krebsforschungszentrums Heidelberg bearbeitet, wobei in kurzer Zeit die „besten" Werte der Parameter ermittelt werden konnten.

Der Ausgangspunkt für unsere Untersuchungen war Tab. 2, die mit geringen Modifikationen aus STOCKS [24] übernommen wurde.

Tabelle 2. *Anzahl der Sterbefälle an Bronchialkrebs in England und Wales in Kohorten von einer Million der Bevölkerung*

Alter bis	1896/1900	1901/1905	1906/1910	1911/1915	gesamt
19	7	10	12	12	41
24	17	21	27	31	96
29	34	46	64	84	228
34	70	116	174	211	571
39	244	384	466	558	1652
44	711	1020	1301	1463	4495
49	1873	2780	3589	3531	11773
54	4626	6590	7656	7688	26560
59	10015	13315	14656	—	37986
64	18007	23183	—	—	41190
69	27932	—	—	—	27932

Diese Tabelle gibt die kumulative Anzahl der Sterbefälle an Lungen- und Bronchialkrebs bei Männern in England und Wales in Kohorten von je einer Million, geboren in den angegebenen Jahrgängen. Da das Modell einen Kohorteneffekt nicht berücksichtigt, wurde die letzte Spalte, die Summe der vier einzelnen Kohorten, zur Grundlage der Approximation gemacht. Diese ist in Abb. 1 noch einmal graphisch dargestellt (ausgezogene Linie). Die ganz darüber verlaufende Linie entspricht der STOCKSschen Annäherung. Die Unstetigkeit zwischen 30 und 40 Jahren ist wohl dadurch entstanden, daß die willkürlich angenommene Altersabhängigkeit von L aus der entsprechenden Altersstufe zu viele Krebsfälle in andere Altersstufen verschoben hat. Die mit $C = 9$ und $C = 13$ bezeichneten Kurven sind zwei Beispiele, die zeigen, daß eine „Erklärung" der Daten durchaus auch mit anderen Parametern möglich ist als mit den von STOCKS gefundenen.

Genauer zeigt dies Tab. 3, aus der gleichzeitig hervorgeht, wie stark der als „der beste" gefundene Wert von C abhängt von der Art der Beurteilung der Approximation. Spalte (1) zeigt die Summe der Abweichungsquadrate der besten Anpassungskurve bei festem Wert von C und variablen L und q. Macht man statt dessen die Summe der absoluten Abweichungen minimal, so erhält man beinahe die gleichen Ergebnisse, und in beiden Fällen ist die Anpassung in den unteren Altersstufen relativ schlecht. In der Hoffnung, dies zu verbessern, wurde in (3) die Anpassung anders beurteilt, und zwar wurden statt der kumulativen Anzahl die Anzahlen der Sterbefälle in den einzelnen Altersklassen approximiert und die auftretenden Differenzen noch mit Gewichten versehen, die den Ein-

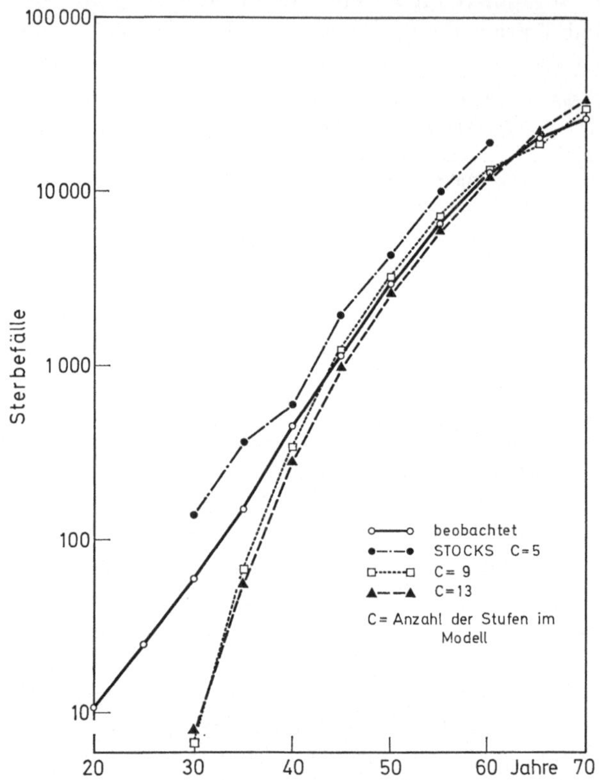

Abb. 1. Sterberaten an Bronchialkrebs in England und Wales

Tabelle 3. *Güte der Anpassung in Abhängigkeit von C*

C	(1)	(2)	(3)
4	13370	9722	163
5	*8131*	*3076*	*99*
6	8262	1775	83
7	8678	*1524*	71
8	6404	1650	63
9	*4662*	1849	59
10	5782	1735	55
11	7813	2024	52
12	8897	2155	50
13	6497	2878	*48*
14	15510	4591	85

fluß der Altersstufen mit großen Sterbezahlen auf die Gesamtapproximation nicht allein bestimmend sein lassen sollten. Spalte (2) zeigt das Ergebnis der Approximation an die Sterberaten, wobei die Summe der absoluten Abweichungen minimalisiert wurde. Die „besten" Approximationen erhält man in Spalten (1), (2) bzw. (3) bei $C = 9$, $C = 7$ bzw. $C = 13$; die zugehörigen Anpassungskurven für $C = 9$ und $C = 13$ sind in Abb. 1 eingetragen.

Tabelle 4. *Beste Approximation in Abhängigkeit von M*

	M	1	6	12	24	60
(1)	C	12	12	9	9	7
	L	7	4	11	7	1
	q	0,0095	0,055	0,085	0,165	0,300
	G	295	292	352	1538	1005
(3)	C	14	14	13	10	7
	L	3	1	1	2	1
	q	0,0110	0,0650	0,120	0,173	0,300
	G	49	48	48	141	88

M = Anzahl der Monate pro Stufe; L = Latenzzeit; G = Güte der Approximation

Die Möglichkeit, mit der Zeitspanne „pro Schritt" zu manipulieren, soll Tab. 4 veranschaulichen. Hier sind die jeweils nach Methode (1) und (3) besten Anpassungen angegeben, wenn man annimmt für jeden Schritt seinen M Monate erforderlich.

Zusammenfassend ist zu sagen: Im Stocksschen Modell sind die Bestandteile nicht mit wirklichen biologischen Größen in Beziehung gesetzt. Es ist nicht einmal der Versuch unternommen worden, eine Isomorphie zwischen Wirklichkeit und Modell herzustellen. Wenn trotzdem das Modell die vorhandenen Daten erklären kann, so ist dies nicht der Richtigkeit des Modells zuzuschreiben, sondern seiner Flexibilität dank seiner vier unabhängigen Parameter. Durch die Möglichkeit des Einsatzes einer elektronischen Datenverarbeitungsanlage konnten wir nachweisen, daß sogar auf mehr als eine Weise die epidemiologischen Daten „zufriedenstellend" approximiert werden können.

Diese Manipulierbarkeit haftet zwar jedem komplexen Modell an; ist jedoch eine solche Isomorphie (wenigstens versuchsweise) hergestellt, d. h. sind die Parameter des Modells mit biologischen Größen identifiziert, so ist es leichter möglich, diese Manipulierbarkeit unter Kontrolle zu bringen.

Literatur

1. ARLEY, N.: Theoretical Analysis of Carcinogenesis. Proc. 4th Berkeley Symposium on Math. Statistics and Probability Vol. IV, 1 (1961).

2. — and R. EKER: Mechanisms of Carcinogenesis. Advanc. biol. med. Phys. 8, 375 (1962).

3. — and S. IVERSEN: On the Mechanism of Experimental Carcinogenesis, III. Acta path. microbiol. Scand. 30, 21 (1951).

4. — — On the Mechanism of Experimental Carcinogenesis, VI. ibid. 31, 164 (1952).

5. — — On the Mechanism of Experimental Carcinogenesis, IX. ibid. 33, 133 (1953).

6. ARMITAGE, P. and R. DOLL: The Age Distribution of Cancer and a Multistage Theory of Carcinogenesis. Brit. J. Cancer 8, 1 (1954).

7. — — A two Stage Theory of Carcinogenesis in Relation to the Age Distribution of Human Cancer. ibid. 11, 16 (1957).

8. — — Stochastic Models for Carcinogenesis. Proc. 4th Berkeley Symposium on Math. Statistics and Probability Vol. IV, 19 (1961).

9. BLUM, H. F.: On the Mechanism of Cancer Induction by Ultraviolet Radiation. J. nat. Cancer Inst. 11, 463 (1950).

10. — Comparable Models for Carcinogenesis by Ultraviolet Light and by Chemical Agents. Proc. 4th Berkeley Symposium on Math. Statistics and Probability Vol. IV, 101 (1961).

11. BÜHLER, W. J.: Mathematische Aspekte der Krebsforschung. Naturwissenschaften 55, 121 (1968).

12. ENGELBRETH-HOLM, J. and S. IVERSEN: On the Mechanism of Experimental Carcinogenesis, II. Acta path. microbiol. Scand. 29, 77 (1951).

13. IVERSEN, O. H. and R. BJERKNES: Kinetics of Epidermal Reaction to Carcinogens. Acta path. microbiol. Scand., Suppl. 165 (1963).

14. IVERSEN, S. and N. ARLEY: On the Mechanism of Experimental Carcinogenesis. Acta path. microbiol. Scand. 27, 773 (1950).

15. — — On the Mechanism of Experimental Carcinogenesis, V. ibid. 31, 27 (1952).

16. KENDALL, D. G.: Birth and Death Processes and the Theory of Carcinogenesis. Biometrika 47, 13 (1960).

17. KLONECKI, W.: A Method for Derivation of Probabilities in a Stochastic Model of Population Growth for Carcinogenesis. Colloquium Math. 13, 273 (1965).

18. KREYBERG, H. J. A.: Empirical Relationship of Lung Cancer to Cigarette Smoking and a Stochastic Model for the Role of Action of Carcinogens. Biometrics 21, 839 (1965).

19. NEYMAN, J.: A two Step Mutation Theory of Carcinogenesis. Bull. int. statist. Inst. 38, 123 (1961).

20. — and E. L. SCOTT: Statistical Aspect of the Problem of Carcinogenesis. Proc. 5th Berkeley Symposium Vol. IV, 745 (1967).

21. NORDLING, C. O.: A new Theory on the Cancer-inducing Mechanism. Brit. J. Cancer 7, 68 (1953).

22. PREHN, R. T.: Clonal Selection Theory of Chemical Carcinogenesis. J. nat. Cancer Inst. 32, 1 (1964).

23. STOCKS, P.: A Study of the Age Curve for Cancer of the Stomach in Connection with a Theory of the Cancer Producing Mechanism. Brit. J. Cancer **7**, 407 (1953).
24. — Recent Epidemiological Studies of the Lung Cancer Mortality, Cigarette Smoking and Air Pollution with Discussion of a new Hypothesis of Causation. Brit. J. Cancer **20**, 595 (1966).
25. TUCKER, H. G.: A Stochastic Model for a Two-Stage Theory of Carcinogenesis. Proc. 4th Berkeley Symposium on Math. Statistics and Probability Vol. IV, 387 (1961).
26. WAUGH, W. A. O'N.: Age Dependence in a Stochastic Model of Carcinogenesis. ibid. Vol. IV, 405 (1961).

Methodische Aspekte einer Krebsstatistik
im Krankenhaus

Von

H. IMMICH

Die Krebsforschung am Menschen kann sich nur auf Beobachtungen stützen. Solche Beobachtungen werden heute im wesentlichen mit vier Verfahren gewonnen:

1. mit der amtlichen Todesursachenstatistik,

2. mit prospektiven epidemiologischen Studien,

3. mit Sektionsstatistiken und

4. mit Krankenhausstatistiken.

Trotz teilweise verschiedener Methodik haben diese vier Verfahren folgendes gemeinsam:

1. die aus Beobachtungsreihen gewonnenen Daten müssen mit wahrscheinlichkeitsstatistischen Methoden ausgewertet werden, bevor man Schlußfolgerungen aus diesen Daten ziehen darf.

2. Schlußfolgerungen, die sich lediglich auf Beobachtungsreihen stützen können, sind weniger zuverlässig als Schlußfolgerungen aus experimentell gewonnenen Daten, selbst wenn wahrscheinlichkeitsstatistische Methoden angewandt worden sind. Sobald man kausale Beziehungen untersuchen will, kann man bei Beobachtungsreihen niemals sicher sein, ob man alle wesentlichen Einflußgrößen oder Faktoren erfaßt hat. Man kann zwar durch verfeinerte Analysen versuchen, auch bei Beobachtungsreihen störende Nebenfaktoren auszuschalten oder zumindest konstant zu halten. Solche Analysen sind aber mühevoll und verursachen im allgemeinen zusätzliche Kosten. Darüber hinaus: Selbst wenn man alle Irrtumsmöglichkeiten ausgeschaltet zu haben glaubt, läßt sich immer noch einwenden, daß möglicherweise eine nicht näher identifizierbare Einflußgröße existiert, die einen kausalen Zusammenhang nur vortäuscht.

Bei Krankenhausstatistiken gibt es aber noch zusätzliche Probleme, durch welche die Schlußfolgerungen aus solchen Statistiken erheblich beeinflußt werden können. Mit diesen Problemen wollen wir uns beschäftigen und aus dieser Beschäftigung Forderungen ableiten, die erfüllt sein müssen, wenn man die Ergebnisse aus Krankenhausstatistiken richtig deuten will.

Weitaus die meisten Krebsstatistiken in Krankenhäusern werden retrospektiv angelegt, d. h. also, zu irgendeinem Zeitpunkt wird angeordnet, die vorhandenen Krankenblätter rückwärts aufzuarbeiten. Dieses Verfahren hat den Nachteil, daß viele Daten, die für das Krebsproblem relevant sein könnten, in den alten Krankenblättern fehlen. Man kann größtenteils nicht mehr feststellen, ob diese Daten fehlen, weil ein Befund normal ausgefallen oder weil eine entsprechende Untersuchung unterlassen worden ist. Die erste Forderung, die an Krebsstatistiken in Krankenhäusern zu stellen ist, lautet demnach:

Die Daten müssen prospektiv nach einem genau festgelegten Plan gesammelt werden.

Ein weiterer schwerwiegender methodischer Mangel bei Krebsstatistiken in Krankenhäusern besteht darin, daß keine Vergleichs- oder Kontrollgruppen mitgeführt werden. Sobald man kausale Beziehungen untersuchen will, muß man prüfen können, wie sich ein als ursächlich angesehener Faktor bei Krebskranken und bei den übrigen Patienten auswirkt. Eine fehlende Vergleichsgruppe verleitet aber auch zur Berechnung der relativen Morbidität mit ihren bekannten fragwürdigen Ergebnissen. Ein Beispiel mag diesen Satz erläutern:

1955 hat eine Krebsstatistik in einem Krankenhaus folgende Zahlen erbracht:

Krebsform	Absolut	%
Bronchial-Ca	10	10,0
Magen-Ca	30	30,0
Übrige Ca	60	60,0
Summe	100	100,0

1965 ergibt die Krebsstatistik im gleichen Krankenhaus:

Krebsform	Absolut	%
Bronchial-Ca	10	13,3
Magen-Ca	5	6,7
Übrige Ca	60	80,0
Summe	75	100,0

Obwohl also die absolute Zahl der Bronchial-Carcinome gleich geblieben ist, hat die prozentuale Häufigkeit dieser Krebsform zugenommen. Man kann diesem Fehlschluß in der Literatur immer wieder begegnen. Dieses Beispiel zeigt, daß man Morbiditätszahlen immer auf die Zahl der Nicht-Krebskranken beziehen muß.

Wird diese Forderung gestellt, dann hört man oft den Einwand, daß man die Zahl der Krebskranken ja nur auf die Gesamtzahl der Patienten in einem Kalenderjahr zu beziehen brauchte. Diese Zahlen könnte man ohne Schwierigkeiten von der Krankenhausverwaltung erhalten. Damit sei eine Vergleichsgruppe entbehrlich.

Dieser Einwand ist nicht stichhaltig. In der Gesamtzahl der Patienten sind nämlich auch diejenigen enthalten, die in einem Kalenderjahr zwei- oder mehrmals stationär aufgenommen worden sind. Werden diese Mehrfachzugänge nicht berücksichtigt, so kann sich beispielsweise folgendes ereignen:

1955 ergibt die Diagnosenverteilung in einem Krankenhaus bei Männern zwischen 55 und 64 Jahren:

Diagnose	Absolut	%
Bronchial-Ca	10	10,0
Emphysem-Bronchitis	50	50,0
Sonstige Krankheiten	40	40,0
Summe	100	100,0

1958 mag im Einzugsgebiet dieses Krankenhauses schlechtes Wetter geherrscht haben. Die Männer mit Emphysem-Bronchitis haben infolgedessen häufige Rückfälle erlitten. Die Jahresstatistik ergibt bei den Männern zwischen 55 und 64 Jahren jetzt folgende Zahlen:

Diagnose	Absolut	%
Bronchial-Ca	10	5,0
Emphysem-Bronchitis	150	75,0
Sonstige Krankheiten	40	20,0
Summe	200	100,0

Wie man sieht, tritt jetzt der umgekehrte Effekt ein; der prozentuale Anteil des Bronchial-Carcinoms nimmt ab, obwohl sich die absolute Zahl nicht geändert hat. Man darf sich also nicht auf die Gesamtzahl aller stationären *Zugänge* in einem Krankenhaus, sondern nur auf die Gesamtzahl aller *Patienten* in einem Beobachtungszeitraum beziehen. Das aber ist nur möglich, wenn man nicht nur die Krankenblätter der Krebskranken, sondern die Krankenblätter aller Patienten erfaßt. Daher lautet die zweite Forderung an eine Krebsstatistik im Krankenhaus:

Die Krankenblätter der Krebs- und der Nicht-Krebskranken müssen nach den gleichen Gesichtspunkten erfaßt und ausgewertet werden.

Wird diese Forderung erfüllt, so hat man damit gleichzeitig die
Möglichkeit geschaffen, Vergleichsgruppen nach Bedarf zu bilden. Will
man die Morbiditätsziffern bösartiger Neubildungen unter Krankenhaus-
verhältnissen über mehrere Jahre studieren, so muß man zunächst dafür
sorgen, daß jeder Patient in dem Beobachtungszeitraum nur ein einziges
Mal gezählt wird. Zu diesem Zweck muß man aus mehreren Krankenhaus-
aufenthalten eines und desselben Patienten einen einzigen streng zufällig

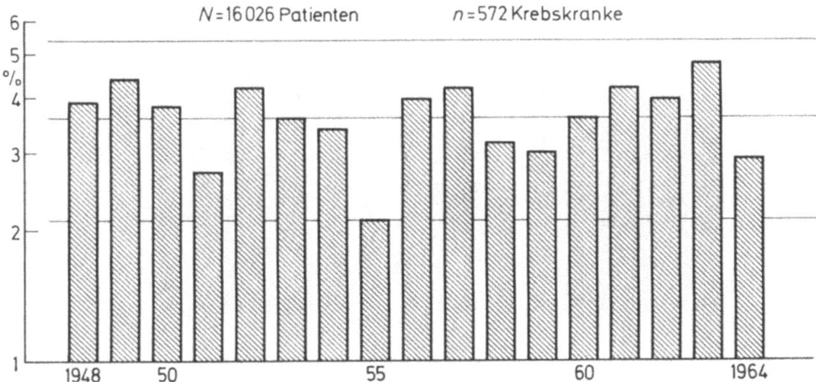

Abb. 1. Prozentuale Häufigkeit von Krebskranken in einer Inneren Abteilung von
1948–1964

auswählen; dieser Krankenhausaufenthalt wird dann bei der Auswertung
gezählt. Damit schafft man eine Beobachtungsreihe, die jeden Patienten
nur in einem zeitlich eng begrenzten Ausschnitt seines Lebens erfaßt.
Diese „Momentaufnahmen" von einer großen Patientenzahl bieten nun
noch den großen Vorzug, selbst in einer Beobachtungsreihe Faktoren
auszuschalten, die bisher jede Schlußfolgerung beeinträchtigt haben.
Diese Faktoren sind:

1. Die Mehrfacherfassung eines und desselben Patienten,

2. Die Umschichtung im Altersaufbau der Bevölkerung,

3. Die Wechselwirkung zwischen diesen beiden Faktoren, d. h. die
Tatsache, daß bei älteren Patienten die Wahrscheinlichkeit, mehrfach
erfaßt zu werden, größer ist als bei jüngeren.

Nicht ausgeschaltet wird dagegen der Einfluß des Faktors Zeit. Diese
Möglichkeit, störende Faktoren in einer Beobachtungsreihe auszuschalten, ist bisher viel zu wenig bekannt und kaum genutzt.
Daher soll jetzt gezeigt werden, welche Vorteile eine verfeinerte
Analyse einer Beobachtungsreihe erbringen kann. Die folgenden Beispiele stammen aus dem Krankengut der Inneren Abteilung des Landes-
krankenhauses Schleswig.

Abb. 1 zeigt die prozentualen Anteile der krebskranken Patienten in den Jahren von 1948–1964. Diese Darstellung stützt sich auf rund 16000 Patienten, von denen rund 23000 Krankenblätter angelegt und dokumentiert worden waren. Der Anteil der Krebskranken schwankt von Jahr zu Jahr; doch zeigt eine wahrscheinlichkeitsstatistische Prüfung auf das Vorliegen einer konstanten Grundwahrscheinlichkeit, daß alle Schwankungen noch im Bereich zufälliger Abweichungen liegen.

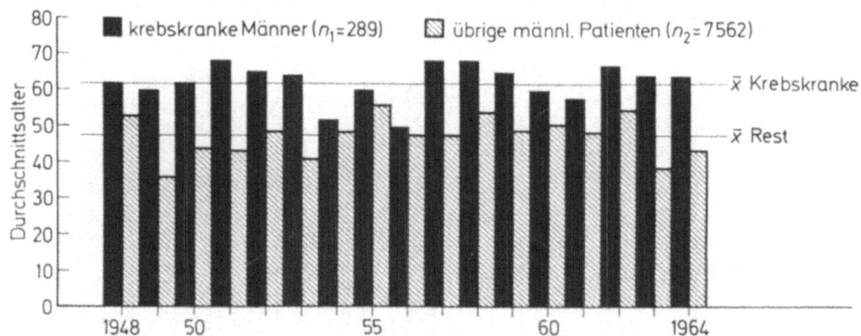

Abb. 2. Durchschnittliches Lebensalter krebskranker und nicht-krebskranker Patienten in den Jahren 1948–1964

Abb. 2 zeigt das durchschnittliche Lebensalter der krebskranken und der nicht-krebskranken Männer in den Jahren von 1948–1964. Der Mittelwert beträgt bei Krebskranken rund 62, bei Nicht-Krebskranken rund 47 Jahre, die Standardabweichung rund 15 Jahre. Auch hier sind die Abweichungen von Jahr zu Jahr nur zufällig. Dagegen sind die Unterschiede zwischen den durchschnittlichen Lebensaltern bei Krebs- und Nicht-Krebskranken statistisch gesichert.

Aus diesen Ergebnissen läßt sich zumindest für die untersuchte Krankenhauspopulation der Schluß ziehen: Eliminiert man rechnerisch die Änderung im Altersaufbau der Bevölkerung von 1948–1964, dann läßt sich keine Zunahme von Krebskrankheiten in diesem Beobachtungszeitraum nachweisen.

Abb. 3 zeigt den Anteil der Magen-, Bronchial- und der übrigen Krebskranken an den männlichen Patienten in den Jahren von 1948 bis 1964. Wie man sieht, geht die prozentuale Häufigkeit des Magenkrebses ab 1953 zurück; dieses Ergebnis läßt sich statistisch sichern. Dagegen ist – wie bei den übrigen Krebsformen auch – bei der prozentualen Häufigkeit des Bronchialkrebses kein zeitlicher Trend zu erkennen; die Schwankungen von Jahr zu Jahr liegen noch im Bereich zufälliger Abweichungen.

Während also die Abnahme der relativen Häufigkeit des Magenkrebses mit den Ergebnissen der amtlichen Todesursachenstatistik über-
einstimmt, weichen die Morbiditätsziffern an Bronchialkrebs in dieser
Krankenhauspopulation von den amtlichen Zahlen ab. Das kann verschiedene Gründe haben. Der nächstliegende ist auch hier die künstliche
Ausschaltung der Altersumschichtung. Dieser Annahme würden die
Zahlen der amtlichen Todesursachenstatistik nicht widersprechen, denn
diese Statistik ist auf die Altersstruktur der Wohnbevölkerung von 1950
standardisiert; seither hat sich aber die Altersstruktur erheblich ge-
wandelt.

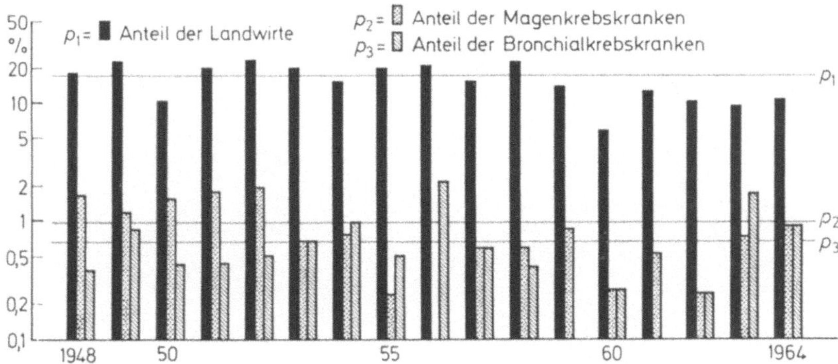

Abb. 3. Relative Häufigkeit bestimmter Krebsformen und des Anteils der Landwirte im Patientenkollektiv der Jahre 1948–1964

Es sei aber noch eine Erklärungsmöglichkeit angeführt, die in der
epidemiologischen Forschung eine besondere Rolle spielt: Die Berufs-
disposition landwirtschaftlicher Berufe. Früher wurde die Ansicht ver-
treten, in dieser Berufsgruppe kämen Magenkrebse gehäuft vor; heute
sagt man, daß Landwirte seltener an Bronchialkrebs erkranken als
andere Berufe. In Abb. 3 ist daher auch der Anteil der Landwirte und der
landwirtschaftlichen Arbeiter am männlichen Patientenkollektiv dargestellt. Der Häufigkeitsanteil dieser Berufe ist von 1948–1959 ziemlich
konstant; ab 1960 ist eine statistisch gesicherte Abnahme zu erkennen.
Wie man weiter sieht, ist weder die Abnahme der Magenkrebshäufigkeit
noch die relative Häufigkeit des Bronchialkrebses mit dem Anteil der
Landwirte korreliert.
Interpretationen allein aus relativen Häufigkeiten sind in der Krebsstatistik zwar verbreitet, gestatten aber keine schlüssigen Aussagen.
Aber auch bei Durchführung eines sinnvollen wahrscheinlichkeitsstatistischen Tests mit Zuordnung jedes einzelnen Probanden zu den beiden

Alternativmerkmalen ,,Landwirt: ja–nein‘‘, ,,Krebs: ja–nein‘‘ läßt sich kein Zusammenhang zwischen landwirtschaftlichen Berufen und Krebslokalisation erkennen.

Somit muß aus den erreichbaren Daten und für das erfaßte Kollektiv auch beim Bronchial-Carcinom der Schluß gezogen werden, daß nach Ausschaltung des Faktors Altersumschichtung keine eindeutige Zunahme des Bronchial-Carcinoms mehr festzustellen ist.

Auswertungsergebnisse bei Mammatumoren
der Chirurgischen Universitätsklinik Heidelberg

Von

G. Ott, K. Hochberg, M. Nuri und C. Köhler

Der Brustkrebs der Frau war der wichtigste Lehrmeister der Krebs-
diagnostik, mehr noch, der Krebstherapie seit Anbeginn der Krebs-
lehre. – Heilung durch Excision, Leidensverschlimmerung durch un-
radikales Vorgehen, Ätzung und Brenneisen, erweiterte radikale Chirurgie
unter Mitentfernung der regionalen Lymphknoten, die Bedeutung des
Stadiums für die Prognose, eine antihormonelle Therapie und manches
andere sind Erkenntnisse, die erstmals beim Mammacarcinom gewonnen
wurden.

Trotz der Kenntnisse vom Brustkrebs über rund vier Jahrtausende ist
unser ärztliches Vorgehen in vieler Hinsicht umstritten. Eine Standardi-
sierung der Behandlung ist bis heute nicht erreichbar gewesen, weil die
bisher vorgelegten ärztlichen Erfahrungen in vielen Fragen nicht miteinander vergleichbar und durchaus widersprüchlich waren.

Erst jetzt sind von der UICC Voraussetzungen geschaffen, um auf
breiter Basis auch beim Mammacarcinom vergleichbare Ergebnisse zu
erarbeiten.

Wir haben in einer retrospektiven Erhebung an der Chirurgischen
Universitäts-Klinik Heidelberg versucht, die von der UICC vorgelegten
Dokumentationsrichtlinien beim Mammacarcinom für klinische Belange
zu testen. Zudem war es unser Anliegen, mit ihrer Hilfe Aussagen zur
Prognose und Therapie zu erhalten.

Unsere Befunde wurden in einem lochkartengerechten Erhebungs-
bogen erfaßt und verschlüsselt, wobei neben den Personaldaten insgesamt 50 Merkmale von jedem Patienten erfaßt wurden. Nach einer
gründlichen Zuverlässigkeitsprüfung der Fälle erfolgte die Auswertung
der Daten mit Hilfe der elektronischen Datenverarbeitungsanlage des
Deutschen Krebsforschungszentrums Heidelberg. Nur wenige Auswer-
tungen werden hier beispielhaft vorgelegt*.

---

* Die statistischen Aussagen wurden mit Hilfe des χ^2-Tests bei einer Irrtums-
wahrscheinlichkeit von 5% ($\alpha = 0,05$) geprüft.

Die Chirurgische Universitätsklinik Heidelberg stand 1943–1962 unter Leitung von K. H. BAUER, seit 1962 unter Leitung seines Schülers LINDER.

Vorangestellt sei eine Übersicht über die beobachteten Fälle (Tab. 1):

Die Seltenheit von Brustgeschwülsten beim Manne entspricht der überwiegend dekorativen Funktion und rudimentären Anlage des Brustdrüsengewebes beim männlichen Geschlecht.

Tabelle 1. *Stationär behandelte Patienten mit Tumoren der Brustdrüse* (Chirurgische Universitätsklinik Heidelberg 1943–1964)

Maligne Tumoren der Frau	1762
Benigne Tumoren der Frau	767
Maligne Tumoren des Mannes	25
Benigne Tumoren des Mannes	68
Insgesamt	2622 Fälle

Unter insgesamt 2622 Tumoren der Brustdrüse finden sich *1762 Brustkrebsfälle* der Frau. Das Spätschicksal dieser Fälle wurde in immerhin 91% erhellt. Die überlebenden Patientinnen wurden einer nachgehenden Krebsfürsorge zugeführt. Für diese und einige andere Organkrebse wurden an der Chirurgischen Universitätsklinik Heidelberg in den letzten Jahren spezielle Sprechstunden eingerichtet, welche sich bereits vielfältig bewährt haben.

Die *Altersverteilung* unserer Brustkrebsfälle zeigt einen Häufigkeitsgipfel zwischen dem 45. und 50. Lebensjahr. Dieses scheinbare Prädilektionsalter wird oft in Beziehung zu Besonderheiten des Klimakteriums gesetzt. Tatsächlich zeigen aber die bereinigten Krebssterbeziffern der Bundesrepublik Deutschland, daß es kein derartiges Prädilektionsalter gibt. Die Gefährdung steigt mit dem Alter an. Die Chance, an einem Brustkrebs zu erkranken, ist für die 70jährige höher als für die 50jährige Frau. Die abnehmenden Zahlen der im eigenen Beobachtungsgut erfaßten Fälle sind die Folge der geringeren Bevölkerungszahl in den höheren Altersgruppen; sie sind zudem Folge der selteneren chirurgischen Behandlung älterer Frauen. Beim Brustkrebs findet sich bei unseren Untersuchungen kein statistischer Hinweis für eine ursächliche Bedeutung des Klimakteriums.

Auch in unserem chirurgischen Beobachtungsgut ist, ähnlich einer geringeren Zunahme in der Todesursachenstatistik, ein deutlicher *Anstieg der erstbeobachteten Fälle* zu verzeichnen. Nicht nur die Absolutzahlen der Neuaufnahmen haben zugenommen, auch der prozentuale Anteil an den Gesamtaufnahmen der Klinik ist angestiegen. Bemerkenswert ist dabei, daß trotz der Zunahme der durchschnittlichen Lebenserwartung der Frau sich in den letzten 20 Jahren die Altersverteilung der beobachteten Fälle praktisch nicht verändert hat (Abb. 1).

1905 hat der Stuttgarter Chirurg STEINTHAL seine für die Prognose bedeutungsvolle Einteilung der Brustkrebserkrankungen in verschiedene Stadien mitgeteilt. Über 50 Jahre wurde der Brustkrebs nach dieser Stadieneinteilung klassifiziert. Diese Einteilung wurde inzwischen durch ein Klassifizierungsprinzip abgelöst, das eine detailliertere Befundbeschreibung zuläßt, das sogenannte TNM-System. Hierbei werden die Merkmale des Primärtumors unter T gesondert von den Befunden des regionalen Abflußgebietes unter N und dem Nachweis eventueller Fernmetastasen unter M erfaßt. Dieses von der UICC vorgelegte System hat

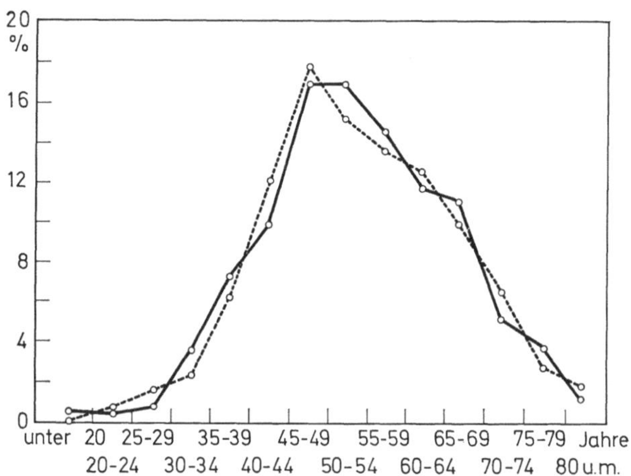

Abb. 1. Prozentuale Altersverteilung der Brustkrebspatientinnen in zwei Jahrzehnten (o----o = 1945–1954, o——o = 1955–1964)

den großen Vorteil, daß es auf andere Organkrebserkrankungen übertragbar ist. Bestimmte Richtlinien für einzelne Organkrebse wurden inzwischen von einer Kommission der UICC ausgearbeitet, weitere sind in Bearbeitung.

Eine so differenzierende Klassifikation läßt für die Erhebung einer einzigen Klinik, auch mit relativ hohen Beobachtungsziffern, nicht für alle Stadien eine ausreichende Fallzahl erwarten. Auch bei unseren Beobachtungen können nur für einzelne, besonders häufige TNM-Stadien gesicherte Aussagen gemacht werden. Erst Sammelerhebungen verschiedener Kliniken werden weitere Ergebnisse ermöglichen.

Bedeutungsvoll ist die Frage, ob im Laufe der letzten zwei Jahrzehnte prognostisch günstigere *Frühstadien* zur chirurgischen Behandlung

kommen. Hier müßte sich eine Bevölkerungsaufklärung, eine statt-
gehabte Vorsorgeuntersuchung, eine bessere ärztliche Betreuung der
Bevölkerung u. a. auswirken. Die Analyse unserer Fälle (Abb. 2) zeigt,
daß hier wahrscheinlich eine Verschiebung stattgefunden hat. Das
T_{1-2} N_0 M_0-Stadium, der gut operable Primärtumor ohne regionale
Metastasen, stellte vor 1954 nur 25% aller beobachteten Patientinnen, in
dem Jahrzehnt danach erhöhten sich diese Fälle auf 35%. Leider verhindert der nicht unerhebliche Anteil der Kranken, in denen die Unterlagen keinerlei Angaben über das Krankheitsstadium enthalten (im
Kollektiv des 1. Nachkriegsdezennium sind es immerhin rund 25%), eine
statistische Absicherung dieser wichtigen Feststellung. Die Dokumentation der Stadien hat sich inzwischen wesentlich gebessert.

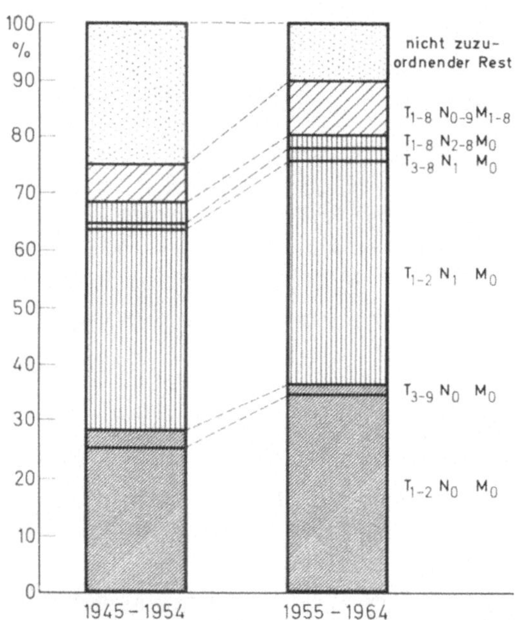

Abb. 2. Vergleich der Stadienverteilung in zwei Jahrzehnten

Will man nicht nur zwei, sondern drei oder mehr Faktoren in ihrer
wechselseitigen Abhängigkeit untersuchen, so ist dies mit den üblichen
konventionellen Methoden, etwa im Strichlistenverfahren, beinahe un-
durchführbar. In solchen Fällen ist eine elektronische Auswertung loch-
kartengerecht dokumentierter Daten weit überlegen. Drei Faktoren
waren beispielsweise im Spiel bei unserer Untersuchung der *Stadienverteilung in verschiedenen Altersgruppen und Beobachtungszeiträumen*
(Abb. 3). Die so gegliederte Analyse zeigt, daß der Anteil der Frauen, die

erst mit bereits feststellbaren Fernmetastasen zur Behandlung kommen, unabhängig vom Lebensalter in beiden Beobachtungszeiträumen mit ca. 8% annähernd konstant geblieben ist. Der Anteil der Früherfassungen scheint dagegen in den letzten 10 Jahren zugenommen zu haben. Für uns

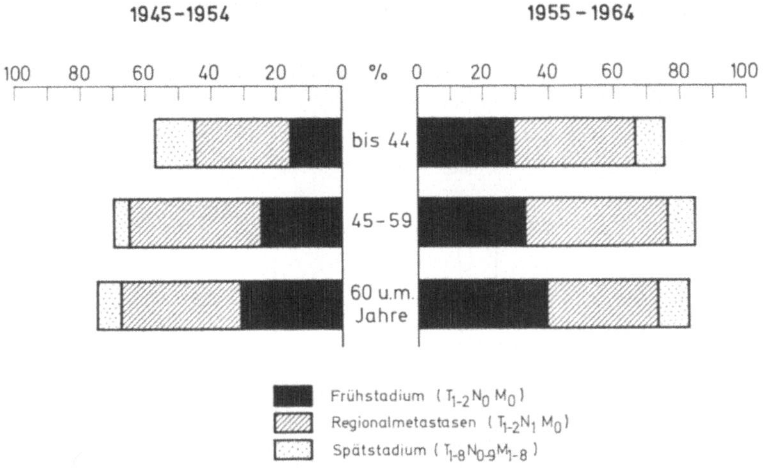

Abb. 3. Stadienverteilung in Abhängigkeit vom Alter in zwei Jahrzehnten

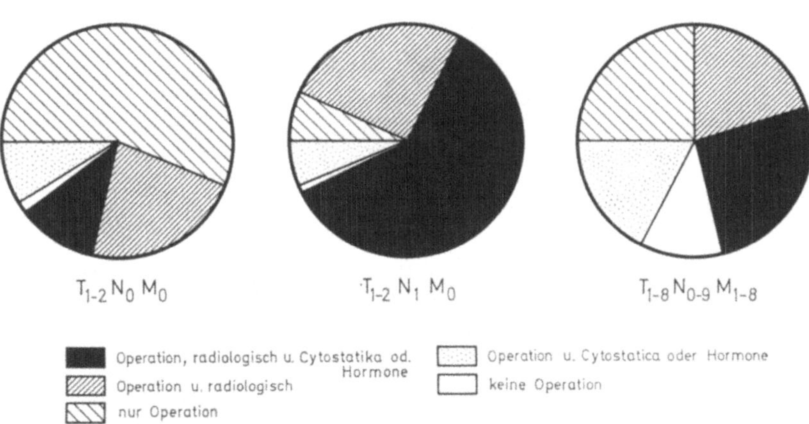

Abb. 4. Therapie und Stadium des Brustkrebses (1943–1964)

unerwarteterweise zeigt sich auch ein gewisser Trend zur früheren Erfassung mit steigendem Lebensalter, was vielleicht dadurch zu erklären ist, daß sich ältere Frauen hinsichtlich des Vorliegens von Krebs-Frühzeichen sorgfältiger beobachten als jüngere, und daß die öfters atrophische Brust leichter eine Früherkennung durch Selbstbeobachtung zuläßt.

Die beiden letzten Aussagen sind allerdings nur Vermutungsaussagen, da sie sich statistisch noch nicht absichern lassen. Immerhin werden sie uns Anlaß sein, hierauf in Zukunft sorgfältiger zu achten als bisher.

Wie wurden die Patientinnen behandelt?

Unabhängig vom Lebensalter wurde ein etwa gleich großer Anteil der Patientinnen nur operiert, operiert und nachbestrahlt bzw. zusätzlich antihormonell behandelt.

Wie Abb. 4 erkennen läßt, richtet sich die *Art des therapeutischen Vorgehens* im wesentlichen nach dem jeweils vorliegenden Tumorstadium. Fälle ohne nachweisbare Metastasen wurden zu über 50% nur operiert; Fälle mit regionalen Metastasen erhielten zu 90% eine Zusatztherapie.

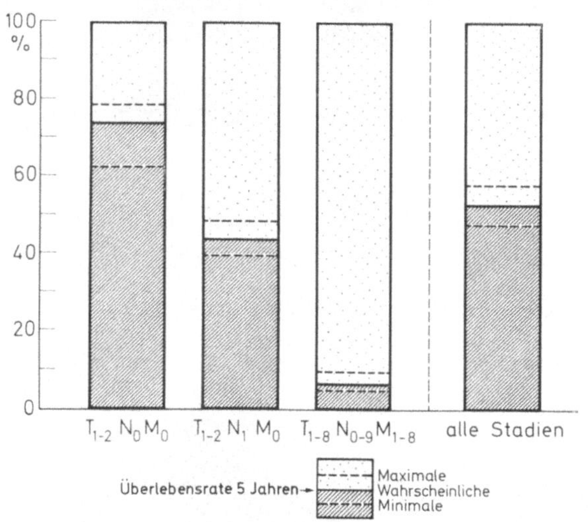

Abb. 5. 5-Jahresüberlebensraten von Brustkrebs in verschiedenen Stadien

Selbstverständlich hat das *Stadium* auch eine entscheidende Bedeutung für die *Prognose* (Abb. 5). So konnten wir bei gut operablen beweglichen Primärtumoren ohne Regionalmetastasen eine wahrscheinliche 5-Jahresüberlebensziffer von immerhin 73,7%, bei Regionalmetastasen von noch 43,4% beobachten. Beim Nachweis von Fernmetastasen aber läßt sich nur noch eine 5-Jahresüberlebensziffer von 5,8% erzielen. Alle Tumorstadien zusammengenommen, erreichten wir bei diesem Organkrebs in den letzten 20 Jahren eine 5-Jahresüberlebensrate von 52,2%. Welcher Fortschritt in nicht einmal 100 Jahren! 1878 teilt v. WINIWARTER, Assistent bei BILLROTH in Wien, in einer der ersten klinischen Krebsstatistiken überhaupt eine 3-Jahresheilziffer beim Brustkrebs von nur 4,7% mit. Zu dieser Zeit galt der Brustkrebs noch als inkurabel. 4,7% waren der erste Hoffnungsschimmer, die lebensrettenden Operationen bei Krebs unter Einhaltung der soeben von Lister erarbeiteten Antisepsis weiter zu entwickeln.

Was erbringt eine *zusätzliche Strahlenbehandlung* beim Mammacarcinom?

Zur ersten Orientierung untersuchten wir das Tumorstadium $T_{1-2} N_1 M_0$, also Fälle mit beweglichem Primärtumor und nachweisbaren, gut beweglichen Achsellymphknoten (Abb. 6). In diesem Stadium wurden unsere Patientinnen überwiegend nachbestrahlt. Bei den nur Operierten betrug die 5-Jahresüberlebensziffer 40,5%, bei den zusätzlich bestrahlten Patientinnen 43,7%. In der Summe der Fälle ist danach

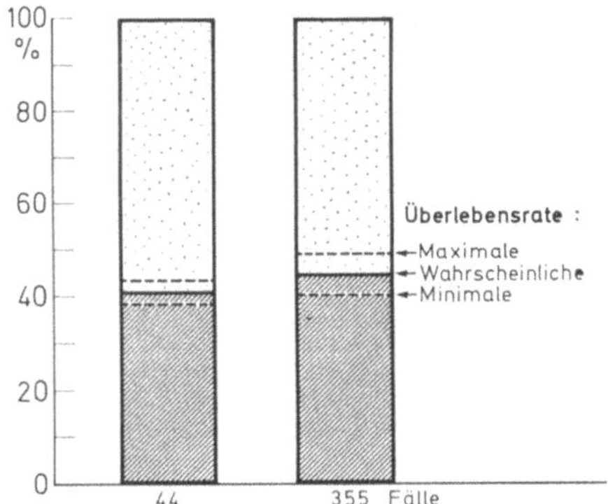

Abb. 6. 5-Jahresüberlebensrate beim Brustkrebs im Stadium $T_{1-2}N_1M_0$ mit und ohne Strahlenbehandlung

durch eine zusätzliche Bestrahlung in diesem Stadium keine wesentliche, statistisch beweisbare Verbesserung der Prognose festzustellen. Damit ist natürlich keine Aussage zu machen über einen eventuellen Effekt der Bestrahlung zur Verhütung rein lokaler Rezidive.

Die *Hypophysenausschaltung* mit Radiogold nach K. H. Bauer beim fortgeschrittenen Mammacarcinom mit Fernmetastasen zeigt in einem beachtlichen Prozentsatz eine palliative Besserung. Dieser weitgehend ungefährliche, in wenigen Minuten durchführbare Eingriff bedeutete daher eine Bereicherung im Behandlungsrüstzeug des Chirurgen. Insbesondere bei osteolytischen Skelettmetastasen finden wir nach dieser Operation oftmals eine Recalcifizierung der befallenen Skelettabschnitte. Bislang ist aber die Frage nicht beantwortet, ob die Hypophysenausschaltung auch einen lebensverlängernden Effekt hat. Von allen verstorbenen Patientinnen haben wir hier nur diejenigen erfaßt, welche vom ersten Tag der Diagnosestellung an in unserer Klinik behandelt wurden (Abb. 7). Es wurden die Absterbekurven dieser Patientinnen

ohne und mit Hypophysenausschaltung verglichen. In beiden Kollekti-
ven war bei der Diagnosestellung die Häufigkeit der einzelnen Stadien
nicht unterschiedlich. Es kann somit ausgeschlossen werden, daß wir in
der Gruppe der Patientinnen mit Hypophysenausschaltung etwa primär
prognostisch ungünstigere Tumorstadien erfaßten.

Insgesamt gesehen bringt die Hypophysenausschaltung zwar eine von
den Patienten dankbar erlebte Minderung der Beschwerden, vorwiegend
bei Skelettmetastasen, jedoch keine Lebensverlängerung.

Unsere Untersuchungen bei dem doch so vielfältig bearbeiteten
Brustkrebs der Frau an Hand einer umfangreichen klinischen Krebsstatistik zeigen, daß eine Vielzahl von standardisierten, international

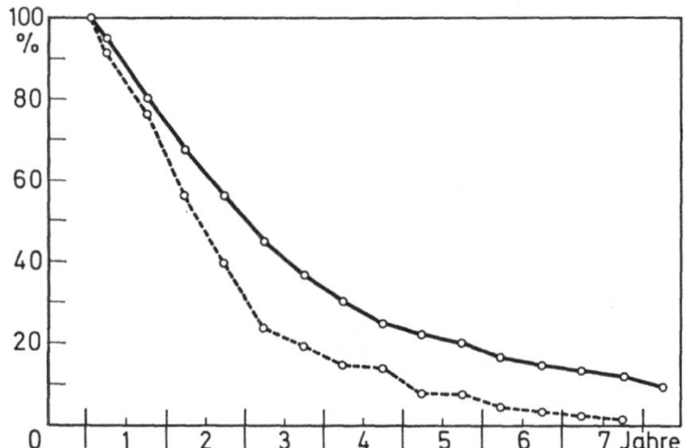

Abb. 7. Absterbekurve von Brustkrebspatientinnen (gerechnet vom Tag der ersten
Diagnosestellung) mit (o-- -o) und ohne (o——o) Hypophysenausschaltung

verbindlichen Klassifizierungsbestimmungen notwendig ist, um zu vergleichbaren Aussagen verschiedener Kliniken zu kommen. Beim Mammacarcinom ist das Stadium nach dem *TNM*-System zu klassifizieren; die
Histologie ist nach dem Vorschlag der UICC aus dem Jahre 1965 zu
erfassen; die Berechnung der Heilziffern muß vergleichbar sein. Die von
der UICC vorgelegten Richtlinien sind beim Mammacarcinom für die
Klinik brauchbar.

Eine Vielfalt von Faktoren sind im Krankheitsablauf von Krebs-
geschwülsten bedeutungsvoll. Therapeutische Maßnahmen sind in jedem
Falle komplexer Natur; sie differieren zudem stets in ihrem zeitlichen
Ablauf. Auch für derartige klinisch-statistische Untersuchungen stellen
die Möglichkeiten einer elektronischen Datenverarbeitung einen un-
schätzbaren Gewinn dar.

Sammelerhebungen zahlreicher Kliniken über lange Zeiträume sind
erforderlich, um verbindlich Zahl und Maß ärztlicher Erfahrungen zur
Richtschnur des zukünftigen therapeutischen Vorgehens zu machen.

C.

3. wissenschaftliche Sitzung am Dienstag, den 26. 9. 1967

Vorsitz: E. Boyland

In Vitro Studies on Cell Transformation
by Oncogenic Viruses

By

I. MacPherson

The basic questions in cancer research are: what causes a cell to become cancerous, and what properties does its progeny possess that distinguishes it from normal cells?

I would like to discuss the advantages of studying the neoplastic process as manifested in the transformation of cells *in vitro* by oncogenic viruses, and describe some of the results from our own work.

We were attracted to this study because it promised to provide a system in which the early events of the neoplastic process were amenable to controlled analysis. As experimental carcinogens, oncogenic viruses have the advantages of rapidity and directness of action. If cloned lines of cells could be prepared and studied in parallel with their transformed derivatives, meaningful comparisons could be made to reveal changes in cell function that are associated with virus-induced transformation. Transformed cells can be recognized and studied within a few generations of their inception and before the progression of secondary changes obscure the characteristics of the primary event.

Before embarking on such studies it is necessary to be satisfied that virus-induced transformation is a valid indicator of the neoplastic change. We know that only oncogenic viruses produce transformations *in vitro* and that cultures of tumour cells induced *in vivo* by a particular virus closely resemble the transformed cells it induces *in vitro*. However, some cells are very weakly tumourigenic shortly after they are transformed [1] and only become highly tumourigenic after they have been passaged for some time in culture. Although transformed cells eventually become neoplastic it is not possible to ensure that this characteristic is always immediately associated with the morphological changes we call transformation.

The ideal system for the study of virus transformation *in vitro* would be one in which a combination of genetically pure stocks of cells and virus resulted in the rapid transformation of all cells.

This ideal has not been achieved in any system so far. For various reasons all available systems fall short in one way or another.

Our earliest experiments with polyoma were made with new-born hamster kidney cell cultures. Even when these cells were infected with large amounts of virus the proportion of cells giving rise to colonies with transformed morphology was very low ($< 0.1\%$) [12]. The important question of whether this low rate of transformation was due to a small proportion of the cells being genetically competent or to some other factor could not be answered with these cells, since their cloning efficiency was extremely low, and they have a growth potential of only a few generations. The latter property would not have permitted the accumulation of sufficient cells with which to carry out the experiments required to settle this point.

Table 1. *Characteristics of BHK 21 cells compared to those of BHK 21 cells transformed by polyoma virus*

Character	BHK 21 cells	Polyoma transformed cells
1. Loss of contact inhibition of movement	—	+
2. Mean generation time *in vitro* [6]	12 hr.	12 hr.
3. Karyotype [6]	44	44 unstable
4. Growth in agar suspension [9]	—	+
5. Relative glycolytic capacity [11]	1	2
6. Increased negative charge [3, 4]	—	+ or —
7. Polyoma specific antigens	—	+
8. Relative transplantability	1	10,000

An important advance in our work was the development of a line of hamster fibroblasts which had spontaneously acquired a high degree of autonomy *in vitro*. This line, called BHK 21, has a rapid growth rate in vitro and can be cloned by micromanipulation. When the polyoma-induced transformation rates of several clones were estimated it was found that they all had approximately the same low value similar to that obtained with the uncloned parent strain [10]. This result showed that genetic heterogeneity in the cells was not responsible for the low rate of transformation.

Since the BHK 21 cells could be readily cloned it was possible to transform a cloned stock and study the changes that were associated with this transformation.

These studies have shown that morphological transformation, as detected by piled up growth of the cells was associated with a number of other properties. These are summarized in Table 1.

The method of plating infected BHK 21 cells and examining the proportion of cells forming transformed colonies has certain limitations.

Since the BHK 21 cells grow as well as the transformed cells there is no selection for the transformed colonies and in experiments in which a low rate of transformation is expected a large number of platings have to be made to obtain an accurate result. The discovery that polyoma-transformed BHK 21 cells can form colonies when freely suspended in soft agar medium has formed the basis of a selective assay [9]. Since small transformed cell colonies of up to 10 cells appear in the agar within 48 hrs. of seeding infected cells it seems that the ability to grow without being in contact with a solid surface is rapidly acquired by a transformed cell.

The agar suspension assay has enabled us to make accurate measurements of the dose response curve of BHK 21 cells to polyoma-induced transformation. The dose response curve had one hit characteristics up to the point where the cells were infected with 10^4 plaque forming units of virus per cell. At higher virus doses no further increase in the transformation rate was obtained and a maximum of 4–5% of the infected cells plated formed colonies. This result has been obtained several times but so far no satisfactory explanation has been found for this effect.

The clear difference between BHK 21 cells and their transformed derivatives with respect to their growth in agar, and the rapidity with which this new property was acquired, prompted an investigation into the possibility that other oncogenic viruses may be able to transform cells in this way.

It was found that both the Schmidt-Ruppin (SR-RSV) [7] and the Bryan (B-RSV) [8] strains of Rous sarcoma virus were able to induce BHK 21 cells to form colonies in agar suspension culture. The transformation rates were very low ($< 0.1\%$) with the virus stocks available. Unlike the colonies induced by polyoma virus, which are smooth, spherical and compact, the colonies induced by the RSV strains diffused into the agar and the individual cells were discernable. When cultured on glass substrates it was of interest to find that the SR-RSV and B-RSV transformed cells resemble chick-embryo fibroblasts transformed by the same virus strains. In the case of SR-RSV these are loose randomly growing networks whereas the B-RSV cells are heaped up epithelioid or round cells.

An unexpected finding in the work with SR-RSV-transformed cells was the discovery that colonies of normal morphology arose in cultures of transformed cells, suggesting a reversion of the transformed phenotype. To prove that these "revertants" were derived from the transformed cells, single transformed cells were isolated by micromanipulation, grown up and plated to produce discrete colonies. Again colonies of cells with well marked parallel orientation were found among the transformed colonies. Revertant clones were isolated and compared in parallel with clones of transformed cells. The results are shown in Table 2. It will be seen that the revertant cells seem to have lost the virus genome or at least it has become undetectable in these cells. The fact that it is possible to re-transform the revertant cells suggests that the virus genome is not simply repressed. Since reversion proceeds at a rapid rate in some transformed clones it may be that the virus genome is lost from the cells by simple dilution from the cytoplasm. The combination of a poorly replicating virus genome with a rapidly growing cell may make this possible. Certainly reversion has not been found in B-RSV transformed cells and the Bryan strain of RSV is more efficient at replicating itself in chicken cells than SR-RSV.

Attempts to transform the BHK 21 cells with the oncogenic viruses simian virus 40 and adenovirus 12 have been unsuccessful. We have however made use of another hamster cell line with properties very similar to those of BHK 21. This line is called NIL 2 and was derived

Table 2. *Loss of SR-RSV induced characteristics in revertant cells derived from SR-RSV transformed BHK 21*

Character	Transformed Cells	Revertant Cells
1. Growth in soft agar medium	+	—
2. Growth on glass	Random	Parallel orientation
3. Induction of RSV in chick embryo fibroblasts	+	—
4. Production of virus releasing tumours in chickens	+	—
5. Avian leukosis group specific antigen	+	—

from hamster embryo cells by DIAMOND [2]. Clones of these cells have been transformed by polyoma, SR-RSV and adenovirus type 12 [5].

Adenovirus type 12 even at very high multiplicities only produces a very low rate of transformation in agar suspension. When grown on glass the agar colony cells grow in tightly packed clumps of rounded or epithelial cells quite unlike the cells transformed by the other oncogenic viruses described here.

With clones of BHK 21 cells transformed by polyoma and two strains of RSV, and also clones of NIL 2 cells transformed by polyoma, RSV and adenovirus type 12, we are continuing comparative studies in the search for common characteristics possessed by all these different trans-formed cells. Common characteristics are likely to be those with the greatest relevance with respect to their behaviour as transformed cells. These in turn are likely to be of importance in determining the cells' neoplastic potential.

The nature of the primary change in virus-induced transformations is obscure. The fact that reversion in SR-RSV transformed cells is associated with cessation of virus gene function suggests that these functions are required to maintain the transformed condition. There is also evidence from a number of sources that at least some of the genes of small oncogenic DNA viruses persist in the cells they transform. If their presence can be shown to be required for the maintenance of the transformed condition in a cell then the task of identifying the required virus function(s) seems feasible in viruses such as polyoma and SV40 which only have enough DNA to code for about 10 proteins. If all the virus gene functions can be identified it should then be possible to discover which activities are required to produce transformation *in vitro* and consequently suggest how the neoplastic change is imposed on a cell.

References

1. DEFENDI, V. and J. M. LEHMAN: Transformation of hamster embryo cells *in vitro* by polyoma virus. J. cell. comp. Physiol. **66**, 351 (1965).
2. DIAMOND, L.: Two spontaneously transformed cell lines derived from the same hamster embryo culture. Int. J. Cancer **2**, 143 (1967).
3. FORRESTER, J. A., E. J. AMBROSE, and I. A. MACPHERSON: Electrophoretic investigations of a clone of hamster fibroblasts and polyoma-transformed cells from the same population. Nature (Lond.) **196**, 1068 (1962).
4. — — and M. G. P. STOKER: Microelectrophoresis of normal and transformed clones of hamster kidney fibroblasts. Nature (Lond.) **201**, 945 (1964).
5. MCALLISTER, R. M. and I. MACPHERSON: Transformation of a hamster cell line by Adenovirus type 12. J. gen. Virol. **2**, 99 (1968).
6. MACPHERSON, I.: Characteristics of a hamster cell clone transformed by polyoma virus. J. nat. Cancer Inst. **30**, 795 (1963).
7. — Reversion in hamster cells transformed by Rous sarcoma virus. Science **148**, 1731 (1965).
8. — Malignant transformation and reversion in virus infected cells. Recent Results in Cancer Research, Vol. VI, p. 1. Berlin, Heidelberg, New York: Springer 1966.
9. — and L. MONTAGNIER: Agar suspension culture for the selective assay of cells transformed by polyoma virus. Virology **23**, 291 (1964).
10. — and M. STOKER: Polyoma transformation of hamster cell clones — an investigation of genetic factors affecting cell competence. Virology **16**, 147 (1962).
11. PAUL, J., M. M. BROADFOOT, and P. WALKER: Increased glycolytic capacity and associated enzyme changes in BHK 21 cells transformed with polyoma virus. Int. J. Cancer **1**, 207 (1966).
12. STOKER, M. and I. MACPHERSON: Studies on transformation of hamster cells by polyoma virus in vitro. Virology **14**, 359 (1961).

Viruswirtszellbeziehungen bei Infektionen mit dem tumorerzeugenden Virus SV40

Von

K. MUNK, W. BRÜMMER und H. FISCHER

Bei Infektionen mit tumorerzeugenden Virusarten beeinflußt die Wirtszelle die Auseinandersetzung zwischen Virusinfektion und Zellprozessen. Alle an diesen Wechselwirkungen beteiligten Vorgänge spielen sich auf molekularbiologischer Ebene ab, denn es handelt sich um ein Wechselspiel zwischen Syntheseprozessen, die einerseits vom Virus, andererseits von der Zelle induziert werden. Wir beschäftigen uns in unseren Experimenten mit den Fragen, welche Prozesse in der Wirtszelle die vom Virusgenom induzierten Vorgänge bei der Infektion mit dem DNS-haltigen onkogenen Virus SV40 beeinflussen können.

Es ist zu erwarten, daß eine große Zahl von Faktoren an diesem Geschehen beteiligt ist. Unser Ziel war es, zumindest einen Faktor durch unsere Experimente aufspüren zu können.

Wir gingen bei unseren Versuchen von der Überlegung aus, daß die hier in Frage kommenden Vorgänge auf einer Wechselwirkung zwischen den Funktionen des Zellgenoms und denen des Virusgenoms beruhen müssen. Nach früheren Untersuchungen [9] über die DNS-Synthese in SV40 infizierten Cercopithecus-Affennierenzellen beobachteten wir diese Wechselbeziehungen an dem Auftreten virusspezifischer Antigene in den infizierten Zellen [4, 7]. Wir untersuchten diese Prozesse in Zellen einmal während der exponentiell wachsenden, zum anderen während der stationären Phase. Außerdem wählten wir zur Analyse der Vorgänge das Actinomycin D als Inhibitor der DNS-abhängigen RNS-Synthese und untersuchten die Vorgänge vor allem während der ersten Stunden des SV40 Vermehrungscyclus. Zur Bestimmung der in den Zellen entstehenden virusspezifischen Antigene als Ausdruck der virusinduzierten Funktionen wendeten wir die Methode der Immunofluoreszenz an. Wir verfolgten in den infizierten Zellen einmal unter Verwendung von Affenrekonvaleszentenserum das Auftreten eines Antigens, das den Proteinanteilen des Virions, dem sogenannten Virushüllprotein-Antigen (V-Antigen), entspricht. Das Entstehen dieses Antigens ist nur in virusproduzierenden Zellen zu beobachten. Zum anderen untersuchten wir die infizierten Zellen auch mit Hilfe eines virusspezifischen Antiserums, das gegen ein Antigen gerichtet ist, das vom Virusgenom in der Zelle induziert wird, das aber nicht mit dem Virushüllprotein selbst identisch ist. Dieses Virusantigen kann in Zellen beobachtet werden, in denen eine Virusvermehrung stattfindet. Es wird aber auch in allen Zellen gefunden, die von diesem Virus zu Tumorzellen transformiert worden sind. Seine Entstehung ist in einer noch nicht bekannten Weise mit der Zelltransformation verbunden. Der Virologe bezeichnet dieses Antigen als Tumorantigen (T-Antigen).

Zur Auswertung und Beurteilung unserer Ergebnisse war es zunächst notwendig, die besonderen Eigenschaften des Cercopithecus-Zellsystems, an dem wir unsere Untersuchungen vorgenommen hatten, genau zu bestimmen.

Untersuchungen zur Definition der exponentiellen und stationären Zellkulturen

Eine Zellkultur wird als weitgehend stationär betrachtet, wenn ihr Zellrasen unter dem Mikroskop konfluent, d. h. geschlossen erscheint. Eine derartige Zellkultur, in der die Zellen einem Wachstumsregulationsfaktor, der Kontaktinhibition, unterliegen, sollte eine konstante, stark reduzierte DNS-Syntheserate in den Zellen aufweisen.

Die Tab. 1 zeigt den Verlauf der Nucleinsäuresynthese in primären Cercopithecuszellen während eines Zeitraumes von 25 Tagen.

Nach dem Anlegen der Zellkulturen wurde das Nährmedium vom 3. Tag an täglich gewechselt. Vom 5. Tag an wurden die Zellkulturen, beginnend mit der 3. Std nach dem Mediumwechsel 60 min lang mit 0,5 μC/ml ³H-Thymidin und ³H-Uridin markiert. Am Ende des Radionuclidpulses wurden die Zellen geerntet und in 3 ml 0,02 M KPO$_4$-Puffer, pH 7,2 suspendiert. Die Ermittlung der spezifischen Radioaktivität der Nucleinsäuren erfolgte in aliquoten Probeanteilen. Hierzu wurde die Nucleinsäure in Gegenwart von Trägerprotein mit Trichloressigsäure gefällt. Der Niederschlag wurde auf Glasfaserplättchen gesammelt, gewaschen, getrocknet, in Probengläschen mit Scintillations-Flüssigkeit überschichtet und im Tricarb-Scintillationsspektrometer ausgezählt. Die DNS wurde nach der Methode von BURTON-DISCHE [1], die RNS nach der abgewandelten Methode von SCHMITT-TANNHAUSER [3] bestimmt.

Das Ergebnis dieser Untersuchung zeigte, daß die Nucleinsäure-Syntheserate vom 16. Tag an nach dem Anlegen der Zellkulturen konstant blieb (Tab. 1). Bemerkenswert war jedoch, daß der Zellrasen dagegen schon vom 8. Tag an mikroskopisch geschlossen erschien. Das weist auf die Diskrepanz in der Beurteilung des stationären Zustandes einer Zellkultur zwischen dem mikroskopischen Befund und zwischen den viel exakteren biochemischen Werten der Nucleinsäure-Syntheseraten hin. Deshalb bezeichnen wir Zellkulturen 5 Tage nach der Aussaat als exponentiell wachsend. Für die Experimente, die wir an den als stationär definierten Zellkulturen durchführten, verwendeten wir Kulturen vom 16. Tag nach der Aussaat ab.

Tabelle 1. *Übergang einer exponentiellen Cercopithecus-Nierenzellkultur in den stationären Zustand. DNS- und RNS-Synthese-Aktivität nach Aussaat der Zellen*

Tage nach Aussaat	^{3}H-Thymidin Aufnahme cpm/10 μg DNS	DNS-Synthese-Aktivität %	^{3}H-Uridin Aufnahme cpm/10 μg RNS	RNS-Synthese-Aktivität %
5	2400	100	2940	100
8	1700	71	2230	76
10	—	—	1840	63
11	1200	50	1690	58
13	900	38	1400	48
14	—	—	1260	43
17	—	—	1050	36
18	360	15	—	—
20	280	12	1000	34
22	240	10	990	34
25	220	9	980	33

Bestimmung der Actinomycin D-Wirkung auf Cercopithecuszellen

Zur Beurteilung unserer Ergebnisse war es weiterhin notwendig, die Wirkung der geeigneten Konzentration und Einwirkungsdauer des Actinomycins auf die Cercopithecuszellen zu bestimmen. Die Verträglichkeit von Actinomycin ist bei verschiedenen Zellarten unterschiedlich [8, 11]. Unter dauernder Einwirkung von 1,0 μg/ml Actinomycin zeigen primäre Mäuse-Fibroblasten noch 48 Std lang ein normales Zellverhalten, während HeLa-Zellen bei gleicher Actinomycinkonzentration bereits nach 8 Std eine deutliche Zellschädigung zeigen. Primäre Hühnerembryozellen und KB-Zellen sind bei gleicher Actinomycineinwirkung schon nach 4 Std cytotoxisch verändert.

Wir bestimmten daher in unserem Zellsystem die erforderliche Konzentration und Einwirkungsdauer des Actinomycins, die einen ausreichenden Effekt erzielt und die vor allem wieder reversibel ist, d. h. die Zelle nicht schädigt. Hierzu wurde der Effekt sowohl verschiedener Actinomycinkonzentrationen im Nährmedium als auch unterschiedlicher Einwirkungsdauer an dem Ausmaß der ^{3}H-Uridinaufnahme, d. h. an der RNS-Syntheseaktivität, gemessen. Die Tab. 2 gibt den Prozentsatz der RNS-Synthese, gemessen am Einbau von ^{3}H-Uridin nach 30 und

60 min Einwirkung verschiedener Actinomycinkonzentrationen auf die Cercopithecus-Affennierenzellen an. Bei diesen Untersuchungen wurden die Zellkulturen am Ende der entsprechenden Actinomycinbehandlung einmal mit Hanksscher Lösung gewaschen und in neues vorgewärmtes Nährmedium übertragen. 30 min nach diesem Mediumwechsel wurde für 30 min ein ^{3}H-Uridinpuls (0,5 μC/ml) gegeben. Die Zellen wurden unmittelbar danach aufgearbeitet und die spezifische Radioaktivität in der säureunlöslichen Fraktion der Zell-RNS ermittelt.

Tabelle 2. *Wirkung verschiedener Konzentration und Einwirkungsdauer von Actinomycin D auf Cercopithecus-Nierenzellkulturen, gemessen an der Hemmung der RNS-Synthese*

Actinomycin D (μg/ml)	% RNS-Synthese	
	30 min Actinomycin-Einwirkung	60 min Actinomycin-Einwirkung
0	100	100
0,2	42	23
0,5	21	13
1,0	12	9

Tabelle 3. *RNS-Synthese in exponentiellen Cercopithecus-Affennierenzellen nach 30 min Actinomycin D-Behandlung (0,5 μg/ml)*

Stunden nach Beginn der Actinomycin-behandlung	Tritium-Uridin Aufnahme cpm/10 μg RNS	RNS-Synthese Aktivität %
unbehandelte Kontrolle	750	100
1,25	240	32
3	270	36
5	730	97
7	750	100
9	750	100
15	750	100

Das Ergebnis zeigte, daß eine 30-minütige Einwirkung von 0,5 μg/ml Actinomycin die RNS-Synthese bis auf 20% der Kontrolle herabsetzt (Tab. 3). Eine Erhöhung der Actinomycinkonzentration oder eine Verlängerung der Einwirkungsdauer ergab eine nur geringe Steigerung der RNS-Synthesehemmung.

Zum Beweis der Reversibilität des Effektes bestimmten wir Zeitpunkt und Umfang des Wiederbeginns der inhibierten RNS-Synthese in den behandelten Zellen. Wie aus der Tab. 3 zu erkennen ist, begann nach einer 30-minütigen Einwirkung von 0,5 μg/ml Actinomycin in den Cercopithecuszellen nach 5–6 Std eine erneute RNS-Synthese (gemessen an der ^{3}H-Uridinaufnahme).

Diese Ergebnisse zeigen, daß eine niedrige und kurzzeitige Actinomycineinwirkung auf primäre Cercopithecus-Nierenzellen reversibel ist. Das gleiche Phänomen hatten wir früher bei HeLa-Zellen beobachtet [10]. Für unsere Experimente bedeutete das weiterhin, daß eine RNS-Synthese in der SV40-infizierten Zelle, die $2^1/_2$–3 Std p.i. mit Actinomycin behandelt wurde, zu dem Zeitpunkt wieder aktiv ist, wenn die viralen Transcriptionsvorgänge zu erwarten sind.

Die Actinomycin-D-Wirkung auf die T- und V-Antigen-Synthese

In unseren Experimenten, in denen wir das Auftreten virusspezifischer Antigene in den Zellen infizierter Cercopithecus-Nierenzellkulturen verfolgten, wählten wir eine niedrige Infektionsdosis und hielten die Kulturen nach 2-stündiger Adsorptionszeit unter ständiger Gegenwart von SV40 Antiserum, um sekundäre Infektionen zu verhindern. Unter dieser Bedingung wird nicht in allen Zellen der Kultur Virusantigen synthetisiert. Die Zahl V- und T-Antigen produzierender Zellen diente als Parameter. Sie wurde in allen Versuchsansätzen 50 Std p.i. ermittelt. Vorversuche hatten ergeben, daß sich die Zahl antigenproduzierender Zellen unter den gegebenen Versuchsbedingungen später als 50 Std p.i. nicht mehr erhöht.

Wir bestimmten in parallelen Versuchsansätzen fluoreszenzimmunologisch den Prozentsatz der antigenproduzierenden Zellen 50 Std p.i.:

1. in exponentiellen Zellkulturen,

2. in exponentiellen Zellkulturen, die $2^1/_2$–3 Std p.i. für einen Zeitraum von 30 min Actinomycin in einer Konzentration von 0,5 μg/ml erhalten hatten,

3. in stationären Zellkulturen,

4. in stationären Zellkulturen, die in gleicher Weise wie die exponentiellen Zellkulturen für 30 min $2^1/_2$–3 Std p.i. mit Actinomycin behandelt worden waren.

Diese Versuche zeigten, daß in den parallelen Versuchsansätzen die Zahl der fluoreszierenden, V- und T-Antigen produzierenden Zellen zu den verschiedenen Zeitpunkten p.i. bei den stationären Zellkulturen stets höher war als bei den exponentiellen Zellkulturen. Außerdem hatte eine 30-minütige Actinomycineinwirkung, welche $2^1/_2$–3 Std p.i. erfolgte, eine Zunahme der Zahl antigenproduzierender Zellen sowohl bei den exponentiellen als auch bei den stationären Zellkulturen zur Folge (Tab. 4).

Tabelle 4. *Wirkung von Actinomycin D in der frühen Phase der SV40-Vermehrung (0,5 µg/ml, 2¹/₂ Std p.i.) auf die Synthese von V- und T-Antigen in Cercopithecus-Affennierenzellkulturen*

| Cercopithecus Zellkultur | Std p.i. | Prozent antigenproduzierender, fluorescierender Zellen | | | |
| | | V-Antigen | | T-Antigen | |
		ohne Actinomycin-einwirkung	mit Actinomycin-einwirkung	ohne Actinomycin-einwirkung	mit Actinomycin-einwirkung
im	15	0	0	0	0
exponentiellen	20	0	0	0,4	1,7
Stadium	25	1,0	1,2	5,0	5,6
	40	9,2	14,8	10,8	21,4
	50	9,8	15,5	16,4	23,2
im stationären	15	0	0	0	0
Stadium	20	0	0	8,0	21,0
	25	9,9	17,4	15,4	41,2
	40	33,5	46,0	31,0	63,6
	50	38,7	59,3	44,7	73,3

Diskussion

Aus diesen Ergebnissen sollte die Frage beantwortet werden, ob die Wirtszelle Funktionen des Virusgenoms beeinflussen kann. Deshalb wurde die DNS- und RNS-Synthese in SV40-infizierten Cercopithecus-Affennierenzellkulturen im exponentiellen und im stationären Zustand mit Actinomycin D inhibiert. Vergleichende Untersuchungen über die SV40-Vermehrung in exponentiellen und stationären Zellkulturen haben CARP und GILDEN [2] durchgeführt. Allerdings wurden dort die Zellkulturen als „stationär" bezeichnet, wenn sie mikroskopisch „konfluent, kontakt-inhibiert" erschienen. Aus unseren Untersuchungen, bei denen wir den stationären Zustand einer Zellkultur nach dem Ausmaß der DNS- und RNS-Syntheserate definierten, zeigte es sich, daß die bisher angewandten Kriterien keineswegs befriedigend sind; denn die Nucleinsäuresynthese-rate beginnt erst vom 16. Tag an nach Aussaat der Kultur konstant niedrig zu werden, während der Zellrasen schon vom 8. Tag nach der Aussaat an mikroskopisch geschlossen erscheint. Wir führten also unsere Experimente einmal mit aktiv sich teilenden, logarithmisch wachsenden Zellkulturen durch, zum anderen in dem kontaktinhibierten Stadium, in welchem die Nucleinsäuresyntheserate einen konstant niedrigen Wert er-reicht hatte.

Die unter diesen Voraussetzungen gewonnenen Ergebnisse lassen erkennen, daß sich genetische Funktionen des Virus wirksamer in stationären Kulturen ausdrücken können als in Zellkulturen, die sich im exponentiellen Wachstumsstadium befinden. Das heißt, wir fanden in stationären Zellkulturen in einem größeren Umfange virusantigen-produzierende Zellen als in exponentiell wachsenden Zellkulturen. Das gleiche Ergebnis fanden wir auch in Zellkulturen, die in der frühen Phase nach der Infektion, d. h. $2^1/_2$–3 Std p.i., mit Actinomycin D behandelt worden waren. Für die Actinomycinbehandlung wurde eine Konzentration und Einwirkungsdauer gewählt, die sich nach Vorversuchen zum einen als wirksam, zum anderen als reversibel erwiesen hatte. Die Zunahme der antigenproduzierenden Zellen nach Actinomycineinwirkung wurde sowohl in exponentiellen als auch in stationären Zellkulturen beobachtet.

Virusspezifische Veränderungen, wie das Auftreten von T-Antigen, sind zu dieser frühen Zeit noch nicht nachzuweisen (KIT u. Mitarb. [5, 6]). Es wird also vermutlich durch das Actinomycin D in diesem frühen Stadium vorwiegend die Zell-DNS-abhängige RNS-Synthese gehemmt.

Die Zunahme der Zahl virusantigenproduzierender Zellen in den Kulturen nach Actinomycinbehandlung weist auf einen wichtigen Befund hin. Es gibt in SV40-infizierten Cercopithecus-Affennierenzellkulturen, die mit einer geringen Multiplizität beimpft worden waren, Zellen, in denen virusgenetische Funktionen nur zum Ausdruck kommen können, wenn die zellulären Transcriptionsvorgänge kurz nach dem Eindringen des Virus in die Zelle durch Actinomycin D inhibiert werden. Der Mechanismus dieser Vorgänge könnte in einer Konkurrenz der zellulären RNS mit der viralen RNS um die in der Zelle vorhandenen Ribosomen zu sehen sein. Mit dieser Konkurrenzreaktion glauben wir zumindest einen Faktor aufgespürt zu haben, mit dem die Wirtszelle die Vorgänge nach der Infektion mit dem onkogenen Virus SV 40 beeinflussen kann.

Die experimentellen Arbeiten wurden mit dankenswerter Unterstützung der Deutschen Forschungsgemeinschaft und des Vereins zur Förderung der Krebsforschung in Deutschland e. V. durchgeführt.

Literatur

1. BURTON, K.: A Study of the Conditions and Mechanism of the Diphenylamine Reaction for the Colorimetric Estimation of Deoxyribonucleic Acid. Biochem. J. **62**, 315 (1956).
2. CARP, R. I. and R. V. GILDEN: A Comparison of the Replication Cycles of Simian Virus 40 in Human Diploid and African Green Monkey Kidney Cells. Virology **28**, 150 (1966).
3. FLECK, A. and D. BEGG: The Estimation of Ribonucleic Acid using Ultraviolett Absorption Measurement. Biochim. biophys. Acta (Amst.) **108**, 333 (1965).
4. FISCHER, H., A. DANN, and K. MUNK: Effect of Actinomycin D on the Synthesis of Viral Antigen in Cercopithecus Kidney Cells infected with SV 40. J. gen. Virology **1**, 253 (1967).
5. KIT, S., D. R. DUBBS, P. M. FREARSON, and J. L. MELNICK: Enzyme Induction in SV 40-infected Green Monkey Kidney Cultures. Virology **29**, 69 (1966).

6. KIT, S., D. R. DUPPS, L. J. PIEKARSKI, R. A. DE TORRES, and J. L. MELNICK: Acquisition of Enzyme Function by Mouse Kidney Cells Abortively infected with Papovavirus SV 40. Proc. nat. Acad. Sci. (Wash.) **56**, 463 (1966).
7. MUNK, K. and H. FISCHER: Early Cell-Virus Interactions in Cercopithecus Cells infected with SV 40. In: Subviral Carcinogenesis Monograph of the 1st International Symposium on Tumor Viruses, p. 176 (1967).
8. REICH, E. and J. H. GOLDBERG: Actinomycin and Nucleic Acid Function. In: Davidson J. N. and Waldo E. Cohn (Ed.): Progress in Nucleic Acid Research and Molecular Biology, Vol. 3 p. 183–234. New York and London: Academic Press 1964.
9. SAUER, G., H. FISCHER, and K. MUNK: The Effect of SV40 Infection on DNA Synthesis in Cercopithecus Kidney Cells. Virology **28**, 765 (1966).
10. —, H. D. ORTH, and K. MUNK: Interference of Actinomycin D with the Replication of the Herpes Virus DNA. Biochim. biophys. Acta **119**, 331 (1966).
11. WONG, K. T., S. BARON, H. B. LEVY, and TH. G. WARD: Dactinomycin: Relative Resistance of Green Monkey Kidney Cell Cultures to its Action. Proc. Soc. exper. Biol. (N.Y.) **125**, 65 (1967).

Fluororganische Verbindungen
und ihre Bedeutung für die Krebsforschung

Von

M. SCHLOSSER

Körpereigene Verbindungen werden durch Fluorierung sterisch minimal, chemisch-biologisch jedoch grundlegend verändert. Der Organismus läßt sich durch die sterische Ähnlichkeit täuschen und akzeptiert das Fluor-Analogon, wodurch dieses als Antimetabolit in die Lebensvorgänge eingreifen kann. Bekannt ist die außerordentliche Giftigkeit der Fluoressigsäure, die an Stelle der Essigsäure in den Fettsäure-Cyclus eintritt und diesen blockiert. Nach dem Prinzip ,,Antimetabolit-Bildung durch Fluorierung" wurde 1957 von HEIDELBERGER [5] und Chemikern der amerikanischen Hoffmann-La Roche-Werke das 5-Fluoruracil entwickelt, das als verhältnismäßig selektiver Tumorinhibitor Eingang in die Chemotherapie des Krebses gefunden hat. Das 5-Fluoruracil besetzt in der Zelle dem Uracil zustehende Plätze am RNS-Strang, unterbindet die Synthese des Thymins und damit letztlich die Weiterteilung des Zellkerns.

Sicherlich ist es nach dem Erfolg des 5-Fluor-uracils sinnvoll, nicht nur weitere Pyrimidine, sondern auch Purine, Fettsäuren, Aminosäuren, Sterine und andere Stoffwechselprodukte selektiv zu fluorieren und hinsichtlich ihrer Wirkung auf das Zellwachstum zu prüfen. Für den Chemiker stellt sich hier die Frage: Gibt es genügend leistungsfähige Verfahren, um Fluor gezielt in ein Molekül einzuführen? Bis vor kurzem kannte man kein einziges zuverlässiges und allgemeingültiges Verfahren, um ein einzelnes Fluoratom an einen gesättigten Kohlenstoff zu binden. Die altbewährte Praxis, Chlor, Brom oder Jod durch Einwirkung eines entsprechenden anorganischen Säurehalogenids auf einen Alkohol einzuführen, ließ sich im Bereich der Fluor-Chemie nicht so einfach wiederholen. Erst in der zweiten Hälfte der 50er Jahre wurden Methoden entwickelt, um Alkohole in Alkylfluoride zu überführen. Den Anfang machte eine indirekte Methode: man verwandelte zuerst den Alkohol in einen Sulfonsäureester, speziell den p-Toluolsulfonsäureester, und verdrängte dann mit Kaliumfluorid in siedendem Äthylenglycol den Tosylat-Rest durch Fluor [2]. Dieses inzwischen schon klassischen

Verfahrens bedienten sich kürzlich LETTRÉ u. WOELCKE im Zuge einer eleganten Synthese des racemischen $\omega.\omega'$-Difluor-valins [10]. Dabei wurde 2-Allyl-propandiol(1.3) tosyliert und mit Kaliumfluorid in 74%iger Ausbeute in das 2-Allyl-1.3-difluor-propan übergeführt. Entsprechend der skizzierten Reaktionsfolge (Schema 1) schlossen sich als weitere Schritte die Ozon-Oxidation zur Carbonsäure an, die Bromierung des zugehörigen Säurebromids und die Substitution des α-ständigen Broms durch die Aminogruppe. Ganz analog gelang es, $\omega.\omega'$-Difluor-leucin darzustellen [10].

$$
\begin{array}{c}
\text{ROOC} \\
\quad\quad \text{CH}_2 \\
\text{ROOC}
\end{array}
\rightarrow
\begin{array}{c}
\text{ROOC} \\
\quad\quad \text{CH–CH}_2\text{–CH=CH}_2 \\
\text{ROOC}
\end{array}
\rightarrow
\begin{array}{c}
\text{HOCH}_2 \\
\quad\quad \text{CH–CH}_2\text{–CH=CH}_2 \\
\text{HOCH}_2
\end{array}
$$

$$
\begin{array}{c}
\text{F–CH}_2 \\
\quad\quad \text{CH–CH}_2\text{–COOH} \\
\text{F–CH}_2
\end{array}
\leftarrow
\begin{array}{c}
\text{FCH}_2 \\
\quad\quad \text{CH–CH}_2\text{–CH=CH}_2 \\
\text{FCH}_2
\end{array}
\leftarrow
\begin{array}{c}
\text{TsOCH}_2 \\
\quad\quad \text{CH–CH}_2\text{–CH=CH}_2 \\
\text{TsOCH}_2
\end{array}
$$

$$
\begin{array}{c}
\text{F–CH}_2 \\
\quad\quad \text{CH–CH–COBr} \\
\text{F–CH}_2 \quad\quad\;\; |\\
\quad\quad\quad\quad\;\; \text{Br}
\end{array}
\rightarrow
\begin{array}{c}
\text{FCH}_2 \\
\quad\quad \text{CH–CH–COOH} \\
\text{FCH}_2 \quad\quad\;\; |\\
\quad\quad\quad\quad\;\; \text{NH}_2
\end{array}
\qquad
\text{d, l-}\omega, \omega'\text{-Difluor-valin}
$$

Schema 1

Der direkte Austausch einer Hydroxylgruppe gegen Fluor ist erst seit kurzem möglich. 1960 wurde mit dem Schwefeltetrafluorid SF_4 ein geeignetes Reagens aufgefunden [4, 17, 18]. Freilich sind immer noch recht robuste Reaktionsbedingungen erforderlich: man arbeitet im Autoklaven, bei erhöhten Temperaturen und mit Fluorwasserstoff als Katalysator. Ein weit milderes Fluorierungsmittel wurde mit dem β-Chlor-$\alpha.\alpha.\beta$-trifluor-äthyl-diäthylamin $ClFCH-CF_2-N(C_2H_2)_5$ entdeckt [1, 7, 19]. Dank der anionischen Lockerung seiner α-ständigen Fluoratome reagiert es mit Alkoholen bereits bei Temperaturen zwischen 0 und 50° glatt und geht dabei in das energiearme Säureamid über. Chlor-trifluor-triäthylamin überträgt Fluor auf primäre Alkohole, wie das von LETTRÉ u. EGLE [8] erstmals präparierte 19-Fluor-cholesterin belegt, auf sekundäre Alkohole (meist unter Konfigurationsumkehr) und auch auf die S_N2-inaktiven tertiären Carbinole, wofür die Darstellung des 25-Fluor-cholesterins durch LETTRÉ u. MEHRHOF [9] ein Beispiel bietet (Schema 2).

Ebenfalls erst vor wenigen Jahren wurde Perchloryl-fluorid $FClO_3$ in die präparative Praxis eingeführt [6]. Es wirkt gegenüber carbanionischen Verbindungen wie Alkali-enolaten, Lithiumorganylen oder Phosphor-Yliden als Fluordonator. Während man es anfänglich bevorzugt

                          M. Schlosser

in alkoholischer Lösung zur Einwirkung brachte und dann störende
Sekundärgleichgewichte und Nebenreaktionen in Kauf nehmen mußte,
ließ sich später zeigen, daß in Äther, Tetrahydrofuran, Benzol und anderen aprotischen Solventien besonders saubere Fluorierungen möglich sind.
Beispielsweise wurde von ROBERTS et al. [3] Cyclooctatetraenyllithium in
das Fluor-cyclooctatetraen übergeführt (Schema 3).

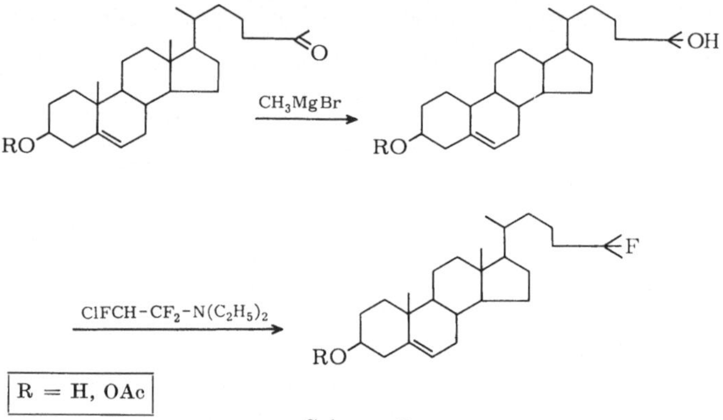

$$CH_3MgBr$$

$$ClFCH-CF_2-N(C_2H_5)_2$$

R = H, OAc

Schema 2

Eine Reihe entsprechender Lithium-Fluor- oder Magnesium-Fluor-
Substitutionen wurden von uns untersucht [16]; sie sind in der folgenden
Tabelle zusammengestellt (Schema 4).

Einen variationsfähigen Zugang zu Monofluorolefinen eröffnete die
Einwirkung von Perchlorylfluorid auf sog. Betain-Ylide. Betain-Ylide [13]
werden gewonnen durch lithium-organische α-Metallierung von Phosphor-
Betainen, die ihrerseits aus der Vereinigung von Phosphor-Yliden und
Aldehyden oder Ketonen hervorgehen. Die Betain-Ylide vermögen in der

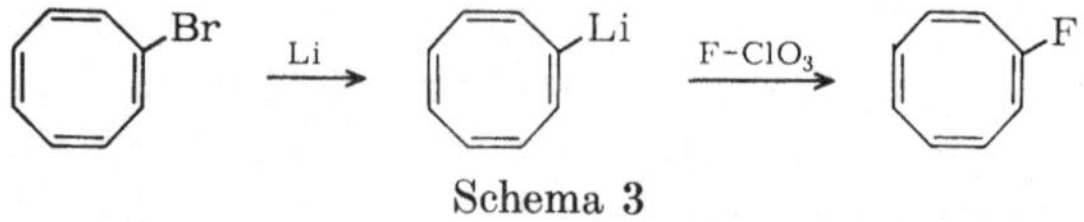

$$Br \xrightarrow{Li} Li \xrightarrow{F-ClO_3} F$$

Schema 3

α-Stellung zum Phosphor zahlreiche Elektrophile anzulagern, beispiels-
weise Fluor, wenn mit Perchlorylfluorid behandelt. Es resultiert ein
α-Fluor-Phosphor-Betain, das beim Erwärmen auf Raumtemperatur zu
Triphenylphosphin-oxid und zu einem Monofluor-olefin zerfällt [12].
Ausgehend von Triphenylphosphonium-methylid und Benzaldehyd ge-
langt man auf diese Weise in 60%iger Ausbeute zu cis- und trans-
Styrylfluorid (Schema 5).

In der folgenden Tabelle (Schema 6) sind eine Reihe weiterer Fluor-
olefine zusammengestellt, die mit Hilfe der geschilderten Varianten der

Wittig-Reaktion, der α-substituierenden Olefinierung, präpariert werden konnten. Wie ersichtlich, fallen nur Vinylfluoride vom Typ R–CH=CH–F als cis-trans-Isomerengemische an; Fluor-olefine mit mittelständiger Doppelbindung werden stereoselektiv aufgebaut [14]. Auch wenn an

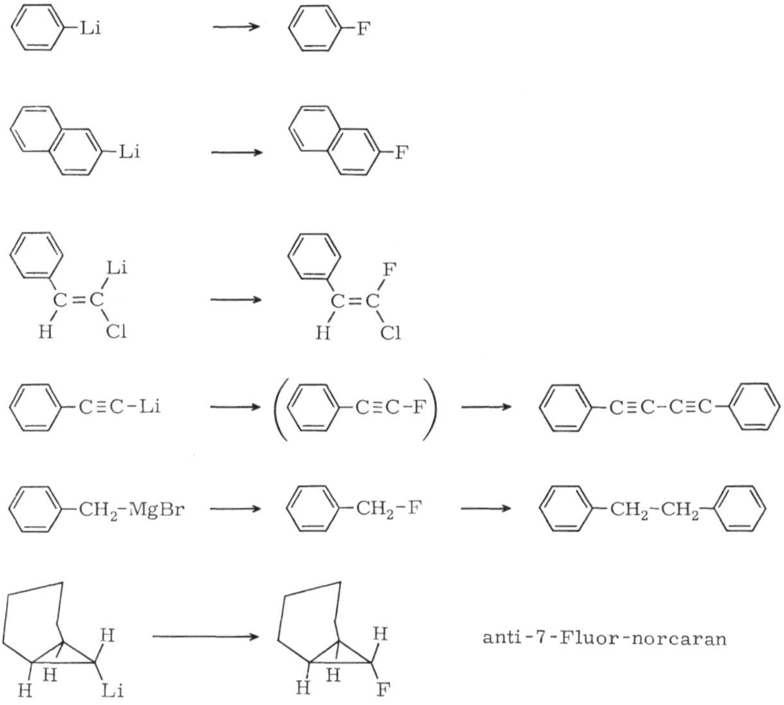

anti-7-Fluor-norcaran

Schema 4

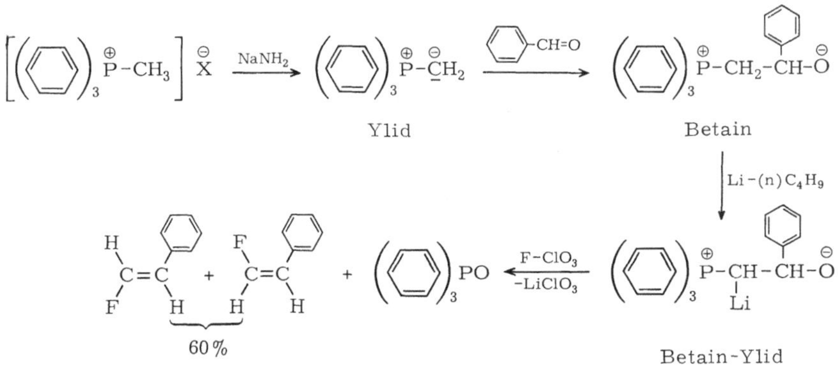

Ylid

Betain

Li–(n)C$_4$H$_9$

60%

Betain-Ylid

Schema 5

152   M. Schlosser

Stelle des Aldehyds ein Keton eingesetzt wird, dessen Carbonyl-Funktion
von einem kleinen und einem sehr großen Rest flankiert ist, wie etwa das
Tetrahydropyranylpregnenolon (Schema 7), entsteht ganz überwiegend

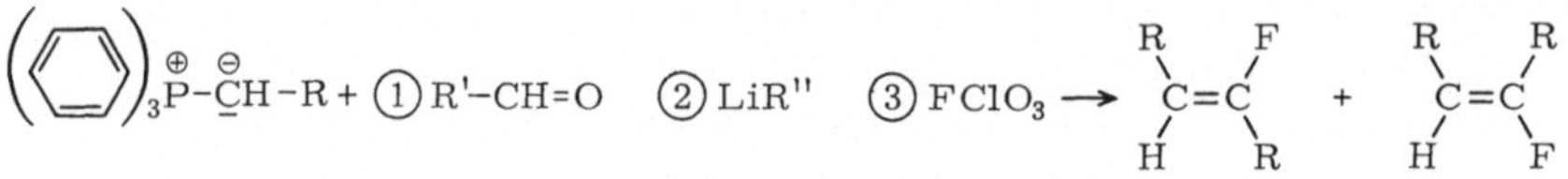

R	R'	Fluorolefin		Ausb.
H	(phenyl–CH=CH–CH$_3$)	(Phenyl–CH=CH–CH=CHF)	+	25%
CH$_3$	(phenyl)	(Phenyl–C(CH$_3$)=CHF isomer)		37%
(n)C$_3$H$_7$	C$_2$H$_5$	(H$_5$C$_2$–C(F)=CH–CH$_2$CH$_2$CH$_3$)		22%

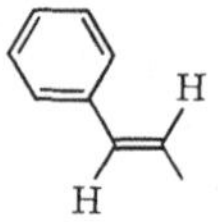

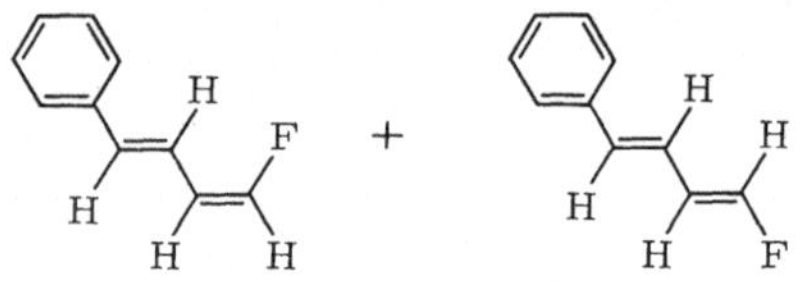

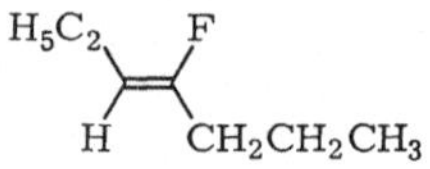

Schema 6

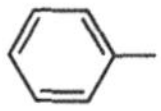

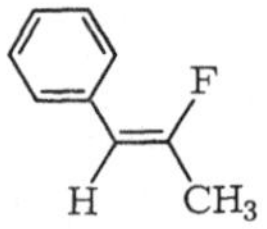

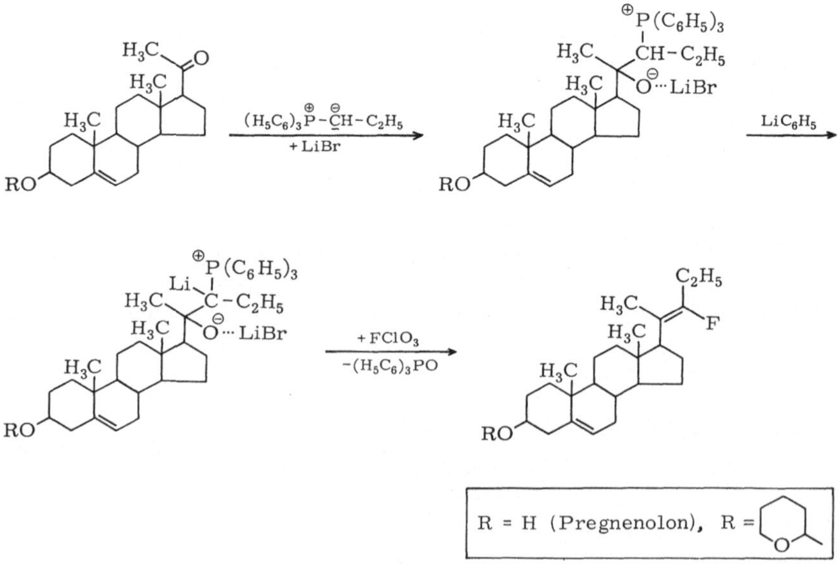

Schema 7

R = H (Pregnenolon), R = (Tetrahydropyranyl)

dasjenige olefinische Produkt, in dem das vicinale Paar der größeren Alkylgruppen trans-ständig an der Doppelbindung angeordnet ist [12].

Das präparative Repertoire des Fluor-Chemikers wurde in jüngster Zeit schließlich durch ganz spezielle „Fluorierungsmittel" bereichert, nämlich durch fluorierte Carbene. Durch Anlagerung von Chlor-fluor-carben an Olefine entstehen Chlor-fluor-cyclopropane [11]. Es ließ sich

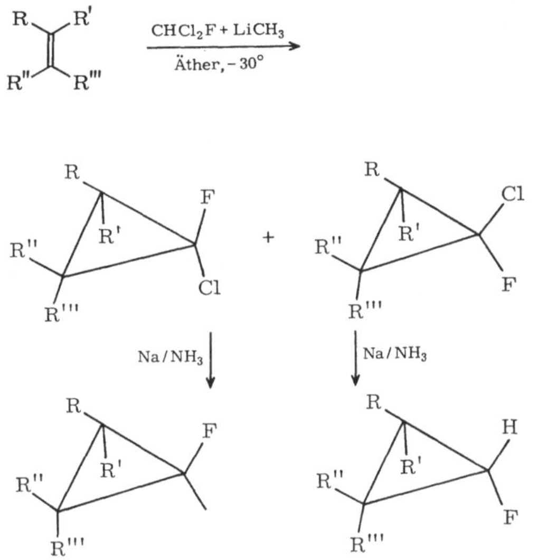

$$CHCl_2F + LiCH_3 \xrightarrow{\ \text{Äther, } -30°\ }$$

Schema 8

nun zeigen, daß diese Chlor-fluor-cyclopropane mit Natrium in flüssigem Ammoniak in guten Ausbeuten und stereospezifisch zu den entsprechenden Fluor-cyclopropanen reduziert werden können [15] (Schema 8). Monofluor-cyclopropane sind somit auf einem Umweg gut zugänglich geworden, wogegen es bislang noch nicht gelungen ist, Monofluor-carben in präparativem Maßstab zu erzeugen und an Olefine anzulagern. Überdies ist zu hoffen, daß man ausgehend von den Fluor-cyclopropanen durch kationische, anionische oder thermische Ringöffnung zu anderen Typen selektiv fluorierter Verbindungen vordringen kann.

Literatur

1. Ayer, D. E.: A new Method for the Preparation of Fluoro Steroids. Tetrahedron Letters **1962**, 1065.
2. Edgell, W. F. and L. Parts: Synthesis of Alkyl and Substituted Alkyl Fluorides from p-Toluenesulfonic Acid Esters. J. Amer. chem. Soc. **77**, 4899 (1955); E. D. Bergmann and I. Shaakh: Transformation of Toluene-p-sulphonates into Fluorides. Chem. and Ind. **1958**, 157.

3. GWYNN, D. E., G. M. WHITESIDES, and J. D. ROBERTS: Nuclear Magnetic Resonance Spectroscopy: Temperature Dependence of the Spectrum of Fluoro-cyclooctatetraene. J. Amer. chem. Soc. **87**, 2862 (1965).
4. HASEK, W. R., W. C. SMITH, and V. A. ENGELHARDT: The Chemistry of Sulfur Tetrafluoride II: The Fluorination of Organic Carbonyl Compounds. J. Amer. chem. Soc. **82**, 543 (1960).
5. HEIDELBERGER, C., N. K. CHAUDHURI, P. DANNEBERG, D. MOOREN, L. GRIES-BACH, R. DUSCHINSKY, R. J. SCHNITZER, E. PLEVEN, and J. SCHEINER: Fluorinated Pyrimidines, A new Class of Tumor-inhibitory Compounds. Nature **179**, 663 (1957).
6. INMAN, C. E., R. E. OESTERLING, and E. A. TYCZKOWSKI: Reactions of Per-chloryl Fluoride with Organic Compounds II: Fluorination of Certain Active Methylene Compounds. J. Amer. chem. Soc. **80**, 6533 (1958).
7. KNOX, L. H., E. VELARDE, S. BERGER, D. CUARDRIELLO, and A. D. CROS: The Reactions of Steroidal Alcohols with 2-Chloro-1.1.2-trifluoro-triethyl-amine. Tetrahedron Letters **1962**, 1249.
8. LETTRÉ, H. u. A. EGLE: unveröffentlicht (1966–1967).
9. — u. W. MEERHOF: unveröffentlicht (1965–1966).
10. — u. U. WOELCKE: Fluor-Derivative biogener aliphatischer Aminosäuren. Liebigs Ann. Chem. **708**, 75 (1967).
11. PARHAM, W. E. and R. R. TWELVES: Formation of Naphtalenes from Indenes III: Substituted Methanes as Carbene Precursors. J. org. Chemistry **22**, 730 (1957).
12. SCHLOSSER, M.: unveröffentlicht (1966).
13. — u. K. F. CHRISTMANN: Trans-selektive Olefinsynthesen. Angew. Chemie **78**, 115 (1966).
14. — — unveröffentlicht (1965–1967).
15. — u. G. HEINZ: Fluorcyclopropane durch reduzierende Entchlorierung von Chlorfluorcyclopropanen. Angew. Chemie **79**, 617 (1967).
16. — — unveröffentlicht (1960–1967).
17. SMITH, W. C.: The Chemistry of Sulfur Tetrafluoride VIII: The Synthesis of Phenylfluorophosphoranes and Phenylarsenic(V)fluorides. J. Amer. chem. Soc. **82**, 6176 (1960).
18. TULLOCK, C. W., F. S. FAWCETT, W. C. SMITH, and D. D. COFFMAN: The Chemistry of Sulfur Tetrafluoride I: The Synthesis of Sulfur Tetrafluoride. J. Amer. chem. Soc. **82**, 539 (1960).
19. YAROVENKO, N. N. u. M. A. RAKSHA: Fluorierung mit α-fluorierten Aminen. Zhur. Obshchei Kim. **29**, 2159 (1959); C.A. **54**, 9724 h (1960).

Über die Verätherung des Phorbols

Von

G. Kreibich und E. Hecker

Berenblum entdeckte 1941 die cocarcinogenen oder tumorrealisierenden Eigenschaften des Crotonöls, das durch Auspressen der Samen des tropischen Wolfsmilchgewächses Croton tiglium L. gewonnen wird.

Tabelle 1. *„Berenblum-Experiment" zur Definition der tumorrealisierenden Eigenschaften*

Applikation	Tumoren
1. DDD . . . . .DDD	+
2. D	−
3. 0CC CCC	−
4. DCC CCC	+

D = 9,10-Dimethyl-1,2-benzanthracen (carcinogen)
C = Crotonöl (cocarcinogen)
0 = Lösungsmittel allein

Die Anlage eines sogenannten Berenblum-Experiments, das den Begriff der tumorrealisierenden Eigenschaften definiert, ist in Tab. 1 schematisch dargestellt. Im Versuch 1 führt eine fortgesetzte Applikation des Carcinogens 9,10-Dimethyl-1,2-benzanthracen zum Auftreten von Tumoren. Die Einzeldosis ist dabei so niedrig gewählt, daß im zweiten Versuch, bei nur einmaliger Applikation des Carcinogens, keine Tumoren auftreten. Im Versuch 3 wird zweimal wöchentlich eine verdünnte Lösung von Crotonöl appliziert; es treten im Idealfall keine Tumoren auf. Der entscheidende Versuch 4, die Kombination der Versuche 2 und 3, zeigt, daß durch fortgesetzte Crotonölbehandlung nach einer einmaligen DMBA-Applikation Tumoren erhalten werden. Dieses Experiment macht es wahrscheinlich, daß die Carcinogenese der Mäusehaut in mindestens zwei Stufen abläuft: im ersten Schritt werden normale Zellen in potentielle Tumorzellen umgewandelt, die im zweiten Schritt durch tumorrealisie-

156   G. Kreibich und E. Hecker

rende Substanzen zu Tumoren entwickelt werden. Diese Substanzen, auch *Cocarcinogene* genannt, sollen selbst keine oder nur schwache carcinogene Wirkung haben.

In unserem Arbeitskreis konnten durch konsequente Anwendung einer Kombination von multiplikativen Verteilungsverfahren mit verschiedenen chromatographischen Methoden erstmals die reinen entzündlichen und tumorrealisierenden Wirkstoffe aus Crotonöl isoliert werden [4]. Es handelt sich um 12,13-Diester des polyfunktionellen Grundalkohols Phorbol mit der Bruttoformel $C_{20}H_{28}O_6$ (Abb. 1), der im Gegensatz zu seinen 12,13-Diestern biologisch unwirksam ist. Er enthält neben einer α,β-ungesättigten Carbonylgruppe noch fünf alkoholische Hydroxylgruppen:

1. an C-20 eine primäre allylische Hydroxylgruppe,
2. an C-12 eine sekundäre Hydroxylgruppe,
3. an C-4, C-9 und C-13 je eine tertiäre Hydroxylgruppe.

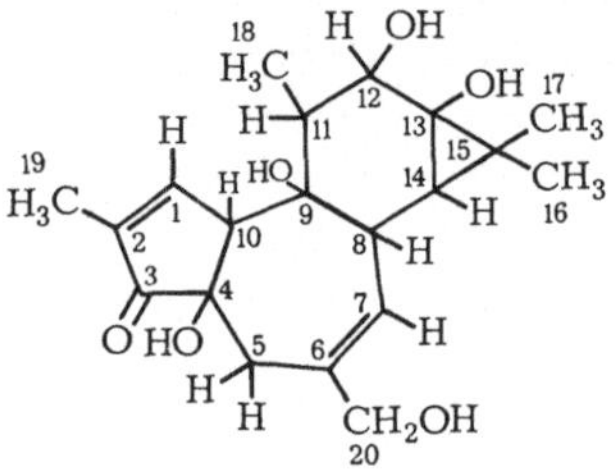

Abb. 1. Strukturformel des Diterpens Phorbol $C_{20}H_{28}O_6$

Die Hydroxylgruppe an C-13 steht an einem Cyclopropanring und ist Teil einer α-Glykolgruppe; die Hydroxylgruppe an C-4 ist Teil eines α-Ketols oder Acyloins.

Phorbol reduziert Fehlingsche Lösung und Tollens Reagens [2, 4, 7]. Die drei Hydroxylgruppen an C-12, C-13 und C-20 sind mit Acetanhydrid in Pyridin veresterbar. Man erhält ein Phorbol-12,13,20-triacetat, das mit Acetanhydrid und p-Toluolsulfonsäure peracetyliert werden kann [4, 12].

Versuche zur Verätherung des Phorbols wurden mit dem Ziel unternommen, die Hydroxylgruppen für chemische Reaktionen selektiv zu schützen und für Untersuchungen über die Zusammenhänge zwischen Struktur und biologischer Wirkung geeignete Derivate herzustellen.

Da Phorbol sowohl hitze- als auch basen- und säureempfindlich ist, schied ein großer Teil der üblichen Verätherungsmethoden aus. Unter milden Bedingungen konnten wichtige Ätherderivate dargestellt werden, die in Abb. 2 aufgeführt sind.

Die primäre allylische Hydroxylgruppe setzt sich in Pyridin mit Triphenyl-chlormethan zum Phorbol-20-trityläther (I) um [8]. Die Abspaltung des Tritylrests gelingt durch kurzzeitiges Erhitzen in Eisessig.

Erhöht man die Acidität der Hydroxylgruppen mit einer Lewissäure wie Al-i-propylat [10], so ist mit Diazomethan neben der primären Hydroxylgruppe auch das tertiäre Cyclopropanhydroxyl methylierbar (II). Das sekundäre Hydroxyl der α-Glykolgruppe des Phorbols ließ sich auf diese Weise nicht methylieren

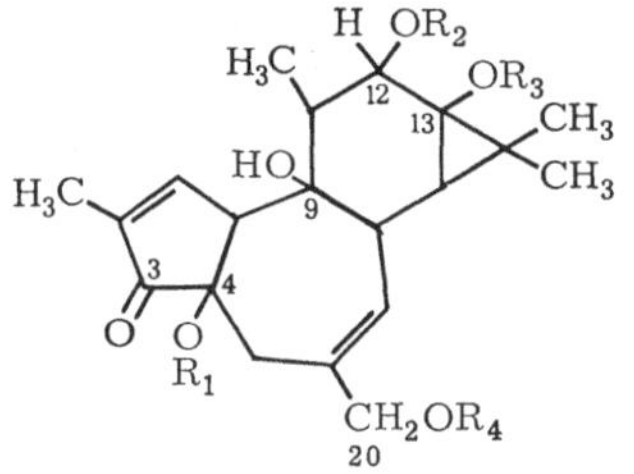

$$\text{[Strukturformel Phorbol]}$$

I	R_1, R_2, R_3	= −H;	R_4	= −C[φ]$_3$	
II	R_1, R_2	= −H;	R_3, R_4	= −CH$_3$	
III	R_1, R_3	= −H;	R_2	= −C$_2$H$_5$; R_4	= −C[φ]$_3$
IV	R_1, R_2	= −H;	R_3	= −C$_2$H$_5$; R_4	= −C[φ]$_3$
V	R_1	= −CH$_3$;	R_2, R_3, R_4	= −COCH$_3$	
VI	R_1, R_3	= −CH$_3$;	R_2, R_4	= −COCH$_3$	
VII	R_1	= −CH$_3$;	R_2	= −H;	R_3, R_4 = −COCH$_3$

Abb. 2. Die wichtigsten Ätherderivate von Phorbol

Setzt man in einer analogen Reaktion Phorbol-20-trityläther mit dem reaktionsfähigeren [1] Homologen Diazoäthan um, so entstehen nebeneinander sowohl der 12- als auch der 13-O-Äthyläther im Verhältnis 1:3 (III + IV). Ein 12,13-Di-O-äthyläther wird nicht gebildet. Offenbar verbieten die sterischen Verhältnisse der α-Glykolgruppe die weitere Umsetzung des benachbarten Hydroxyls, sobald das erste der beiden veräthert ist.

Die tertiäre Hydroxylgruppe an C-4 kann mit Methyljodid und Silberoxyd in Dimethylformamid [9] methyliert werden, wenn die Hydroxylgruppen an C-12, C-13 und C-20 durch Acetatreste geschützt sind (V). Der Versuch, durch Verlängerung der Einwirkungszeit des Methylierungsmittels auf Phorbol-12,13,20-triacetat auch die Hydroxylgruppe an C-9 zu veräthern, ergibt − neben zahlreichen nicht identifizierten Nebenprodukten − unter Verdrängung der 13-O-Acetylgruppe das 4,13-Di-O-methyl-phorbol-12,20-diacetat (VI). Die Hydroxylgruppe an C-9 ist also unter diesen Bedingungen nicht verätherbar.

Versucht man, in Phorbol-13,20-diacetat die sekundäre Hydroxylgruppe an C-12 mit Methyljodid/Silberoxyd in Dimethylformamid zu methylieren, so wird nur die tertiäre Hydroxylgruppe an C-4 veräthert (VII).

Die Methylierung der primären Hydroxylgruppe mit Methyljodid/ Silberoxyd gelingt, wenn man als Lösungsmittel statt Dimethylformamid Essigester verwendet, und wenn die Hydroxylgruppe an C-13 blockiert ist. Verwendet man Phorbol-12,20-diacetat mit ungeschütztem Cyclopropan-Hydroxyl an C-13 als Ausgangsmaterial für diese Reaktion, so wird der Cyclopropanring in bemerkenswerter Reaktion dehydrierend gesprengt. Es entsteht ein Derivat des Bisdehydrophorbols (Abb. 3). Diese Verbindung wird im Vortrag von GSCHWENDT u. HECKER ausführlicher behandelt.

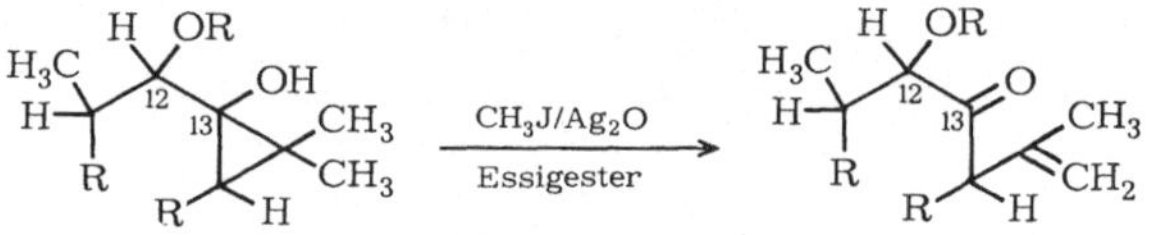

Abb. 3. Die dehydrierende Öffnung des Cyclopropanols mit CH_3J/Ag_2O in Essigester

Auf Grund des Befundes, daß Phorbol und seine Ester positive Fehling- und Tollens-Reaktionen zeigen, wurden die von uns nachgewiesenen Partialstrukturen (1) und (2) des Phorbols [4] zunächst in einem ersten Strukturvorschlag (Abb. 4) zu einem sekundären Acyloin verknüpft [3].

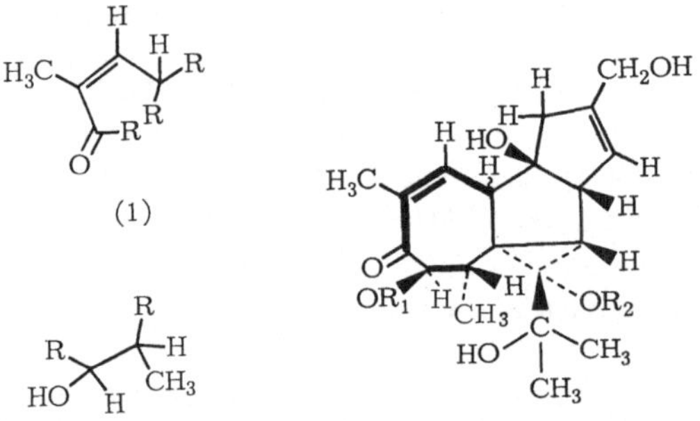

Abb. 4. Erster Strukturvorschlag für Phorbol. Verknüpfung der Teilstrukturen (1) und (2) zu einem sekundären Acyloin

Mit Hilfe geeigneter Ätherderivate des Phorbols können dessen reduzierende Eigenschaften nunmehr eindeutig dem tertiären Cyclopropanhydroxyl zugeordnet werden. In Abb. 5 sind die in diesem Zusammenhang getesteten Ätherderivate aufgeführt. Schon die positive Tollens- und Fehling-Reaktion des in 3-Stellung reduzierten Phorbols – des Phorbol-3-ols – das man durch Behandlung von Phorbol mit Natriumborhydrid erhält, ist mit einer sekundären Acyloingruppe nicht zu vereinbaren. Man sieht weiter, daß die Tollens- und Fehling-Reaktion nur dann negativ ausfällt, wenn das Cyclopropanhydroxyl wie beim 13-O-Äthylphorbol-20-trityläther blockiert ist. Um auszuschließen, daß ein eventuell bei der oxydativen Ringsprengung entstehendes sekundäres Acyloin wie das Bisdehydrophorbol reduzierend wirkt, wurde auch der 12-O-Äthylphorbol-20-trityläther getestet. Da die reduzierenden Eigenschaften durch die Äthylierung des an C-12 stehenden sekundären Hydroxyls nicht beeinflußt werden, kann nur das tertiäre Cyclopropanhydroxyl für diese Reaktion verantwortlich sein. – Unabhängig von uns [6] ist kürzlich eine analoge Reaktion an einfachen, tertiären Cyclopropanolen gefunden worden [11].

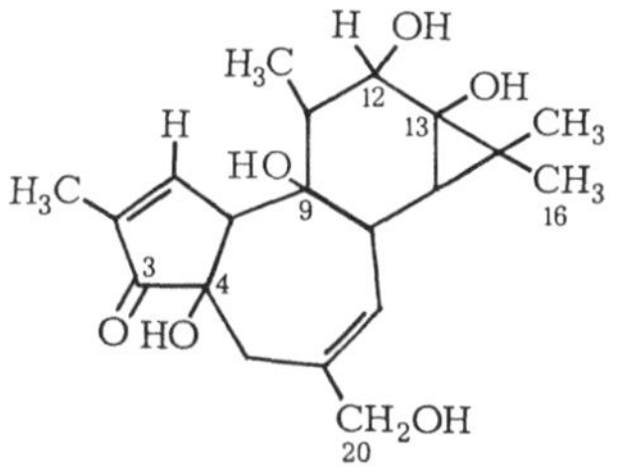

Derivat	Tollens-Reaktion	Fehling-Reaktion
Phorbol	+	+
Phorbol-3-ol	+	+
13-O-Äthyl-phorbol-20-trityläther	-	-
12-O-Äthyl-phorbol-20-trityläther	+	+
Phorbol-12-trityläther	+	+

Abb. 5. Die reduzierenden Eigenschaften einiger Ätherderivate des Phorbols gegenüber Fehlingscher Lösung und Tollens Reagens

Phorbol enthält aber dennoch eine Acyloingruppe (Abb. 1), worauf schon die Verätherbarkeit des Hydroxyls an C_4 hinweist, und wie in den nachfolgenden Vorträgen u. a. auf Grund von Daten verätherter Phorbolderivate gezeigt wird. Sie ist aber tertiär und gibt sich daher mit Fehling- und Tollens-Reagens nicht zu erkennen.

Um Beziehungen zwischen Struktur und biologischer Wirkung aufzuklären, wurden die Äthyläther 12-O-Tetradecanoyl-phorbol-(13)-äthyläther (III) und 12-O-Äthylphorbol-(13)-tetradecanoat (IV) synthetisiert (Abb. 6). Sie entsprechen in ihrer Struktur dem hochaktiven Wirkstoff A_1, einem 12-O-Tetradecanoyl-phorbol-13-acetat (I) bzw. dem inversen Phorbolester (II). Sie enthalten also an Stelle der Acetylgruppen Äthyläthergruppen.

Getestet wurde bisher die Verbindung III auf ihre entzündliche Wirkung am Mäuseohr durch Ermittlung der entzündlichen Dosis 50 (ED_{50}) [5]. Die tumorpromovierenden Eigenschaften werden im eingangs beschriebenen Berenblum-Experiment an 28 Mäusen getestet. Die einmalige, initiale Dosis des Carcinogens DMBA ist 0,1 μMol. Von den zu prüfenden Verbindungen werden zweimal wöchentlich 0,02 μMol auf die Rückenhaut der Mäuse aufgetragen.

Während der Wirkstoff A_1, das 12-O-Tetradecanoylphorbol-(13)-acetat (I) und das isomere 12-O-Acetylphorbol-(13)-tetradecanoat eine ED_{50} von 0,01 μg/Ohr zeigen, liegt die ED_{50} des (I) entsprechenden Ätherderivats (III) um den Faktor $2,5 \cdot 10^3$ höher (Abb 6).

	R_1	R_2
I:	$-CO-(CH_2)_{12}-CH_3$;	$-CO-CH_3$
II:	$-CO-CH_3$;	$-CO-(CH_2)_{12}-CH_3$
III:	$-CO-(CH_2)_{12}-CH_3$;	$-CH_2-CH_3$
IV:	$-CH_2-CH_3$;	$-CO-(CH_2)_{12}-CH_3$

		Entzündliche Dosis am Mäuseohr ED_{50} [μg/Ohr]	Tumorpromovierende Wirkung nach 12 Wochen*)	
			% Tiere mit Tumoren	Tumoren/ Tiere
I	12-O-Tetracanoyl-phorbol-(13)-acetat (A_1)	0,01 : 1,3	82	3, 6
II	12-O-Acetyl-phorbol-(13)-tetradecanoat	0,01 : 1,2	54	1, 7
III	12-O-Tetradecanoyl-phorbol-(13)-äthyläther	25 : 1,3	0	0
IV	12-O-Äthyl-phorbol-(13)-tetradecanoat	Versuche noch nicht abgeschlossen		

*)   0, 1 μMol DMBA einmalig
     0, 02 μMol Tumorpromotor 2x wöchentlich

Abb. 6. Entzündliche und cocarcinogene Wirkung einiger Phorbol-Ester und -Äther

Im Tumor-Promotionstest zeigen bei Behandlung mit A_1 (I) und der isomeren Verbindung (II) nach 12 Wochen 82 bzw. 54% der Tiere Tumoren. Die Tumorausbeuten sind 3,6 bzw. 1,7 Tumoren/Tier. Im Gegensatz dazu ist beim 12-O-Tetradecanoyl-phorbol-(13)-äthyläther (III) keine tumorpromovierende Wirkung feststellbar. Auch nach 36 Wochen traten keine Papillome auf. Die vorhandenen Ergebnisse zeigen bereits, daß der Ersatz einer Acetylgruppe in I durch die entsprechende Äther-gruppe zu einem Verlust der biologischen Wirkung führt. – Die entsprechen-den Versuche mit den inversen Äther (IV) sind noch nicht abgeschlossen.

Literatur

1. ADAMSON, D. W. and J. KENNER: Improved Preparation of Aliphatic Diazo-Compounds and Certain of Their Properties. J. chem. Soc. **322**, 1551 (1937).

2. FLASCHENTRÄGER, B.: Über den Giftstoff im Krotonöl. Festschrift Heinrich Zangger, II. Teil, S. 857. Zürich, Leipzig und Stuttgart: Verlag Rascher u. Cie., A.G. 1935.

3. HECKER, E. et al.: Phorbol – ein neues tetracyclisches Diterpen aus Crotonöl. Tetrahedron Letters **23**, 1837 (1965); Die Cocarcinogene des Crotonöls. In Doerr-Linder-Wagner (Hrsg.): Aktuelle Probleme aus dem Gebiet der Cancerologie, S. 121. Berlin-Göttingen-Heidelberg: Springer 1966.

4. — et al.: Kombination wirksamer Trennverfahren mit modernen analytischen Methoden in der Naturstoffchemie. Z. analyt. Chem. **221**, 424 (1966); Über die Wirkstoffe des Crotonöls, VII. – Phorbol. Z. Naturforsch. **21** b, 1204 (1966).

5. —, H. IMMICH, H. BRESCH u. H. U. SCHAIRER: Über die Wirkstoffe des Croton-öls – VI. Entzündungsteste am Mäuseohr. Z. Krebsforsch. **68**, 366 (1966).

6. — et al.: Structure and Stereochemistry of the Tetracyclic Diterpene Phorbol from Croton Tiglium L. Tetrahedron Letters **1967**, 3165

7. KAUFFMANN, T. u. H. NEUMANN: Über die reduzierende Gruppe des Phorbols. Chem. Ber. **92**, 1715 (1959).

8. KUBINYI, H.: Isolierung, Struktur und Partialsynthese biologisch aktiver Naturstoffe aus Crotonöl. Dissertation Univ. München 1964.

9. KUHN, R., H. TRISCHMANN u. J. LÖW: Zur Permethylierung von Zuckern und Glykosiden. Angew. Chem. **67**, 32 (1955).

10. POPELAK, A. u. G. LETTENBAUER: Rauwolfia-Alkaloide IX; Über die Ver-ätherung der Yohimban Alkaloide mit Diazomethan. Arch. Pharm. **295**, 427 (1962).

11. SCHAAFSMA, S. E., H. STEINBERG, and TH. J. DE BOER: Isomerisation and Oxidative Dimerisation of 1-substituted Cyclopropanols. Recueil Trav. chim. Pays-Bas **85**, 73 (1966).

12. v. SZCZEPANSKI, CH., H. U. SCHAIRER, M. GSCHWENDT u. E. HECKER: Zur Chemie des Phorbols, III. – Mono- und Diacetate des Phorbols. Liebigs Ann. Chem. **705**, 199 (1967).

Circulardichroismus und Röntgenstrukturanalyse
des Phorbols

Von

H. Bartsch und E. Hecker

Das tetracyclische Diterpen Phorbol bietet wegen der besonderen
Anordnung funktioneller Gruppen und der Stereochemie des Kohlenstoff-
gerüsts eine Reihe interessanter Meßergebnisse im Circulardichroismus.

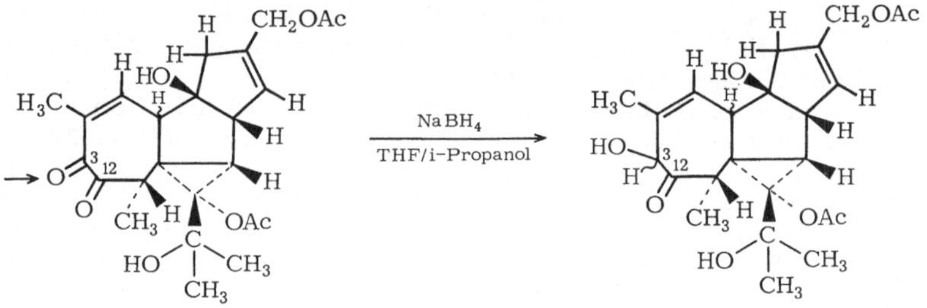

Abb. 1. Reduktion von Phorbol-12-on-13,20-diacetat zum
Neophorbol-13,20-diacetat

Für Phorbol, dessen Fettsäurediester starke entzündliche und tumorpromovierende Eigenschaften aufweisen [5], konnte 1964 in unserem
Arbeitskreis eine erste Strukturformel vorgeschlagen werden [6], die mit
allen damals bekannten chemischen und physikalischen Daten in Einklang stand (vgl. Abb. 4 des Vortrags von Kreibich u. Hecker), jedoch
der späteren Überprüfung durch chemische Reaktionen und durch CD-
Messungen nicht standhielt [8].

So entsteht z. B. durch Oxydation der sekundären Hydroxylgruppe
an C-12 ein Diketon, das Phorbol-on [6], in dem sich die bereits im Phorbol
vorhandene Carbonylgruppe an C-3 mit NaBH$_4$ selektiv zur sekundären
Alkoholfunktion reduzieren läßt (Abb. 1). Auf diese Weise entsteht ein
mit Phorbol isomeres Monoketon, das als Neophorbol bezeichnet wird [10].

In Abb. 2 sind die CD-Kurven der 13,20-Diacetate von Phorbol (I), von
Neophorbol (II) und von Phorbol-on(Diketon) (III) aufgetragen. – Auf die
anomale Bande der Phorbolderivate, in I bei 272 mμ, wird weiter unten

noch eingegangen. Addiert man die Dichroismen der isomeren Monoketone I und II, so erhält man eine Kurve – in Abb. 2 durch Dreiecke
gekennzeichnet – die im Rahmen der erzielten Meßgenauigkeit mit der
gemessenen CD-Kurve des Diketons identisch ist.

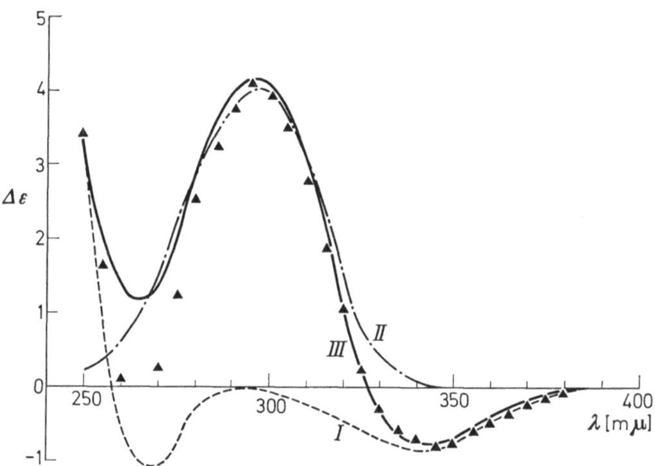

Abb. 2. CD-Kurven von Phorbol-13,20-diacetat (I), Neophorbol-13,20-diacetat (II)
und Phorbol-12-on-13,20-diacetat (III); weitere Erläuterungen im Text

Aus diesem additiven Verhalten der CD-Kurven I und II läßt sich
eine α-ständige Anordnung der Ketogruppen, wie sie nach der für das
Phorbol-on zuerst vorgeschlagenen Struktur zu fordern wäre, ausschließen. Im Siebenring des ersten Strukturvorschlages steht nämlich die
Sequenz der Kohlenstoffe C-3,12 im Widerspruch zur Regel der „Addi-
tivität der Chromophore“.

In diesem Falle, d. h. bei 1,2-Diketonen, hätte der Dichroismus nichts
mehr mit der Summenkurve der entsprechenden Monoketone gemein, da
die elektronische Wechselwirkung der Oscillatoren eine völlig veränderte
Kurvenform verursacht [15, 16]. Aus dem gleichen Grund ist eine 1,3-
Diketogruppierung unmöglich [12], was nach der zugrundegelegten
Phorbolstruktur einer Anordnung der Carbonyle in verschiedenen Ringen
gleichkommt. Damit kann also auch auf diesem Wege eine sekundäre
Acyloingruppe im Phorbol ausgeschlossen werden.

Als benachbarter Partner des Carbonyls C-3 im Phorbol konnte eine
tertiäre Hydroxylgruppe nachgewiesen werden, wie aus dem Vergleich
der Dichroismen verschiedener Phorbolacetate und -Äther [10] mit den
entsprechenden unveresterten und unverätherten Derivaten hervorgeht.

In Abb. 3 sind die CD-Kurven des Phorbol-12,13,20-triacetats I,
seines an C-4 verätherten Derivats II und seines 4-Acetats III dargestellt.

Ausschließlich bei der Veresterung oder Verätherung der *einen* OH-Gruppe an C-4 treten im CD Vicinaleffekte auf. Aus der hypsochromen Lageverschiebung des Maximums kann auf eine axiale α-Acetoxygruppe

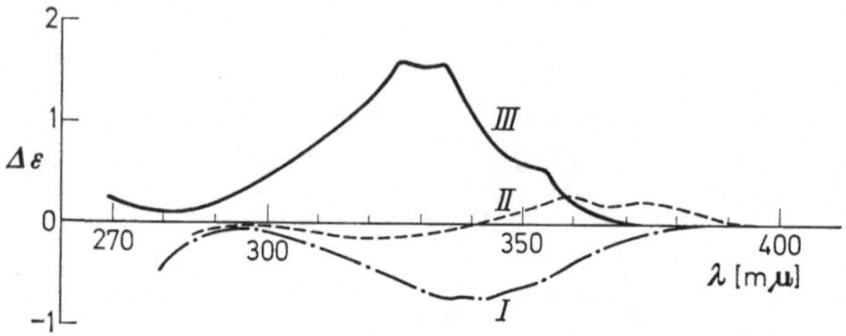

Abb. 3. CD-Kurven von Phorbol-12,13,20-triacetat (I), Phorbol-4-methyläther-12,13,20-triacetat (II), Phorbol-4,9,12,13,20-pentaacetat (III)

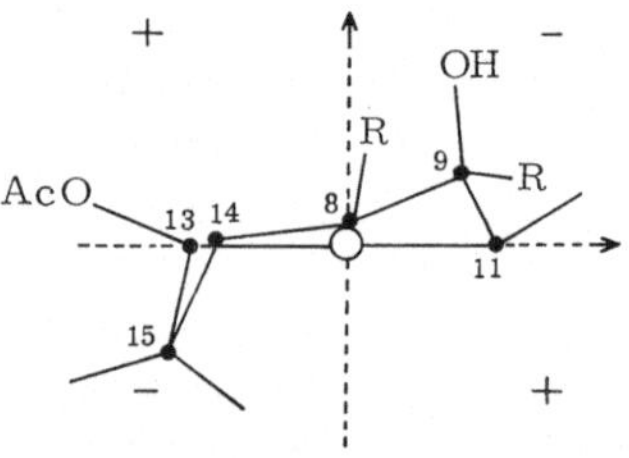

Abb. 4. Octantenprojektion des Sechsrings mit α-ständigem Dreiring in Neo-phorbol-13,20-diacetat

geschlossen werden [2, 3]. Bei II und III wird zudem eine Vorzeichen-umkehr der R-Bande des Enons beobachtet, die beim verätherten Derivat aus einem positiven und einem negativen Anteil besteht.

Die Erklärung für alle Phänomene bietet eine zum Carbonyl α-ständige, tertiäre Hydroxylgruppe, wie sie der modifizierte Struktur-vorschlag für Phorbol ausweist [8, 10] (siehe Abb. 1 bei KREIBICH u. HECKER).

Außerdem findet man in der neuen Formel die oben geforderte Anordnung der zwei Carbonylgruppen in verschiedenen Ringen: Im Phorbol-on steht das zweite Carbonyl in Position C-12.

Nach Untersuchungen von SNATZKE, DJERASSI, KLYNE und anderen [2, 4, 14] bestimmt bei α,β-Cyclopropylketonen – eine derartige Gruppe liegt im Neophorbol vor – die *Absolutkonfiguration des Dreirings* das Vorzeichen des Cottoneffekts.

Wendet man die für diese Verbindungstypen gültige „inverse Octantenregel" auf Neophorboldiacetat an (Abb. 4), so erhält man diejenige Absolutkonfiguration, die nach der Octantenprojektion einen gemessenen positiven CD ergibt, der hier $\Delta\varepsilon =$ plus 4 beträgt. Daraus

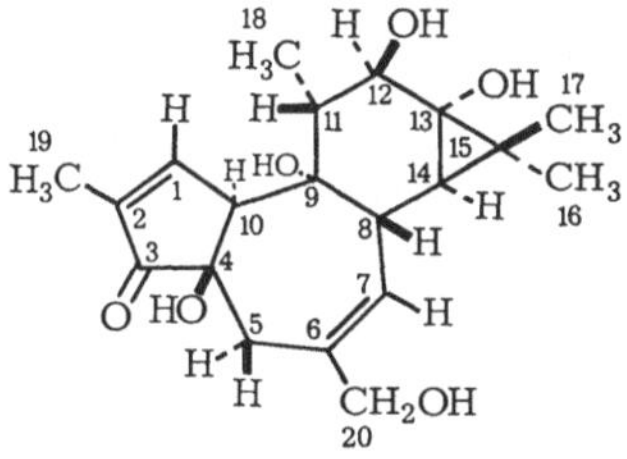

Abb. 5. Absolute Konfiguration des Phorbols

resultiert für Neophorbol – wie aus dem Bild zu ersehen – ein α-ständiger Dreiring. Die Größe der dichroitischen Absorption steht überdies in Übereinstimmung mit der Halbsesselkonformation des Sechsrings, die im Neophorbol und auch im Phorbol vorliegt, wie es chemische und spektrale Daten ausweisen.

Die Röntgenstrukturanalyse ermittelt dagegen für Neophorbol und damit auch für Phorbol das Spiegelbild (Abb. 5) der auf diese Weise abgeleiteten Absolutkonfiguration [11].

Die allgemeine Gültigkeit der Regel für α,β-Cyclopropylketone erfährt daher durch den Chromophor des Neophorbol-13,20-diacetats – ein α,β-Cyclopropylketon mit tertiärem Acetoxyl am Dreiring – eine Einschränkung. Bisher ungeklärt ist auch das Auftreten der bereits zu Anfang erwähnten dritten CD-Bande des Phorbols bei 272mμ, die gleiches Vorzeichen wie die R-Bande des Enons bei 343 mμ aufweist [9].

Nach BRAGG [1] verstärken die Röntgenstrahlen unseren Gesichtssinn um mehr als das 10000fache, so daß wir sogar einzelne Atome und Moleküle „sehen" können. Für diesen „Sehvorgang", der sich bei der Röntgenstrukturanalyse auf die Elektronendichteverteilung im Molekül bezieht, ist allerdings ein erheblicher rechnerischer Aufwand nötig. Dieser kann erst in jüngster Zeit mit den modernen elektronischen Rechenanlagen getrieben werden, wie sie z. B. dem Deutschen Krebsforschungszentrum im Institut für Dokumentation, Information und Statistik zur Verfügung stehen. Dazu müssen im Röntgenbeugungsdiagramm eines Kristalls, das üblicherweise photographisch aufgenommen wird, die Intensitäten der Reflexe – gewöhnlich mehrere Tausend – visuell geschätzt oder photometrisch bestimmt werden.

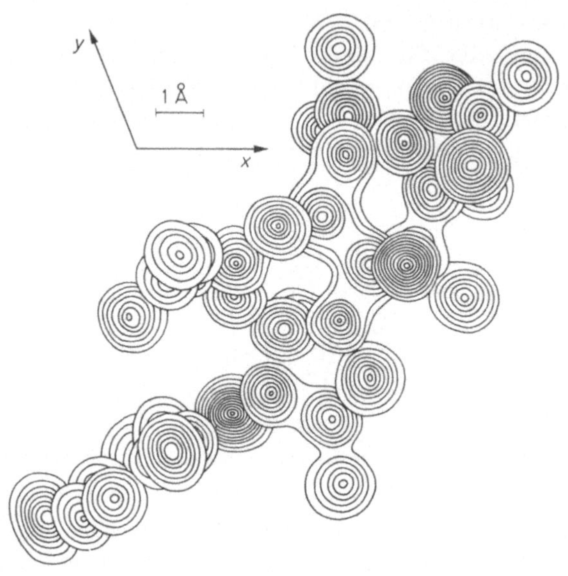

Abb. 6. Elektronendichteverteilung in der Umgebung der Atome von Neophorbol-13,20-diacetat-3-[p-brombenzoat]. Leichtatome: Linienabstand 1e/Å³. Brom: 1 Linie 2e/Å³, Abstand der übrigen Höhenlinien 5e/Å³

Die oben angedeuteten umfangreichen Berechnungen verlangen die Summation einer Fourier-Reihe, deren Glieder die Amplituden und Phasen der Reflexe des Röntgendiagramms beschreiben. Beide hängen von der Lage der Atome im Kristall ab; in gewöhnlichen Kristallen lassen sich jedoch nur die Amplituden leicht messen.

Führt man dagegen an einer definierten Stelle des untersuchten Kristalls ein schweres Atom wie z. B. Brom oder Jod ein, so wird dadurch die direkte Berechnung der *Phasenwinkel* möglich.

Unsere Bemühungen, ein derartiges kristallines Schweratomderivat des Phorbols darzustellen, begegneten zunächst ungewöhnlichen Schwierigkeiten. So blieben viele der synthetisierten Derivate amorph oder kristallisierten in Zwillingskristallen, die für die Röntgenstrukturanalyse ungeeignet sind. Erst vom 3-[p-Brombenzoat] des Neophorbol-13,20-diacetats konnten geeignete Kristalle gezüchtet werden.

Das Ergebnis der Röntgenstrukturanalyse, die von HOPPE u. Mitarb.
am Max-Planck-Institut für Eiweiß- und Lederforschung in München [*11*],
und in jüngster Zeit an einem anderen Phorbolderivat auch von FERGUSON
und PETTERSEN in Glasgow [*13*] durchgeführt wurde, zeigt die Abb. 6.
Die berechnete Elektronendichteverteilung, durch ein System von
Höhenlinien gekennzeichnet, ergibt die Raumkoordinaten der Sauerstoff-
und Kohlenstoffatome des Neophorbols.

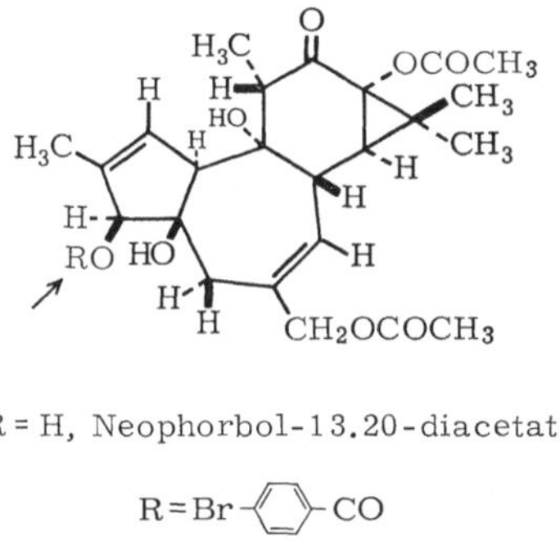

R = H, Neophorbol-13.20-diacetat

Abb. 7. Neophorbol-13,20-diacetat-3-[p-brombenzoat]: Schweratomderivat zur
Röntgenstrukturanalyse

Die daraus abzulesende Konstitution und Konfiguration ist in Abb. 7
in der üblichen Projektion wiedergegeben. Die Röntgenstrukturanalyse
bestätigt die von uns auf unabhängigem Wege ermittelte Konstitution
des Phorbols und ergänzt sie an einigen Stellen. Damit ist eine zuverlässige
Grundlage für Untersuchungen auf molekularbiologischer Ebene geschaffen.

Die Diester des Phorbols mit Fettsäuren unterschiedlicher Ketten-
länge zeigen stark entzündliche und, sofern DMBA in unterschwelliger
Dosis appliziert wird, tumorpromovierende Wirkung auf der Mäusehaut [5, 7].

Nimmt man funktionelle Veränderungen am Grundalkohol Phorbol
vor, so ändert sich die biologische Aktivität der Fettsäureester. In Abb. 8
werden entzündliche und tumorfördernde Wirkung einiger Fettsäureester
von modifizierten Phorbolabkömmlingen mit dem biologisch aktivsten
Phorbolester, dem Wirkstoff A_1, verglichen. A_1 enthält an der Hydroxylgruppe C-12 des Phorbols einen Tetradecanoyl- und an C-13 einen Acetyl-
rest. Beim Test an Mäusen des Inzuchtstamms NMRI zeigt A_1 eine entzündliche Dosis 50 von 0,01 μg/Ohr. Als tumorpromovierende Wirkung
ergibt sich: 82% Tiere mit Tumoren. Dabei entfallen durchschnittlich
3,6 Tumoren auf ein Tier.

Hydriert man die beiden Doppelbindungen im Phorbol, wobei die Hydroxylgruppe an C-20 eliminiert wird, so zeigt das mit n-Decansäure am Hydroxyl C-12 und Essigsäure am Hydroxyl C-13 veresterte Derivat bei Applikation von 232 μg keinerlei entzündliche Wirkung mehr.

$$R_1 = -CO(CH_2)_{12}CH_3$$
$$R_2 = -COCH_3 (A_1)$$
$$R_{1,2} = H \text{ (Phorbol)}$$

Verbindung	Entzündliche Dosis (ED$_{50}$) am Mäuseohr [μg/Ohr]*)	Tumorpromovierende Wirkung nach 12 Wochen**)	
		% Tiere mit Tumoren	Tumoren/ Tiere
12-O-Tetradecanoyl-phorbol-(13)-acetat (A$_1$)	0,01	82	3,6
12-O-Decanoyl-20-desoxy-tetra-hydrophorbol-(13)-acetat	>232	noch nicht getestet	
13-O-Decanoyl-phorbol-12-on	0,11	4	0,04
3-O-Tetradecanoyl-neophorbol-(13)-acetat (Neo-A$_1$)	0,66	noch nicht getestet	

*) einfache Standard-abweichung : 1,3

**) 0,1 μMol DMBA einmalig
0,02 μMol Tumorpromotor 2x wöchentlich

Abb. 8. Entzündliche und tumorpromovierende Wirkung einiger Fettsäureester von modifizierten Phorbolabkömmlingen im Vergleich zum Wirkstoff A$_1$

Oxydiert man die Hydroxylgruppe des Phorbols an C-12 zum Keton und verestert am Hydroxyl C-13 mit n-Decansäure, so liegt die ED$_{50}$ gegenüber A$_1$ um eine Zehnerpotenz niedriger. Der prozentuale Anteil der Tiere mit Tumoren fällt auf 4, die Zahl Tumoren/Tiere auf 0,04 ab. In der gleichen Größenordnung bewegt sich bei der ED$_{50}$ auch der Wert von Neo-A$_1$, in dem die Hydroxylgruppe an Position 3, die durch Reduktion der Ketogruppe in Phorbol entsteht, mit n-Tetradecansäure, die Position 13 mit Essigsäure verestert ist. Die sekundäre Hydroxylgruppe an

C-12 ist dabei zum Carbonyl oxydiert. Die tumorpromovierende Wirkung ist noch nicht getestet.

Aus diesen Ergebnissen läßt sich naturgemäß noch keine Allgemeinaussage über die Relation zwischen Struktur und biologischer Aktivität bei Phorbolderivaten ableiten. Entsprechende Untersuchungen darüber sind im Gange.

Literatur

1. Bragg, W. H.: Concerning Nature of Things, London: Bell & Sons 1925.
2. Crabbé, P.: Optical Rotatory Dispersion and Circular Dichroism in Organic Chemistry. San Francisco: Holden-Day 1965.
3. Djerassi, C.: Optical Rotatory Dispersion. Application to Organic Chemistry p. 113. New York: McGraw-Hill Book Company 1960.
4. —, W. Klyne, T. Norin, G. Ohloff, and E. Klein: Rotatory Dispersion Curves of Cyclopropyl-ketones and Epoxy-ketones. Tetrahedron 21, 163 (1965).
5. Hecker, E. u. H. Bresch: Reindarstellung und Charakterisierung eines toxisch, entzündlich und cocarcinogen hochaktiven Wirkstoffes. Z. Naturforsch. 20b, 216 (1965).
6. —, H. Kubinyi, Ch. v. Szczepanski, E. Härle u. H. Bresch: Phorbol – ein neues tetracyclisches Diterpen aus Crotonöl. Tetrahedron Letters 1965, 1837.
7. — Die Cocarcinogene des Crotonöls. In Doerr-Linder-Wagner (Hrsg.): Aktuelle Probleme aus dem Gebiet der Cancerologie, p. 121. Berlin-Heidelberg-New York: Springer 1966.
8. — et al.: Kombination wirksamer Trennverfahren mit modernen analytischen Methoden in der Naturstoffchemie. Isolierung und Strukturaufklärung der biologisch aktiven Substanzen aus Crotonöl. Z. analyt. Chem. 221, 424 (1966).
9. — et al.: Über die Wirkstoffe des Crotonöls, VII Phorbol. Z. Naturforsch. 21b, 1204 (1966).
10. —, H. Bartsch, H. Bresch, M. Gschwendt, E. Härle, G. Kreibich, H. Kubinyi, H. U. Schairer, Ch. v. Szczepanski, and H. W. Thielmann: Structure and Stereochemistry of the Tetracyclic Diterpene Phorbol from Croton Tiglium L. Tetrahedron Letters 1967, 3165.
11. Hoppe, W., F. Brandl, J. Strell, M. Röhrl, J. Gassmann, E. Hecker, H. Bartsch, G. Kreibich u. Ch. v. Szczepanski: Röntgenstrukturanalyse des Neophorbols. Angew. Chem. 79, 824 (1967).
12. Moscovitz, A. and A. E. Hansen: Prototypic Systems for Optically Active Helical Polypeptides. Biopolymers, Symposia No. 1, 75 (1964).
13. Pettersen, R. C., G. Ferguson, L. Crombie, M. L. Games, and D. J. Pointer: The Structure and Stereochemistry of Phorbol, Diterpene Parent of Cocarcinogens of Croton Oil. Chem. Communications 1967, 716.
14. Schaffner, K. u. G. Snatzke: Circulardichroitische Messungen an gesättigten und α,β-ungesättigten Cyclopropyl-ketonen. Helvet. chim. Acta 48, 347 (1965).
15. Snatzke, G. and H. W. Fehlhaber: Circulardichroismus-III. Tetrahedron 20, 1243 (1964).
16. Velluz, L., M. Legrand, and M. Grosjean: Optical Circular Dichroism, p. 110–114. Weinheim: Verlag Chemie 1965.

Ermittlung von Partialstrukturen des Phorbols durch Perjodat- und Bleitetraacetatspaltung

Von

M. Gschwendt und E. Hecker

Alle aus Crotonöl in reiner Form isolierten entzündlichen und cocarcinogenen Wirkstoffe sind Fettsäurediester desselben Grundalkohols – Phorbol –, wobei jeweils die beiden Hydroxylgruppen an C-12 und C-13 (vgl. Abb. 1) verestert sind.

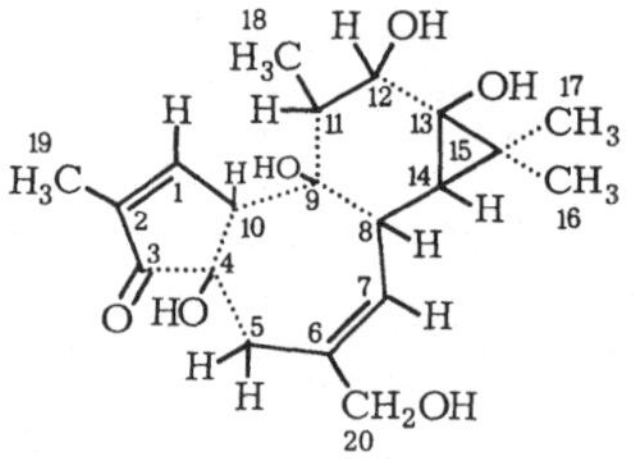

Abb. 1. Ausgezogene Linien: Durch KMR-Messungen mit Spinentkopplung sowie chemische Reaktionen festgelegte Teilstrukturen des Phorbols. Punktiert: Strukturelemente, die auf Grund von physikalischen und chemischen Messungen festliegen und deren Verknüpfung mit den Teilstrukturen zur Struktur des Phorbols führt

Die cocarcinogene oder tumorrealisierende Wirkung der aus Crotonöl isolierten Naturstoffe besteht darin, daß diese imstande sind, eine in einer *Initialphase* durch eine unterschwellige Dosis eines Carcinogens erzeugte latente Tumorkeimanlage in einer *Realisierungsphase* zur Geschwulst zu entwickeln.

Für die Untersuchung dieser Realisierungsphase und damit für die Untersuchung des Wirkungsmechanismus der tumorrealisierenden Wirkstoffe aus Crotonöl ist die Kenntnis der Struktur ihres Grundalkohols Phorbol von entscheidender Bedeutung. Über die Strukturaufklärung von Phorbol mit chemischen und spektrometrischen Methoden soll im folgenden berichtet werden.

Den Ansatzpunkt für Oxydationsversuche an Phorbol bildeten die in unserem Arbeitskreis durch Kernresonanzmessungen mit Spinentkoppelung und chemische Reaktionen festgelegten Teilstrukturen von Phorbol [1]. Sie sind in Abb. 1 durch ausgezogene Linien wiedergegeben.

Wie in dem vorangegangenen Vortrag bereits erwähnt wurde, sprechen mehrere Befunde für das Vorliegen einer nicht reduzierenden tertiären Acyloingruppe im Phorbol, die verätherbar, jedoch mit Acetanhydrid/Pyridin nicht veresterbar ist. Das Vorliegen einer solchen Acyloingruppe und ihre Stellung im Molekül werden durch die in Abb. 2 angegebene Reaktionsfolge bewiesen:

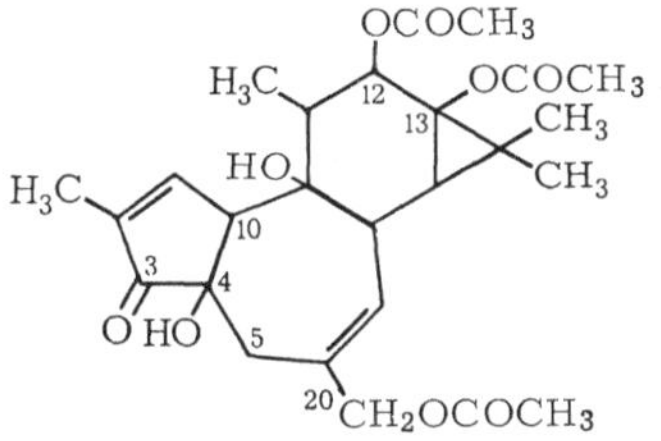

Phorbol-12,13,20-triacetat 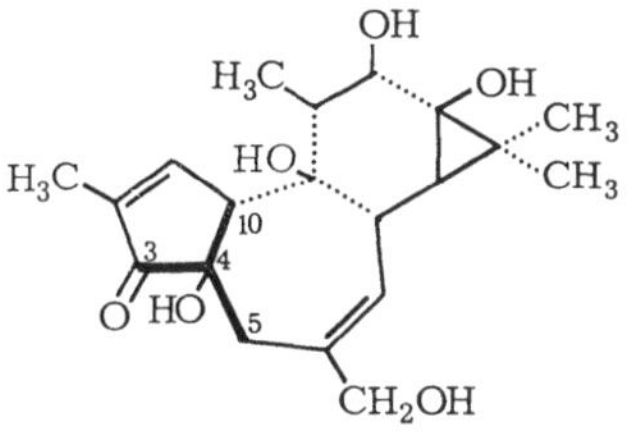   (5)

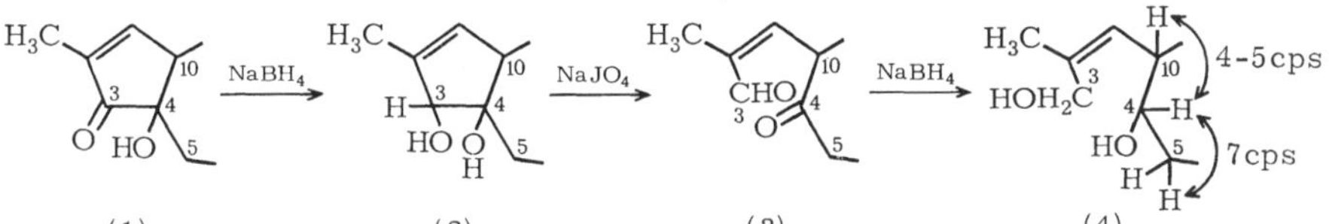

Abb. 2. Beweis für das Vorliegen einer tertiären Acyloingruppe sowie deren Lokalisierung im 5-Ring des Phorbols

Ausgehend von Phorbol-12,13,20-triacetat wird nach Reduktion der tertiären Acyloingruppe (Abb. 2) (1) mit Natriumborhydrid die entstandene sekundär-tertiäre Glykolgruppe (2) mit Natriumperjodat zum Ketoaldehyd (3) gespalten. Reduktion des Ketoaldehyds liefert den primär-sekundären Alkohol (4), in dem die Sequenz C-10, C-4, C-5 durch kernmagnetische Doppelresonanzmessungen eindeutig bewiesen werden kann. Die Kopplungen H-10/H-4 sowie H-4/H-5 sind in Abb. 2 angegeben. Formel (5) zeigt die erweiterten Teilstrukturen von Phorbol, in denen die neuen Verknüpfungen verstärkt gezeichnet sind.

Für die Klärung der Struktur und Lokalisation der α-Glykolgruppe in Phorbol ist seine Oxydation mit Bleitetraacetat und Natriumperjodat von großer Bedeutung.

Die Oxydation von Phorbol mit äquimolaren Mengen Bleitetraacetat (vgl. Tab. 1) liefert neben 16% eines nicht weiter untersuchten Substanzgemisches mit einer Ausbeute von zusammen 70% drei neue Verbindun-

172   M. Gschwendt und E. Hecker

gen: Bisdehydrophorbol (Abb. 3), Tiglophorbol und Phorbolactonhalbacetal. Die Oxydation von Phorbol mit 2 Mol Natriumperjodat liefert ein
weiteres Produkt – Hydroxy-phorbolactonhalbacetal, während Bisdehydrophorbol nicht nachgewiesen werden kann. Die vier Oxydationsprodukte
sind in reiner Form isoliert, charakterisiert und in ihrer Struktur geklärt
worden.

Tabelle 1. *Oxydationsprodukte von Phorbol*

Substanz	Summenformel	Ausbeute in % d. Theorie bei	
		Pb(OAc)$_4$-Oxyd.	NaJO$_4$-Oxyd.
Tiglophorbol	C$_{20}$H$_{26}$O$_6$	37	15
Bisdehydrophorbol	C$_{20}$H$_{26}$O$_6$	25	—
Phorbolactonhalbacetal	C$_{20}$H$_{24}$O$_6$	8	37
Hydroxyphorbolacton- halbacetal	C$_{20}$H$_{26}$O$_7$	—	18
Gemisch		ca. 16	—

Phorbol   Bisdehydrophorbol

(6)   (7)   (8)

Abb. 3. Oxydation des Phorbols mit Bleitetraacetat unter Öffnung des Cyclopropanrings zu Bisdehydrophorbol

Bereits 1959 hatten KAUFFMANN u. Mitarb. [2] bei der Bleitetraacetatoxydation von Phorbol Tiglophorbol und Aceton isoliert. Den
Nachweis von Aceton konnten wir jedoch nicht reproduzieren.

Wegen der Beteiligung eines Cyclopropanols an der α-Glykolgruppe
(Abb. 3) (6) wird diese von Bleitetraacetat, wie auch von Natriumperjodat, nicht in der bekannten Weise zwischen den beiden Hydroxylgruppen gespalten. Vielmehr hat die Öffnung des Cyclopropanringes

Vorrang und führt zu einem Carboniumion (7), für das es mehrere Reaktionsmöglichkeiten gibt. Eine davon führt unter Abspaltung eines Protons aus einer der beiden geminalen Methylgruppen zur Bildung von Bisdehydrophorbol (8).

Der Vergleich der Kernresonanzspektren von Bisdehydrophorbol und Phorbol ergibt eine weitgehende Übereinstimmung beider Strukturen. Allein im Bereich des Cyclopropanringes treten wesentliche Veränderungen auf. Das Verschwinden der Signale des Cyclopropanprotons (das durch seine charakteristische Lage bei besonders hohen Feldstärken auf-

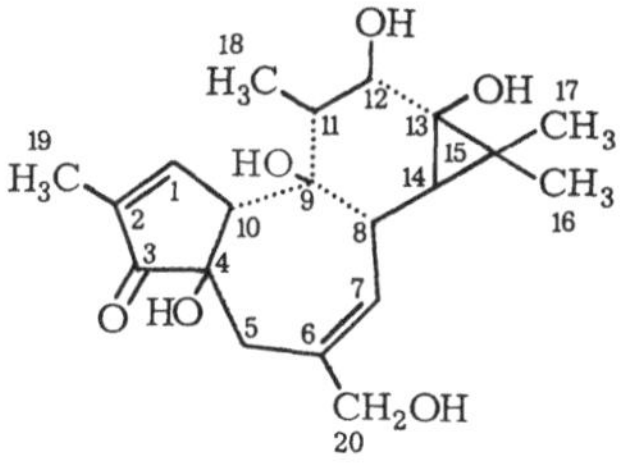

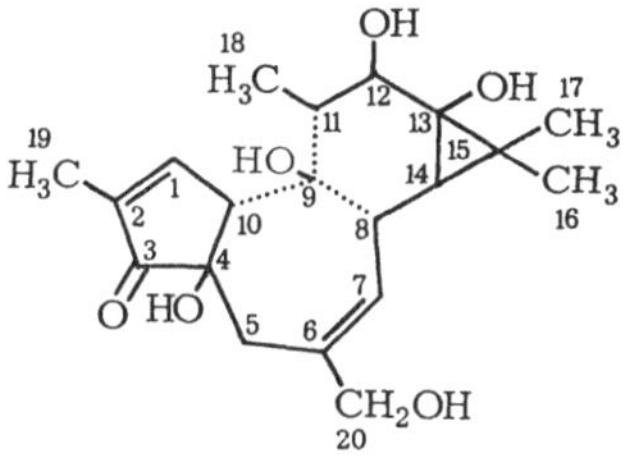

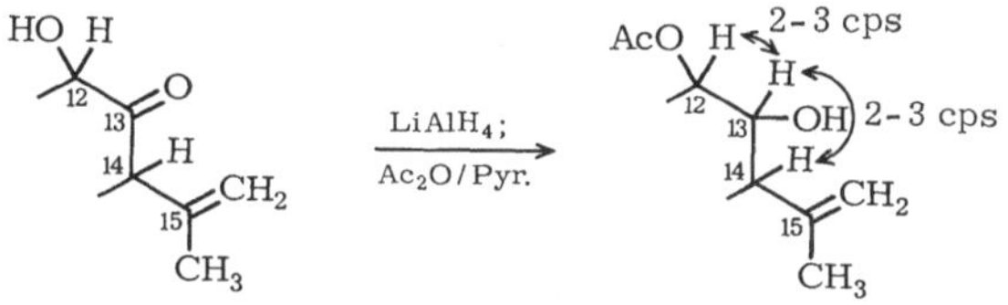

Abb. 4. Beweis für die Verknüpfung des tertiären Cyclopropanhydroxyls mit der sekundären Hydroxylgruppe des Phorbols zur α-Glykolgruppe im Phorbol

fällt) und der beiden geminalen Methylgruppen sowie das Auftreten der Signale einer neuen Methylgruppe an einer Doppelbindung und einer endständigen Methylengruppe führen zur Formulierung einer aus dem Cyclopropanring entstandenen Isopropenylgruppe. Die neue, gesättigte Carbonylgruppe läßt sich nach selektiver Reduktion der α,β-ungesättigten Ketogruppe im Ultraviolett-Spektrum nachweisen. Damit ist die α,α'-Dimethylcyclopropanol-Teilstruktur des Phorbols gesichert.

Noch gibt es mehrere Möglichkeiten, die drei Teilstrukturen des Phorbols (Abb. 4) (9) zu verknüpfen. Bisdehydrophorbol erweist sich als Schlüsselsubstanz für den Nachweis der Verknüpfung von C-12 mit C-13. Nach Reduktion von Bisdehydrophorbol (10) mit Lithiumalanat und anschließender Acetylierung kann man eine Substanz (11) isolieren, die die Hydroxylgruppe an C-12 acetyliert und die aus der Carbonylgruppe entstandene Hydroxylgruppe an C-13 unverestert enthält. Mit Hilfe kernmagnetischer Doppelresonanzmessungen lassen sich die im Bild eingezeichneten Kopplungen nachweisen, womit die Verknüpfung der Kohlenstoffatome 12 und 13 sichergestellt ist. Es gibt nun nur noch eine Möglichkeit, die verbleibenden offenen Bindungen zu schließen, da drei freien Valenzen verschiedener Kohlenstoffatome drei freie Valenzen eines einzigen Kohlenstoffatoms gegenüberstehen (Abb. 4) (9a).

Bildungsweise und Struktur der übrigen Oxydationsprodukte von Phorbol können im Rahmen dieses kurzen Vortrages nicht besprochen werden.

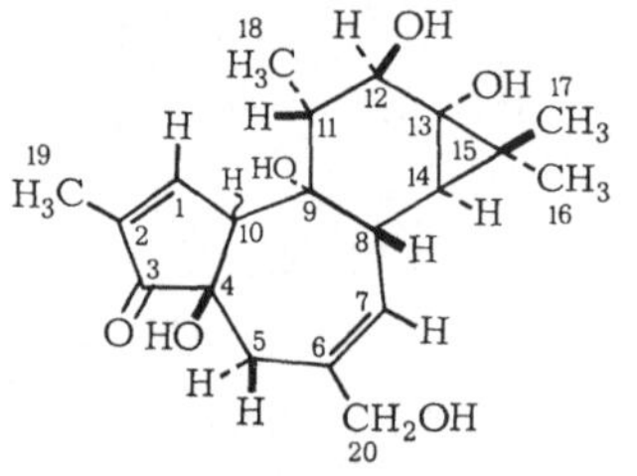

Abb. 5. Relative Konfiguration des Phorbols sowie Konformation des 6-Rings. Die absolute Konfiguration der Asymmetriezentren ist durch Röntgenstrukturanalyse ermittelt

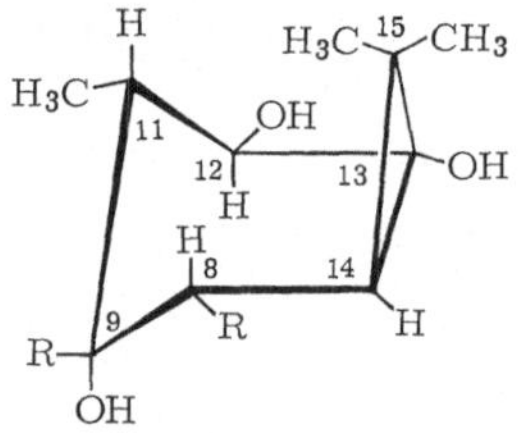

Abb. 5 zeigt die relative Konfiguration von Phorbol (12), soweit sie auf Grund der Strukturen und der Kernresonanzdaten der Oxydationsprodukte von Phorbol abgeleitet werden kann. Mit Ausnahme von C-10 sind alle Asymmetriezentren konfigurativ bestimmt.

Für die Bicyclo-(4.1.0)-heptan-Teilstruktur des Phorbols sind ohne Berücksichtigung der Spiegelbilder vier verschiedene Konformationen denkbar: zwei Halbsessel- und zwei Wannenformen. Da eine trans-diaxiale Verknüpfung von Cyclohexan- und Cycloheptanring nicht möglich ist, und auf Grund der Kernresonanzdaten können drei Möglichkeiten ausgeschlossen werden. Danach liegt im Phorbol die in Abb. 5 (13) gezeigte Halbsesselform vor.

Literatur

1. HECKER, E., CH. V. SZCZEPANSKI, H. KUBINYI, H. BRESCH, E. HÄRLE, H. U. SCHAIRER u. H. BARTSCH: Über die Wirkstoffe des Crotonöls, VII. Phorbol. Z. Naturforsch. **21**b, 1204 (1966).
2. KAUFFMANN, TH., A. EISINGER, W. JASCHING u. K. LENHARDT: Zur Konstitution des Phorbols, II. Über die α-Glykolgruppe des Phorbols. Chem. Ber. **92**, 1727 (1959).

D.

4. wissenschaftliche Sitzung am Mittwoch, den 27. 9. 1967

Vorsitz: G. Wagner

Molecular Units of the Mitotic Apparatus and the Government of Mitosis*

By

D. MAZIA

If it is true that a deeper knowledge of mitosis is one of the roads toward a deeper insight into the cancer problem, the truism is too dilute for practical or heuristic purposes. Mitosis is not a phenomenon of cells but a destiny. Research has to be directed toward phenomena, and it is not self-evident that the relevant phenomenon is the act of mitosis itself, seen as a culmination of the life of a cell.

What aspects of mitosis are most relevant to the cancer problem? On the aspect that I call "organismal" all would agree; that is, we all recognize that the decision of a normal cell to divide or not to divide is under the government of the society of cells that is the "body" and that the student of cancer is concerned with the nature of that government and the escape of some cells from its rule. There is now a good deal of interest in humoral factors and factors of cell contact by which a collective of cells governs the reproductive behavior of its members, and it is not obvious that useful answers to such questions require a deep and detailed knowledge of the process of mitosis itself.

We know that the decisive events which prepare a cell for division – and which do not occur in a cell that is not planning to divide – begin early in interphase [9]. Of these events, the most conspicuous is some change in the chromosomes whereby their DNA can commence to replicate. One can make a very good case for the proposition that research on the commitment of a cell to division should focus on its life early in interphase.

Thus I introduce a discussion of mitosis itself, the transformations of the cell which bring about the separation of the replicated chromosomes, the series of events from the beginning of prophase to the end of telophase, by pointing out that the study of these processes *might* not be so relevant to the control of cell reproduction. But the study of the control

---

* This work was supported in part by grant GM 13882 from the U.S.-Public Health Service, National Institutes of Health, to DANIEL MAZIA.

of division and of the preparations for mitosis tends to be carried out at a rather superficial level, and a deeper level may be accessible through a consideration of the processes that are being controlled or prepared for.

Structure and molecular units of structure in the mitotic apparatus

At first glance, it would seem that the mitotic performance is composed of at least three groups of processes: the cycle of chromosome condensation, the buildup of a mitotic spindle, and the execution of the chromosome movements. As research problems, these processes have in common the fact that they are problems of structure and only indirectly problems of biosynthesis. We shall want to ask whether they have even more in common; at least we can ask whether the problem of the assembly of the mitotic apparatus and problem of the movements it carries out may be the same problem.

When KATSUMA DAN and I isolated the mitotic apparatus back in 1952 [8] by a combination of rather extreme procedures and dissolved the preparations by equally extreme procedures, we came to the following conclusions about its molecular character. First, it was composed largely of one protein, the so-called major protein, for which we obtained a sedimentation constant of about 4s and an estimated molecular weight of the order of magnitude of 45,000 with the limited resources then at our disposal. Second, we concluded that S-S bonds played a large role in the assembly of the proteins into a mitotic apparatus, with the reservation that other types of intermolecular bonding were involved.

The pursuit of the major protein has continued in the intervening years. Some of the findings were: evidence that the protein may be synthesized before the onset of mitosis and assembled during mitosis; evidence of an association of the protein with nucleotides; strong parallelisms of its properties and composition with those of actin from muscle; a variety of confirmations of the original contention that S-S bonds played an important role in intermolecular association (reviewed in [9]). The characterization of the molecular units became satisfactory, in my opinion, with the work of our collaborator SAKAI [14]. The practical problem – and one that I now think may have profound significance – lay in the problem of dissolving the isolated mitotic apparatus down to genuine molecular units. We are dealing with molecules that have a strong tendency to associate spontaneously into states that are extremely difficult to dissolve – behavior which may be important in the formation of stable structures but which has created problems and controversy in the biochemical research. SAKAI's findings were the following. The direct dissociation of isolated mitotic apparatus of sea urchin eggs – the only material on which we have a body of information – permits the isolation of the "major protein" as a particle having a sedimentation constant of 3.5 s, and a molecular weight of about 68,000. The particle is a dimer, composed of 2.5 s subunits having a molecular weight of about 34,000. The monomer subunits, each of which has 4-SH groups, are joined in the dimer by one S-S bond. Thus far, only the dimers (and larger aggregates) have been obtained by direct dissolution of the mitotic apparatus; the monomers are obtained only if the S-S bond is cleaved or reduced. I will use this characterization of the major protein of the mitotic apparatus in the following discussion, recognizing however that future detailed study may modify the picture of the molecule.

Structurally, the mitotic spindle had been thought to be a system of fibers whose arrangements were consistent with their proposed functions. The light microscope had revealed a set of fibers running from chromosomes to poles, which might be thought to contract when the chromosomes move to the poles. A second set of fibers, making up the so-called central spindle, was seen to run from pole to pole, and could be thought to elongate as the pole-to-pole distance increased, as it does late in anaphase in many cases. A debate about the "reality" of these fibers was not alleviated by the earlier attempts to see them with the electron microscope, which were mostly unsuccessful.

An important advance was the discovery that the fibrous elements of the mitotic spindle consist of microtubules, a discovery we owe mainly to DE HARVEN and BERNHARD [4]. But the mitotic apparatus as isolated does not consist entirely of microtubules, for it is a coherent region of the cell that also includes vesicles and ribosomes in varying amounts [3] and may also include material which is not identified by electron microscopy.

All the structural and molecular components of the mitotic apparatus may be of interest, but all our preconceptions direct our first interest to the "spindle fibers". (At this point I am not considering the chromosomes.) The earlier work on the chemistry of the mitotic apparatus was carried out by dissolving the entire structure and characterizing its molecules, and one could not be sure that the "major protein" which was the center of interest from a chemical standpoint was derived from microtubules. Recently, we have presented the evidence that the "major protein" does derive from microtubules [6]. SAKAI had found that 70% of all the protein in the isolated mitotic apparatus was dissolved in 0.5 M KCl at pH 8.5, and that the "major protein" was 60% of all the dissolved protein. Thus, the "major protein" represents 40% of all the protein contained in the apparatus as isolated by the method used [10]. Electron microscopic study showed that the dissolution procedure did put the microtubules into solution, and conversely that other material contained in the mitotic apparatus – ribosomes, vesicles, etc. – was found in the undissolved fraction. Thus, we can conclude that the dissolved proteins include the proteins of the microtubules.

The rest of the argument is based on the correspondence between the size of the molecular units of microtubules as observed by high resolution electron microscopy and the size to be expected from the properties of the molecules. The microtubule is generally seen in material fixed, embedded and sectioned as a straight, unbranched body of tubular appearance, about 200 Å in diameter. In favorable cross-sections, 13 linear elements are seen to make up the tubules [7]. In material spread on grids and negatively stained the tubule can easily be resolved as a cylindrical array of filaments, the number of filaments being about 13. Further resolution shows that the filaments are linear arrays of particles. The particles measure about 35–40 Å in diameter in negatively-stained preparations. Comparing the particles seen at high resolution in microtubules from isolated mitotic apparatus with the unit molecules isolated from the same material, we concluded that the molecular unit of the structure of the microtubules of the mitotic apparatus was the "major protein". In our publication [6] we gave arguments in favor of the 2.5 s subunit as the visible unit, although the measurements made by the electron microscope are not really accurate enough to distinguish between the 2.5 s subunit (estimated molecular weight, 34,000) and the 3.5 s unit, the dimer, of twice that weight. At present, the latter is more appealing to me in terms of the theorizing that I will undertake below.

Assembly of the mitotic apparatus

The other issue in the background is the matter of the role of SH-groups in the mitotic apparatus. There is a large body of evidence which can be summarized in this way: experiments designed to ask whether S-S bonds are essential to the formation of the mitotic apparatus always gave positive results. Yet there is an equally valid body of evidence from experiments asking whether the mitotic apparatus is held together by weaker bonds, often referred to in the literature as hydrogen bonds. Such experiments also give positive results: the coherence and orientation of the mitotic apparatus depends on weak bonds. As will be seen, these findings are no longer contradictory; the hypothesis I now make assigns an essential role to both kinds of bonds.

The hypothesis is simple and invokes few unknown facts or unfamiliar concepts. It merely states that the unit of the assembly of the micro-tubule is the dimer which in fact is obtained when one dissolves the microtubule under "mild" conditions. If one adds the hypothesis that the conformational state required for the proper fit of the units exists only in the dimer, then one cannot make a mitotic apparatus without first linking the monomers by an S-S bond. Conversely, the structure may become unstable if the S-S bond is split. But the assembly of the dimeric units into filaments and into the tubules depends on weak bonding between these units, thus the structure of the mitotic apparatus as a whole would always be subject to the conditions for weak bonding. The final assembly of the structure would be governed by those factors which have been studied in other cases of the "spontaneous self-assembly" of relatively small and "globular" proteins, such as the G-F transformation of actin and the assembly of virus coats. These factors, one notes, generally are the factors of the small-molecule environment in which the macromolecules are placed: pH, metallic ions, nucleotides, etc. In a sense, "spontaneous self-assembly" is the counterpart of the allosteric effects now being studied by the students of enzyme regulation. In the latter case, small molecules bring about conformational changes in the proteins which influence their "fit" with substrates; in self-assembly, the conformational changes influence the "fit" of structural protein molecules with other protein molecules of their own kind.

The formation of a mitotic apparatus would, then, involve the following: synthesis of the monomeric subunits; dimerization by formation of S-S bonds; assembly into the microtubules. The synthesis, we know, is completed before prophase. We know little about the dimerization, although we can imagine it to be driven by a cycle of changes in the soluble thiols of the cell such as was first described by RAPKINE [12]. About the final assembly, we can make some speculations. Microtubules of the mitotic apparatus appear to grow from centrioles and at least their orientation is determined by centrioles. It may not help very much to propose that the centrioles function as loci which maintain a small-molecule environment favorable for the self-assembly of microtubules, yet such a proposal will have more meaning when – as I am sure will happen soon in one of the laboratories working on the problem – the conditions for such assembly are defined through successful assembly *in vitro*.

Assembly and movement in the mitotic apparatus

The assembly of the mitotic apparatus leads to its operation; that is, to the movements of chromosomes. These movements begin as soon as the nuclear membrane breaks down. The movements of chromosomes can be described by the shortening and lengthening of the spindle fibers, thus of the microtubules, and I will not debate here whether these changes of length of the fibers actually exert mechanical pull or push or express a guidance device; they would be important in either case and we are pretty sure that mitosis will not be achieved without them. So far as can be judged from electron-microscopic evidence, of which there is a good deal, the changes in the length are changes in mass; that is, the microtubules do not change in thickness as they shorten or lengthen. This has been interpreted, especially by INOUE [5], in terms of an hypothesis that postulates a dynamic equilibrium between the molecules in the oriented form – presumably in microtubules, although this detail has been questioned by BEHNKE and FORER [1], – and a pool of unoriented and presumably unassociated molecules in the background. In my opinion, the evidence for the conclusion that the shortening and lengthening of the microtubules is a subtraction or addition of molecules from the tubules is very good. To the extent that these changes are related in any way to the movements of chromosomes, we can conclude that the formation and the function of the mitotic apparatus are similar processes. If such an analysis of the problem, having gone this far in the identification of the molecules, in the characterization of the microtubular structure into which they are organized and in the description of the visible changes associated with mitotic movements, does not help us answer the question "how are chromosomes moved", the difficulty lies in the failure of our science to have found the basis of *any* kind of movement. The analogy is given by the exhaustively studied case of muscle. There we know the molecules, know their structural arrangements in filaments, possess a remarkably complete description of the visible changes (sliding rather than absolute shortening) – but have no useful theory of how the shortening actually takes place. It is simply that we know a lot about the composition and assembly of structures but have no science dealing with the translation of molecules in space.

I have summarized the work on the chemistry of the mitotic apparatus which has led to a characterization of the classical "spindle fibers" in molecular terms. There are, of course, other kinds of questions. For example, there is very good evidence of the involvement of ATP in mitosis and fair evidence about an ATPase of the mitotic apparatus. There are studies of the association of nucleotides with the structure of the mitotic apparatus, but that picture is not clear. If I have been able to speculate in loose terms about the function of the centrioles, there is even less to say about the important functions of the kinetochores. One can make a neat hypothesis by saying that the processes which lead to the growth of microtubules are located in the centriole while the processes leading to the shortening are located at the kinetochores. Thus we could understand how chromosome-to-pole connection can either lengthen or shorten, while pole-to-pole connections only lengthen. But such a statement only tells us where to look, not what to look for. Finally, it is not so easy to segregate the problem of the cycle of chromosome condensation from the problem of the spindle. While it is true that the chromosome cycle goes on in the apparent absence of a spindle, as in natural endomitosis or in experiments with colchicine-like agents, nevertheless it has to be coordinated closely with the rest of the mitotic process in the normal case.

Interpretation of antimitotic action

Now I return to the question of the control of mitosis in the normal organism and in the organism under treatment. Once more, it must be admitted that the most striking lead we have is one that is not related to the mitotic process itself in an obvious way. This is the fact that the "turning on" of DNA synthesis generally commits a cell to divide, and cells which do not intend to divide do not enter into DNA synthesis. We see this in the normal organism and you who work in therapy use it in your application of antimetabolites such as fluorouracil. However, the conspicuousness of this one important process does not necessarily make it primary or independent. In saying that the turning on of DNA synthesis leads to mitosis we are also saying that all the other preparations which divert the cell from one that is minding its current business to one that is anticipating division are also turned on. Cases where cells make DNA but do not subsequently make a spindle are rare, and even in such cases it could be that the processes leading to a spindle are begun but are aborted. The only important case where cells make a spindle without having doubled their DNA is the special case of the second meiotic division. There must be a deep connection between the chromosomes and the factors responsible for the mitotic apparatus, and we do not know which if any leads the way.

The search for ways to control cell division has included studies of antimitotic agents in the narrow sense of the term: agents that stop mitosis after it has been set into motion. Much of that work has been done in the distinguished laboratory of Professor Lettré here in Heidelberg.

In my opinion, the investigation of this type of antimitotic action – the effect of "spindle poisons" of which colchicine is the prototype – is now subject to a molecular and predictive attack, which derives from our present knowledge of the chemistry of the mitotic apparatus. The first assumption is that the spindle-poisoning action is a prevention of the assembly of the microtubules and – up to a certain point in anaphase when cells in mitosis will complete mitosis – a disruption of the structure of microtubules already present. The microtubules are assembled by self-association of a molecular unit which can now be isolated, and the assembly depends on an exact conformation fit between the molecules. It is now proposed that all the spindle poisons are agents which combine with these molecular units, and that the combination brings about a conformational change which in turn affects the ability of the molecules to associate with the exactness of fit that is necessary to make a proper microtubule. One notes that the agents combine with the unit molecule, before assembly, and thus assembly can be prevented. After assembly has taken place, the agent might act in two ways. It might combine with molecules already assembled, distorting their structure so that the association falls apart. Or one may appeal to the hypothesis [5] that the assembled molecules are in equilibrium with a pool of unassembled molecules. Thus, binding the agent to the unassembled molecules will cause a dissociation of the assembled ones according to ordinary equilibrium considerations. Finally, one can see how the molecules of the microtubules at a certain stage – say anaphase, which can be completed in the presence of spindle-poisons – might be associated so firmly that they would not bind the antimitotic agent; possibly the sites to which the agent would attach are occupied by the interaction of the protein units themselves.

Thanks to the recent work of BORISY and TAYLOR [2], we now have evidence that colchicine does bind specifically to a protein which is a structural unit of microtubules. They show that colchicine is bound to a protein molecule which is present in free form in many kinds of cells and which is also present in the mitotic apparatus and in at least the central microtubules of flagellae. WILSON and FRIEDKIN [16] also have obtained evidence on the existence of a colchicine binding macromolecule.

It is not surprising, of course, that colchicine does bind to a protein, but my point is that the molecule is one that we know and can isolate, that it is the structural unit of the microtubules of the mitotic apparatus, and that it is also present in an unassociated form in cells that do not have a mitotic apparatus. I predict, then, that one can study and test antimitotic agents of the spindle-poison type in an exact way *in vitro*. The first proposition is that the action of such agents is predictable from their tendency to bind to the protein. Moreover, the mysterious fact that the many agents acting like colchicine seem to be very different from colchicine in their structure may be no mystery at all. Their common feature would be their tendency to bind to this particular protein, the structural unit of the microtubules of the mitotic apparatus, a property which might not be evident from the inspection of structural formulas. A second proposition is that the binding alone might not be a quantitative measure of antimitotic action because the binding would be effective only to the extent that it led to a conformational distortion of the protein, interfering with its self-assembly. This might be difficult to measure, for the measurement of conformational change is still a new field in the study of proteins. But it is an active one in which rapid progress can be expected.

It should, in my opinion, now be possible to deal in a very much more precise way with the development of substances which prevent or attack the formation of the mitotic apparatus. One then asks those who have experience with attempts at cancer therapy through antimitotic agents: is there a set of specifications for such an agent that would make it more useful in practice?

Molecular units of cell structure; a generalization

The casual reader of the literature on cancer constantly encounters the idea that there ought to be a fundamental difference between "cancer" and "normal" cells. While such a difference has been sought without spectacular success by comparing supposed prototypes of the two kinds of cells according to most of the biochemical and metabolic criteria known to us, you who work with cancer are compelled daily to make decisions as to differences between cancer and normal cells by criteria of structure. Such criteria are empirical, but in a loose way they do relate to the contrast between cells whose main activity is continuing division and cells whose activity is related to their differentiation, their association into tissues and organs, and in general to the government of the organism.

Naturally, those of us who have worked on the chemistry of mitosis have thought a good deal about the structural character of cells preparing for mitosis – and the molecular basis of that character. The isolation of the mitotic apparatus and the discovery of the "major protein" was followed by the finding which could almost have been guessed by eye – that the mitotic spindle of a dividing cell represented a substantial proportion of all the protein in that cell. If this was mostly of one kind, and if – as is the case – it has to be synthesized before division, then it seemed logical to conclude that a major activity of the interphase cell was the synthesis of a "division protein". Such a synthesis of a large amount of a protein of one kind has, at times, been thought of as a diversion of the biosynthetic activity of the cell from other pathways which would make the proteins which are expressed in differentiation; in any case, it has seemed to be useful to think of a cell preparing for division as one that was synthesizing a "division protein".

I would not take such a position now. I think that the recent study of cell structure – of which the study of mitotic structures has been a part – leads to a more comprehensive view of the molecular basis of all structure. In fact, I think a major and revolutionary insight into the cell is now breaking, having evolved in a patient and piecemeal way in the hands of many cell biologists and having been overshadowed by the seemingly more exciting developments in molecular genetics and the control of biosynthesis.

Improvements of the preparative techniques of electron microscopy first showed that the fibrillar structure of the cilia and flagella and of the mitotic apparatus was based on microtubules. Moreover, the structure of the microtubules, even at high resolution, seems to be the same in the spindle fiber and in the filaments of cilia and flagella.

It is now found that the molecular units are similar. I have described above the molecular unit of the microtubules of the mitotic apparatus, concluding that the unit of assembly was the 3.5 s dimer to which SAKAI assigns a molecular weight of around 68,000. We owe to IAN GIBBONS the basic work on the molecules composing the microtubules of cilia [15], and he finds a unit of molecular weight of around 60,000. So far as I can see, the properties of the molecules from the two sources are similar, though much of the detailed study remains to be done. Recently, I have attempted the next step of isolating the 2.5 s monomer from microtubules from flagella by reduction of S-S bonds and have obtained such units.

Meanwhile, the literature has abounded in excellent descriptions of microtubules in all kinds of cells and in all kinds of structural situations. I cannot attempt to review that large literature. Workers in the field have been interested in the association of microtubular structures with cell movements, as in the microvilli and active projections of cells, in the cortex of streaming plant cells, in melanocytes, in the axopods of heliozoan protozoa, in relation to the saltatory movements so often observed in movies of cells in culture [13]. I wonder if the distinction between structure and movement would be a sharp one if we could observe all kinds of cells while they are alive. There is another class of structure associated with movement, the so-called microfilaments, which some workers are inclined to relate to the microtubules. These filaments, often associated with streaming movement, have the same dimensions (about 40 Å) as the individual filaments whose side-by-side associations make up the microtubules. We owe to KEITH PORTER the important proposal that the microtubules may participate generally in the form and the movements of cells [11].

If all this is so, then the type of molecule which we called the major protein of the mitotic apparatus may in fact be a major protein of cell structure in general. As a promise of that possibility, we have the recent observations of BORISY and TAYLOR [2] who used colchicine binding as a criterion of the microtubule protein. It is interesting that they found nerve cells to be the richest source of the colchicine-binding protein. That would be a surprising result if one correlated the protein with mitosis, but not at all surprising if one correlated it with filamentous and microtubular structure.

In this brief statement of ideas that are just developing, I must acknowledge the reservation that all microtubules may not necessarily be the same. E. g., BEHNKE and FORER [1] have argued that there are several kinds of microtubules because birefringence varies in various

parts of the mitotic apparatus independently of the number of microtubules and because certain other cytological properties vary. BORISY
and TAYLOR distinguish between the central microtubules of flagella
which react with colchicine and the peripheral microtubules which do not.
From my own experience, I would suggest that microtubules may vary a
great deal at the level of intermolecular association, without correspond-
ing differences in the molecular units. For example, the transitory
microtubules of the mitotic apparatus are so unstable that methods of
isolation must be considered to be methods of imposing stability upon
them. We prefer to work with barely stable isolated mitotic apparatus, in
which the microtubules hold together in the isolation medium but can be
dissolved in 0.5 M KCl. But everyone who has worked in the field has
remarked that the microtubules of the mitotic apparatus pass spontaneously into a more stable state in which they can be dissolved only by
drastic means, involving high pH and agents that attack S-S bonds. Yet
the molecules obtained from the stable states seem to be the same as those
obtained from less stable states. In nature, the microtubules of cilia and
flagella are more stable than those of the mitotic apparatus; they appear
to be permanent structures. The peripheral ring of microtubules is
especially stable in isolation and difficult to dissolve. Yet when these
microtubules are dissolved, they give a molecule similar to that obtained
from the mitotic apparatus. We need not expect all formed microtubules
in cells to be the same, yet we may make the hypothesis that they are
composed of the same kinds of molecules.

Thus I am proposing that there is a major protein of cells that is the
structural element not only of the mitotic apparatus but of a wide range
of cell structures. The hypothesis is not a guess, but is admittedly a rather
audacious generalization of a body of fact that is not negligible. In a way,
it has an ancient history, which interestingly enough stems from the
pioneer work on mitosis. When STRASBURGER wrote of a "kinoplasm" and
FLEMMING wrote of an "archoplasm" their proposals had about the same
intent as what I am saying, with the difference that the 19th century
resorted to the rather vague idea of "plasms" while we imagine we are on
a more solid ground with molecules. Since I am speaking of molecules that
do exist and are important, even if my larger generalization is wrong, I
propose the name *tektin* or the generic name *tektins* for these molecules, a
name intended to convey the structural role.

From the standpoint of cancer research, the generalization which I
have been proposing could be fatal to a possibility that has been dis-
cussed a good deal, though perhaps not so much in print. If there is a
"mitotic protein", and if it can be isolated from the mitotic apparatus of a
given organism – say, the human – then it could be used diagnostically to
identify cells which are preparing for division whether they are dividing

or not. For example, such cells could be identified by the use of fluorescent antibodies to the "mitotic protein". Now I think the possibility must be rejected; there is no mitotic protein but there is a protein of microtubule (and perhaps microfilament) structure which is diverted to the making of a mitotic apparatus in cells that are going to divide.

Let us suppose that the cell can use the same kind of molecules to make different structures performing different functions. Given the molecule, how shall we attack the problem of structure? Obviously, there will be efforts to assemble structures *in vitro*. We can investigate the possibility that tektins are molecules that have alternative modes of fitting together and thus have alternative modes of assembling structures. But that does not get us far with the problem of the higher level of structure. For example – and this is now a much-discussed question – why is a flagellum formed in one situation and a mitotic apparatus in the other, when we know that the formation depends in large part on the same kinds of molecules and is even guided by the same kind of commanding particle, the centriole? The problem seems all the more painful in that it tends to wrench us away from the secure ground of the doctrine of molecular genetics, which is best adapted to explain differences in cells as differences in the proteins synthesized by cells. Of course, I do not know the answer but can suggest three directions in which our thinking might go. First, a little reflection tells us that "spontaneous self-assembly" is not, of course, spontaneous; it is the result of the establishment of a well-defined local medium in which the assembly can take place, and one that is no less definite because it involves small molecules. In fact the situation cautions the cell biologist who is concerned with structure to reactivate his interest in the work of his biological colleagues for whom pH, ionic concentrations, ATP concentrations, etc. are anything but trivial even if the molecules are small. Here we encounter a whole world of enzymes, carriers, transport systems, etc. in which the guidance mechanisms for structural assembly could reside. Second – and here I generalize the comments I made earlier about antimitotic agents – the forms of the structural molecules may very well be determined by the direct binding of smaller molecules, and these forms in turn may determine what kinds of assembly are favored. Third, our thinking is returning to the guidance of the assembly of structures by particles in the cell which we sometimes see as centrioles or kinetosomes, sometimes infer when cytological evidence is lacking (as in mitosis in plants). About these particles themselves we know almost nothing.

Summary

The spindle fibers of the mitotic apparatus, which govern the disposition of the chromosomes in mitosis, have been resolved into microtubules, and more recently the microtubules have been resolved to molecular units which in turn appear to be dimers of a subunit of molecular weight of about 34,000. An hypothesis concerning the assembly of the microtubules is proposed. It invokes two processes: (1) the formation of the dimeric structural units by formation of an S-S bond between two monomeric units and (2) the association of the dimeric units, under conditions favoring conformational "fit", by weak bonds, into the microtubule structure. The participation of the microtubules in chromosome movement – observed as lengthening or shortening of microtubules – is interpreted in terms of this hypothesis about the formation of microtubules. The action of antimitotic agents having the properties of "spindle poisons", of which colchicine is the most familiar example, is interpreted, and a way of testing and predicting such antimitotic action is proposed. A review of recent developments suggests that the spindle fiber is only one example of a more general participation of microtubules in cell structure and movement. If this is so, and if the molecular units of microtubules in various kinds of cell structure and movement is the same, the hypothesis that the main protein of the mitotic apparatus is a special "division protein" now has to be abandoned.

References

1. BEHNKE, O. and A. FORER: Evidence for four classes of microtubules in individual cells. J. Cell Sci. **2**, 169 (1967).
2. BORISY, G. G. and E. W. TAYLOR: The mechanism of the action of colchicine. Binding of colchicine-^{3}H to cellular protein. J. Cell Biol. **34**, 525 (1967); The mechanism of the action of colchicine. Colchicine binding to sea urchin eggs and the mitotic apparatus. J. Cell Biol. **34**, 535 (1967).
3. HARRIS, P.: Electron microscope study of mitosis in sea urchin blastomeres. J. biophys. biochem. Cytol. **11**, 419 (1961).
4. HARVEN, E, DE et W. BERNHARD: Etude au microscope electronique de l'ultrastructure du centriole chez les vertébrés. Z. Zellforsch. **45**, 378 (1956).
5. INOUE, S.: Organization and function of the mitotic spindle. In ALLEN, R. D. and N. KAMIYA (Edit.): Primitive Motile Systems in Cell Biology, p. 549. New York: Academic Press 1964.
6. KIEFER, B., H. SAKAI, A. J. SOLARI, and D. MAZIA: The molecular unit of the microtubules of the mitotic apparatus. J. mol. Biol. **20**, 75 (1966).
7. LEDBETTER, M. C., and K. R. PORTER: Morphology of microtubules of plant cells. Science **144**, 872 (1964).
8. MAZIA, D. and K. DAN: Isolation and biochemical characterization of the mitotic apparatus of dividing cells. Proc. nat. Acad. Sci. (Wash.) **38**, 826 (1952).
9. — Mitosis and the physiology of cell division. In BRACHET, J. and A. E. MIRSKY (Edit.): The Cell; Vol. III, p. 77. New York: Academic Press 1961.

10. Mazia, D., J. M. Mitchison, H. Medina, and P. Harris: The direct isolation of the mitotic apparatus. J. biophys. biochem. Cytol. **10**, 467 (1961).
11. Porter, K. R.: Cytoplasmic microtubules and their functions. In: Ciba Foundation Symposium on Principles of Biomolecular Organization, p. 308. Wolstenhome, G. E. W. and M. O'Connor (Edit.): London: J. A. Churchill, Ltd., 1966.
12. Rapkine, L.: Sur les processus chimiques au cours de la division cellulaire. Ann. Physiol. et Physiochim. biol. **7**, 382 (1931).
13. Rebhuhn, L.: Structural aspects of saltatory particle movement. J. gen. Physiol. **50** (pt. 2), 223 (1967).
14. Sakai, H.: Studies on sulfhydryl groups during cell division of sea urchin egg. VIII. Some properties of mitotic apparatus proteins. Biochim. biophys. Acta **112**, 132 (1966).
15. Stevens, R. E., F. L. Renaud, and I. R. Gibbons: Guanine nucleotide associated with the protein of the outer fibers of flagella and cilia. Science **156**, 1606 (1967).
16. Wilson, L. and M. Friedkin: The biochemical events of mitosis. II. The *in vivo* and *in vitro* binding of colchicine in grasshopper embryos and its possible relation to mitosis. Biochemistry **6**, 3126 (1967).

Elektronenmikroskopie der unbeeinflußten und beeinflußten mitotischen Zellteilung

Von

N. PAWELETZ

In den vergangenen fünf Jahren erschien eine Reihe von elektronenmikroskopischen Arbeiten über die Teilung tierischer und pflanzlicher Zellen (Literatur bei ALLENSPACH et al. [2]). ROBBINS et al. [10] beschrieben an Hand von zahlreichen guten Aufnahmen besonders eingehend die frühen Stadien der Teilung bei HeLa-Zellen. Wir haben uns deshalb bei unseren Untersuchungen, die ebenfalls an HeLa-Zellen durchgeführt wurden, zunächst auf die Beobachtung der späteren Mitosestadien beschränkt. Bei einem Teil unserer Versuche wurde die Zahl der Zellen in Teilung durch die Zugabe von Thymidin zum Nährmedium erhöht.

Bei lichtmikroskopischer Beobachtung wird während der Telophase, wenn die Tochterzellen noch durch eine Plasmabrücke miteinander verbunden sind, in der Mitte dieser Brücke ein kleines basophiles Körperchen sichtbar. FLEMMING [5] beschrieb es 1891 als Zwischenkörper (Abb. 1a). Da der Ausdruck Zwischenkörper in der neueren Zeit eine andere Bedeutung erhalten hat (siehe PAWELETZ [9]), soll das Gebilde als „Flemming-Körper" bezeichnet werden, eine Bezeichnung, die ebenfalls häufig gebraucht wird.

Wie entsteht der „Flemming-Körper" und welche Aufgabe hat er bei der Zellteilung?

Während der Anaphase, wenn sich die Chromosomengruppen trennen, erkennt man in elektronenmikroskopischen Aufnahmen mehrere kleine Bündel von Spindelfibrillen, die in einer ca. 0,4 μ breiten Zone von osmiophilem Material umgeben sind; in dieser osmiophilen Region liegen die Spindelfibrillen am engsten nebeneinander. Zwischen den Fibrillenbündeln findet man keine Einzelfibrillen ohne osmiophilen Abschnitt (Abb. 1c).

Durch die Einschnürung des Cytoplasmas zwischen den Chromosomengruppen werden die Fibrillenbündel enger zusammengedrängt, die osmiophilen Regionen vereinigen sich zu einem plattenartigen Gebilde, das im Schnitt als Streifen erscheint (Abb. 1b). Es soll als osmiophiler Streifen bezeichnet werden.

Während der Telophase wird die Plasmabrücke so schmal, daß die Spindelfibrillen zu einem einzigen großen Bündel zusammengedrückt werden (Abb. 1d). Durch ringförmige Einschnürungen zu beiden Seiten der osmiophilen Platte (Abb. 1d, Pfeile) entsteht der linsen- oder kugelförmige „Flemming-Körper", wie er im Lichtmikroskop sichtbar wird.

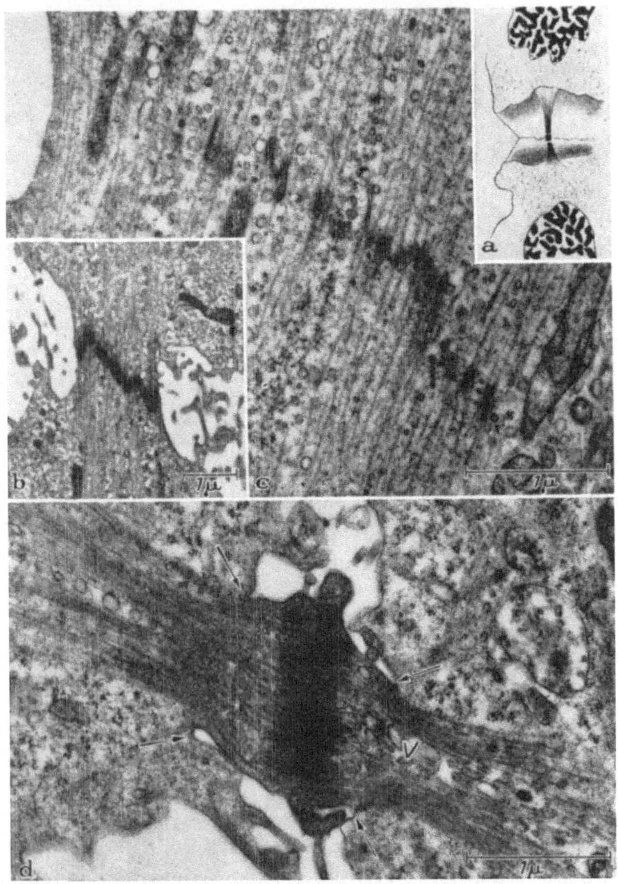

Abb. 1. a Telophase mit dem „Zwischenkörper". (Aus Flemming [5]). b Anaphase. Osmiophile Partien stellenweise zum Streifen vereinigt. c Telophase. Zusammenhängender osmiophiler Streifen in der Plasmabrücke. d Rekonstruktionsphase. „Flemming-Körper" ausgebildet. Ringförmige Einschnürung des Cytoplasmas (Pfeile), Vesikel (V). (Aus Paweletz [9])

Die beiden Tochterzellen bleiben durch die Plasmabrücke, die den „Flemming-Körper" enthält, noch mehrere Stunden nach dem Beginn der Anaphase verbunden (Abramson et al. [1]). In dieser Zeit bilden sich die Spindelfibrillen von den Tochterkernen auf den osmiophilen Streifen hin zurück. Die Plasmabrücke mit dem „Flemming-Körper" löst sich zunächst von einer der beiden Tochterzellen. Einige Zeit nach der Loslösung trennt sich die Plasmabrücke auch von der zweiten Tochterzelle. Der Rest des „Flemming-Körpers" scheint dann zugrunde zu gehen (siehe auch ALLENSPACH et al. [2]).

Der Verlauf einer einzelnen Spindelfibrille läßt sich im voll ausgebildeten „Flemming-Körper" nicht gut verfolgen, da die Fibrillen sehr eng nebeneinander liegen und das osmiophile Material dicht gepackt ist (Abb. 1d). Wenn die kleinen Fibrillenbündel während der Anaphase

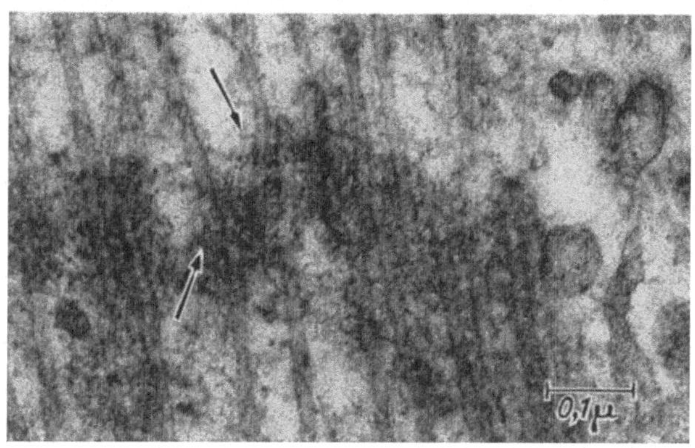

Abb. 2. Vergrößerter Ausschnitt aus Abb. 1b. Die Spindelfasern weichen sich aus (Pfeile), sie enden, von beiden Seiten kommend, im osmiophilen Streifen. (Aus PAWELETZ [9])

jedoch noch nicht zu einem einheitlichen Gebilde zusammengedrängt sind, läßt sich der Verlauf einzelner Fibrillen auch im osmiophilen Streifen leichter verfolgen (Abb. 2): Die Fibrillen, die von beiden Seiten auf den osmiophilen Streifen zulaufen, vereinigen sich nicht, sondern lagern sich ein Stück weit parallel aneinander, manchmal weichen sie sich durch leichtes Umbiegen aus (Abb. 2, Pfeile). Alle Fibrillen enden ungefähr in der Mitte des Streifens oder auf der Gegenseite der Eintrittstelle. Zählt man die Fibrillen zu beiden Seiten und innerhalb des Streifens, dann stellt man fest, daß die Zahl der Fibrillen im Innern des Streifens ungefähr der Summe der Zahl der Fibrillen zu beiden Seiten des Streifens entspricht.

Aus den eben erwähnten Beobachtungen muß man schließen, daß bei HeLa-Zellen die Spindelfibrillen zwischen den Chromosomengruppen der Anaphase nicht ununterbrochen durchlaufen; vielmehr beginnen bzw. enden alle Spindelfibrillen im osmiophilen Streifen.

Das Spindelsystem während der Anaphase besteht bei HeLa-Zellen und vermutlich auch bei allen anderen Zellarten, die einen „Flemming-Körper" besitzen, nicht, wie bisher angenommen wurde, aus einem nahtlosen einheitlichen Gebilde, sondern es setzt sich aus zwei Halbspindeln zusammen, die im osmiophilen Streifen miteinander verkittet sind; als Kittsubstanz dient das osmiophile Material. Beim biochemischen Nachweis von maskierten Lipoiden mit Sudanschwarz B erscheint der „Flemming-Körper" als dunkle Struktur innerhalb der Plasmabrücke; deshalb ist anzunehmen, daß ein großer Teil der Kittsubstanz aus Lipoprotein besteht.

Der voll ausgebildete „Flemming-Körper" fällt natürlich bei lichtmikroskopischer Beobachtung als erstes auf; er ist jedoch nur noch ein Relikt des osmiophilen Streifens, dessen Aufgabe darin besteht, die Spindelhälften während der Anaphase zusammenzuhalten.

Bereits 1929 hatte BELAR [4] eine „äquatoriale Kittstelle" in der Spindel vermutet. Er konnte sich bei seinen Vermutungen natürlich nur auf eine Reihe von „Indizien" stützen.

MAZIA [8] konnte zeigen, daß der isolierte mitotische Apparat von Seeigeleiern in Anaphase leicht in zwei Halbspindeln zerfallen kann. Vermutlich wird durch die Wirkung der Isolierungsflüssigkeiten die Kittstelle verändert, so daß die Spindelhälften auseinanderfallen können. Unsere Befunde haben den Nachweis für BELARS Vermutungen gebracht und sie erklären MAZIAS Ergebnisse.

Mit dem osmiophilen Streifen ist ein weiterer Ort in der Zelle gefunden worden, an dem Mitosegifte angreifen können, um eine regelrechte Verteilung der Chromosomen zu verhindern.

Eines der bekanntesten Mitosegifte ist das Colchicin. Im folgenden sollen einige charakteristische Veränderungen des Zellaufbaus nach Zugabe von Colchicin beschrieben werden:

Während der Metaphase von unbeeinflußten HeLa-Zellen liegen die Chromosomen in einer Platte geordnet. Spindelfibrillen ziehen von den Chromosomen zu den Zentriolen. Der Spindelraum ist frei von Mitochondrien, die Zisternen des endoplasmatischen Retikulums (ER) befinden sich unregelmäßig verteilt in der Randzone der Zelle (siehe ROBBINS et al. [10]).

Ein vollkommen anderes Bild bietet sich bei einer Metaphasezelle, die durch Colchicin arretiert wurde (Abb. 3): Die Chromosomen liegen in einem ungeordneten Haufen meist in der Mitte der Zelle. Spindelfibrillen lassen sich nicht erkennen. Das Membransystem des ER hat sich vergrößert und umgibt den Chromosomenhaufen in mehreren konzentrischen Lagen (siehe auch GEORGE et al. [7]). Die Mitochondrien liegen in der ganzen Zelle unregelmäßig verteilt. Häufig findet man in der Nähe des Chromosomenhaufens eine Ansammlung von Vakuolen, die in sich kleine Bläschen oder kristallartige Gebilde einschließen. Der Vakuolenhaufen wird von den übrigen Strukturen durch Zisternen des ER abgetrennt; solche abgetrennten Anhäufungen findet man in Kontrollpräparaten nicht. Der Inhalt der Vakuolen läßt darauf schließen, daß es sich um Anhäufungen von Speicherprodukten handelt.

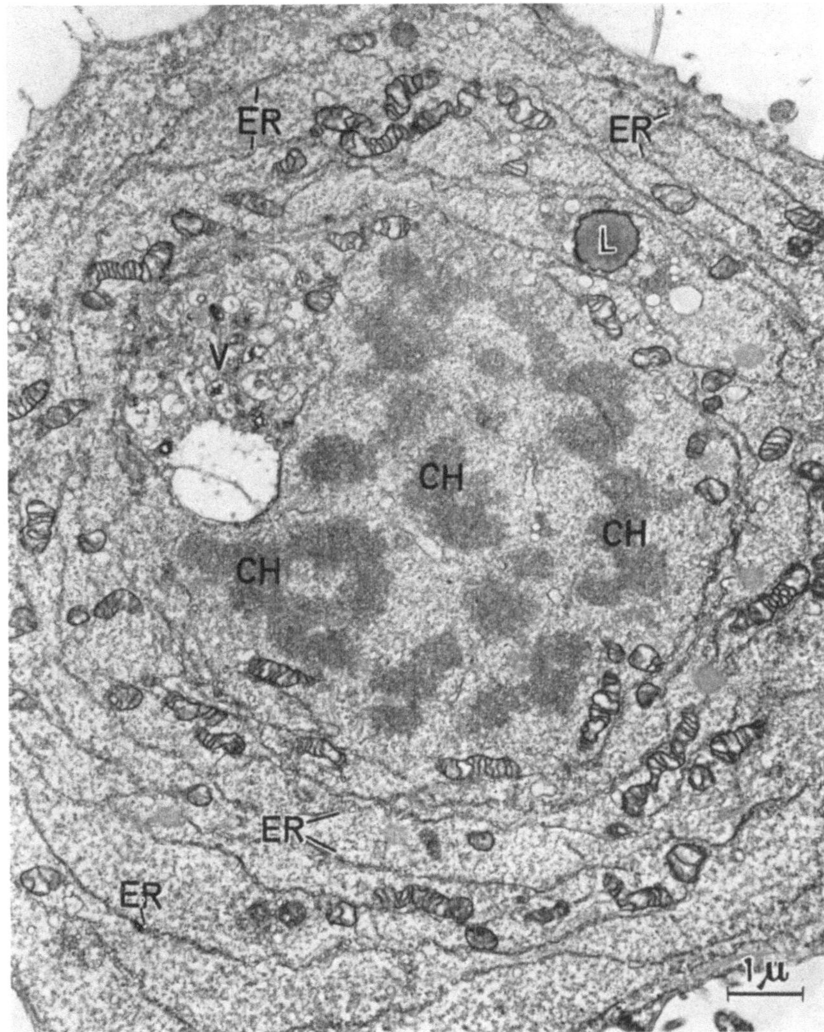

Abb. 3. Durch Colchicin arretierte Metaphase einer HeLa-Zelle. Endoplasmatisches Reticulum (ER), Lipoproteingranum (L), Chromosomen (CH), Vacuolenhaufen (V)

Bei genauer Beobachtung stellt man fest, daß die Zisternen des ER, die zunächst wie ein zusammenhängender Schlauch erschienen, aus einer Reihe von flachgedrückten Bläschen zusammengesetzt sind (Abb. 4b, c ER). Die geordnete Aneinanderreihung der Bläschen deutet darauf hin,

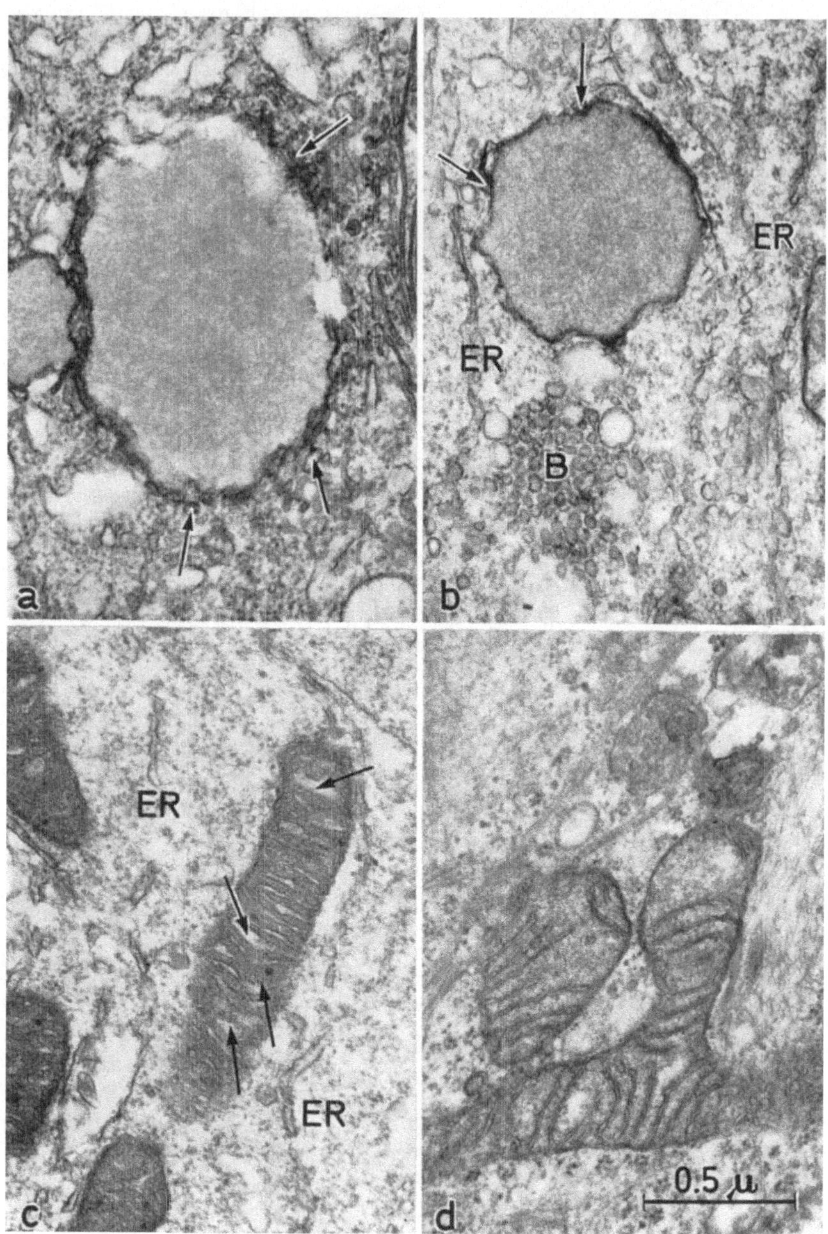

Abb. 4. a Lipoproteingranum eines Hühnerfibroblasten. Die Pfeile weisen auf Bläschen unmittelbar neben dem Granum. b Lipoproteingranum einer HeLa-Zelle. Endoplasmatisches Reticulum (ER), Bläschenhaufen (B). Die Pfeile weisen auf Bläschen unmittelbar neben dem Granum. c Mitochondrium einer arretierten Metaphasezelle. Endoplasmatisches Reticulum (ER). Die Pfeile weisen auf geblähte Cristae. d Mitochondrium einer mit Colchicin behandelten Interphasezelle. c und d HeLa-Zellen

daß sie miteinander in Verbindung stehen: Das gesamte System des ER scheint hier aus doppelwandigen Säcken zu bestehen, die stark durchlöchert sind. Dieses Membransystem dient dazu, die Zelle in bestimmte Räume aufzuteilen, um bestimmte Strukturen voneinander zu trennen.

Colchicin und Vincristin (GEORGE et al. [7]) scheinen die arretierten Zellen zur Bildung von Membranen anzuregen bzw. deren Abbau zu verhindern: Die Membranen des Golgiapparats, die normalerweise während der Prophase verschwinden (ROBBINS et al. [10]), sind in arretierten Metaphasezellen häufig zu finden.

Auffallend sind ca. 1–2 μ große Anhäufungen von unstrukturiert erscheinendem Material (Abb. 3 L, 4a, b): Es handelt sich dabei um Lipoproteingrana. Man findet sie einzeln oder zu mehreren in den meisten arretierten Metaphasen, sowohl bei HeLa-Zellen (Abb. 3 L, 4b) als auch bei Hühnerfibroblasten (Abb. 4a). In Interphasezellen liegen sie in geringer Zahl vor, in Kontrollpräparaten sind sie selten. In der Nähe der Grana erkennt man häufig eine Ansammlung von kleinen Bläschen (Abb. 4a, b B) und Membranen des Golgiapparates. Einige Bläschen liegen unmittelbar neben den Grana (Abb. 4a, b Pfeile). Vermutlich entstehen die Lipoproteingrana dadurch, daß Bläschen des Golgiapparates oder des ribosomenlosen ER ihren Inhalt an bestimmten Stellen ins Cytoplasma entleeren.

Die Lipoproteingrana scheinen unter dem Einfluß von Colchicin vermehrt zu entstehen. Es ist noch nicht geklärt, ob sie den hyalinen Tropfen (GAULDEN et al. [6], ALTMANN et al. [3]), die aus Spindelmaterial bestehen, entsprechen.

Die Mitochondrien von arretierten Metaphasezellen, die mit Glutaraldehyd fixiert wurden, zeigen ein anderes Aussehen als die Mitochondrien von Interphasezellen (Abb. 4c): Die Cristae sind stellenweise gebläht (Pfeile), der Raum, der von den Cristamembranen gebildet wird, wirkt leer, dagegen ist die Mitochondrienmatrix sehr dicht granuliert. Bei den Mitochondrien von colchicinbehandelten Interphasezellen ist wie bei normalen Zellen die Matrix lockerer (Abb. 4d), die Cristae sind nicht gebläht, alle Membranen treten deutlich hervor. Beide Typen kommen in einem Präparat nebeneinander vor. Auf welchen funktionellen Unterschieden diese strukturellen Veränderungen beruhen, müssen biochemische Untersuchungen klären.

In vielen Interphasezellen von HeLa-Zellen und von Hühnchenfibroblasten, zuweilen auch in arretierten Metaphasezellen, findet man kleine Bündel von ca. 70 Å dicken Fibrillen, die ungeordnet im Cytoplasma liegen. Da die Fibrillen in Kontrollpräparaten von HeLa-Zellen selten und von Hühnerfibroblasten nur in kleinen Mengen vorkommen, erhebt sich die Frage, ob die vermehrte Fibrillenbildung auf den Einfluß des Colchicins zurückzuführen ist.

Munk u. Waldeck (persönliche Mitteilung) fanden in HeLa-Zellen, die mit Viren infiziert waren, große Fibrillenbündel, meistens in der Nähe des Kernes. George et al. [7] zeigten Fibrillenbündel nach Einwirkung von Vincristin.

Da die Fibrillen auch nach Einwirkung anderer Mitosegifte und nach Virusinfektion zu finden sind, dürfte es sich nicht ausschließlich um eine Wirkung des Colchicins handeln, vielmehr scheint die Zelle auf verschiedene Schädigungsarten mit der gleichen Reaktion (vermehrte Fibrillenbildung) zu antworten.

Um funktionsfähige Spindelfasern handelt es sich bei den Fibrillen sicher nicht. Roth [11] nimmt an, daß durch bestimmte Einwirkungen (z. B. Mitosegifte) der Zusammenbau der 70 Å dicken Fibrillen zu funktionsfähigen Spindelfasern verhindert wird. Es sollte sich danach um verändertes Spindelmaterial handeln. Nach Wohlfarth-Bottermann [12] dienen gleichaussehende Fibrillen bei Amöben und Schleimpilzen zur Bewegung des Cytoplasmas. Mazia (persönliche Mitteilung) nimmt an, daß die Vorgänge bei amöboider und saltatorischer Bewegung gleich oder sehr ähnlich sind wie bei der Chromosomenbewegung während der Mitose. Danach könnte es sich bei den Fibrillen um Proteine handeln, die sowohl zum Aufbau der Spindel als auch zur Bewegung des Cytoplasmas dienen.

Die vorgelegten Befunde sollten zeigen, daß die Wirkung des Colchicins nicht nur darin besteht, die Spindelbildung zu hemmen oder die schon gebildete Spindel aufzulösen. Es wirkt auch auf andere Organellen der Zelle und verändert dadurch die Struktur der arretierten Metaphasezelle stark.

Literatur

1. Abramson, D. H. and B. Byers: Morphological Changes in HeLa Cells during Late Cytokinesis. J. Cell Biol. **31**, 3 A (1966).
2. Allenspach, A. L. and L. E. Roth: Structural Variations during Mitosis in the Chick Embryo. J. Cell Biol. **33**, 179–196 (1967).
3. Altmann, H.-W. u. J. Haubrich: Über hepatocelluläre Mitosestörungen und Kerneinschlüsse nach wiederholten Colchicingaben. Beitr. path. Anat. **131**, 355–395 (1965).
4. Belar, K.: Beiträge zur Kausalanalyse der Mitose. II. Wilhelm Roux' Arch. Entwickl.-Mech. Org. **118**, 359–484 (1929).
5. Flemming, W.: Neue Beiträge zur Kenntnis der Zelle. II. Theil. Arch. mikrosk. Anat. **37**, 685–751 (1891).
6. Gaulden, M. E. and J. G. Carlson: Cytological Effects of Colchicine on the Grashopper Neuroblast in vitro with Special Reference to the Origin of the Spindle. Exp. Cell Res. **2**, 416–433 (1951).
7. George, P., L. J. Journey, and M. N. Goldstein: Effect of Vincristine on the Fine Structure of HeLa Cells during Mitosis. J. nat. Cancer Inst. **35**, 355–375 (1965).

8. MAZIA, D.: Mitosis and the Physiology of Cell Division. In: J. Brachet u. A. E. Mirsky (Edit.): The Cell, Vol. 3: Meiosis and Mitosis. New York: Academic Press 1961.
9. PAWELETZ, N.: Zur Funktion des „Flemming-Körpers" bei der Teilung tierischer Zellen. Naturwissenschaften **54**, 533–535 (1967).
10. ROBBINS, E. and N. K. GONATAS: The Ultrastructure of a Mammalian Cell during the Mitotic Cycle. J. Cell Biol. **21**, 429–464 (1964).
11. ROTH, L. E.: Electron Microscopy of Mitosis in Amebae. III. J. Cell. Biol **34**, 47–59 (1967).
12. WOHLFARTH-BOTTERMANN, K. E.: Dynamik der Zelle. Vortrag gehalten auf der 13. Tagung der Gesellschaft für Elektronenmikroskopie. 17.–21. Sept. 1967 in Marburg.

Konstitution und Wirkung von Mitosegiften

Von

H. Lettré und Th. J. Fitzgerald

Ehe das eigentliche Thema behandelt wird, soll im Anschluß an die Ausführungen von Prof. Mazia kurz eine Hypothese dargelegt werden, welche den reversiblen Aufbau einer Faser aus Untereinheiten an einem chemischen Modell zu erklären versucht. Ausgangspunkt sind hierbei die

$$
\begin{array}{c}
\quad\;\diagup CH_2 \diagdown \\
CH_2 \quad CH-CH_2-CH_2-CH_2-CH_2-COOH \\
\;\big|\qquad\big| \\
S\!\!-\!\!-\!\!S
\end{array}
$$

$$\updownarrow$$

$$
\begin{array}{c}
\quad\;\diagup CH_2 \diagdown \\
CH_2 \quad CH-CH_2-CH_2-CH_2-CH_2-COOH \\
\;\big|\qquad\big| \\
SH \quad\; SH
\end{array}
$$

<pre>
Formel I: Thioctsäure
Formel II: Dihydro-thioctsäure
</pre>

Experimente von Mazia, aus denen der Übergang von *Disulfid-Gruppen* in intra- und inter-molekularer Bindung in freie Thiolgruppen und umgekehrt als wesentlich für den Aufbau der Spindelfaser abgeleitet wurde [7]. Eine natürlich vorkommende Verbindung mit einer intramolekularen Disulfid-Bindung ist die Thioctsäure (Liponsäure, Formel I) [2]. Durch Hydrierung geht sie in die ringoffene Dithiolform (Formel II) über, aus der sich durch Dehydrierung I zurückbildet. Nach früheren Untersuchungen hat die Thioctsäure eine mitoseanregende Wirkung [4], steht also in irgendeiner Beziehung zu den Faktoren, die am mitotischen Geschehen beteiligt sind. Nimmt man an, daß in ein Protein, welches freie Thiolgruppen enthält, Thioctsäure eingebaut ist, so sind damit die Voraussetzungen für eine polymerisationsfähige Untereinheit gegeben. Durch innermolekulare Wasserstoffverschiebung kann die Disulfidbrücke der Thioctsäure reduktiv geöffnet werden, während durch die Wegnahme des Wasserstoffs von den Thiolgruppen freie Schwefelbindungen entstehen. Hierdurch ist eine Polymerisierung durch Bildung intermolekularer Disulfidbrücken möglich. In Abb. 1 ist dies schematisch dargestellt und weiterhin die Variationsmöglichkeit durch Hydrierung und Dehydrierung bei Monomerem und Polymerem wiedergegeben. Bei dem reversibel polymerisationsfähigen Monomeren ist das Gleichgewicht mit dem Polymeren jedoch nicht von einem anderen Redoxsystem abhängig. Dieses Gleichgewicht sollte von anderen, physikalischen und chemischen, Faktoren abhängen.

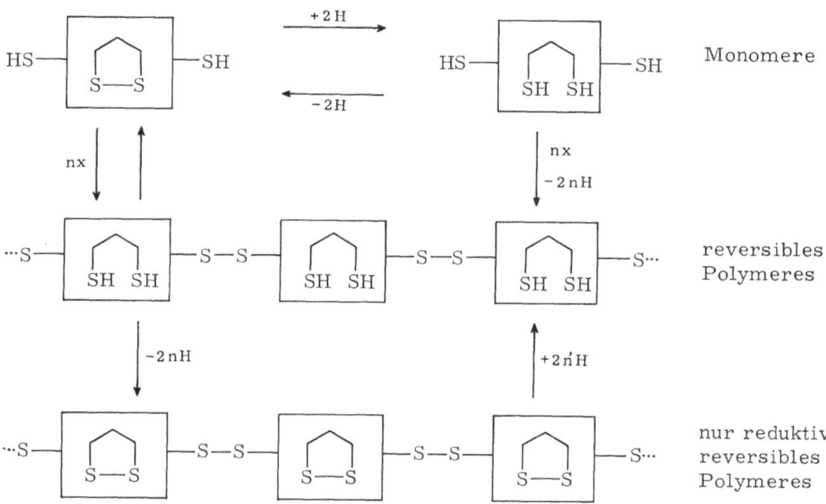

Abb. 1. Schema der Bildung eines reversiblen Polymeren durch intramolekulare Wasserstoffverschiebung

Von SHELANSKI und TAYLOR [10] ist kürzlich ein Protein beschrieben worden, welches eine Untereinheit der die Spindelfasern bildenden Mikroröhrchen darstellt. Dieses Protein hat die Fähigkeit das Mitosegift Colchicin zu binden. Die Autoren nehmen an, daß hierdurch die Fähigkeit dieses Proteins, Mikroröhrchen aufzubauen, unterbunden wird. Die weitere Analyse dieses Proteins wird zeigen können, ob die zuvor entwickelte Hypothese dem Wesen der Eigenschaften der Spindelfaser gerecht wird.

Wir haben uns nicht mit dem Rezeptor beschäftigt, der Colchicin bindet, sondern den Zusammenhang zwischen Konstitution und Wirkung bei dieser Verbindung bearbeitet. Unsere früheren Arbeiten befaßten sich dabei mit den strukturellen Voraussetzungen der Wirksamkeit des Colchicins (Formel III), seiner Derivate und synthetischer Verbindungen als Mitosegifte [3]. Hier sollen nun einige neuere Ergebnisse über die Bedeutung der räumlichen Anordnung in den Molekeln für die Wirksamkeit mitgeteilt werden.

Den ersten Hinweis, daß außer bestimmten strukturellen Voraussetzungen die räumliche Form der Molekel wichtig ist, brachte die Untersuchung einer Verbindung, die wir vor einigen Jahren von dem japanischen Chemiker T. Nozoe erhielten. Es handelt sich bei dieser synthetisch hergestellten Verbindung (Formel IV) um ein Analogon des Colchicins,

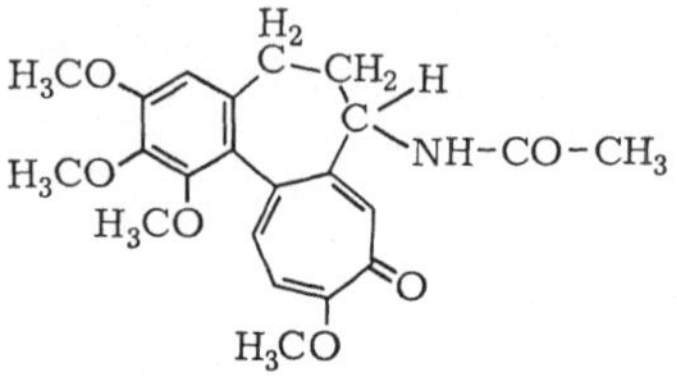

Formel III: Colchicin

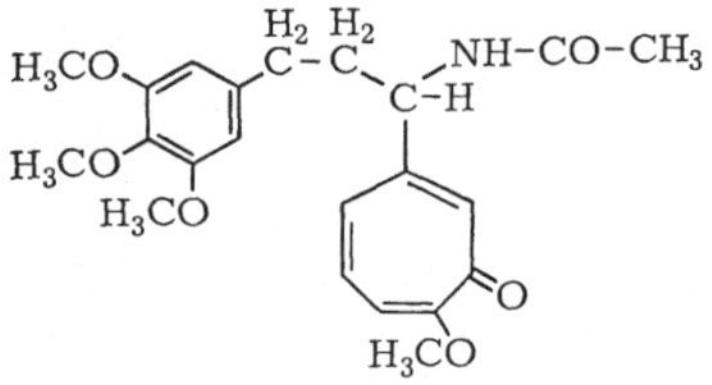

Formel IV: Ringoffenes Dihydrocolchicin (T. Nozoe)

bei dem der mittlere Ring des Colchicins (Formel III) geöffnet ist und die freien Bindungen mit Wasserstoff substituiert sind. Obschon alle Strukturelemente des Colchicins in dieser Verbindung enthalten sind, ließ sich auch mit dem 10000fachen der Dosis, mit der Colchicin wirkt, keinerlei mitosehemmende Wirkung von IV feststellen. Durch die Öffnung der

Tabelle 1. *Wirksamkeit von (—)-Colchicin und Derivaten*

	Wirksamkeit γ/ml	Formel	Molgewicht	Molare Wirksamkeit
(+)-Colchicin	1	$C_{22}H_{25}O_6N$	400	$2,5 \cdot 10^{-6}$
(—)-Colchicin	0,01	$C_{22}H_{25}O_6N$	400	$2,5 \cdot 10^{-8}$
Desacetylamino-Colchicin	0,002	$C_{20}H_{22}O_5$	343	$6 \quad \cdot 10^{-9}$

Bindung zwischen dem aromatischen Ring und dem Tropolonring ist eine freie Drehbarkeit in der Kette der drei C-Atome, welche die Ringe noch verbindet, möglich. Hierdurch kann die Molekel Formen annehmen, die von der des Colchicins abweichen, und wahrscheinlich die dem Colchicin entsprechende gar nicht einnehmen. Bei ähnlichen ringoffenen Verbindungen hatten wir früher mit α,β-Diphenyl-äthylaminen antimitotische

Wirksamkeit feststellen können, während zu IV analoge α,γ-Diphenyl-propylamine keine Wirksamkeit besaßen. Die Konformation, d. h. die räumliche Form, spielt neben strukturellen Voraussetzungen eine Rolle.

Ein eigentlich stereochemisches Problem behandelt die Untersuchung der optischen Antipoden des Colchicins. Aus dem natürlichen links-drehenden Colchicin haben CORRODI u. HARDEGGER [1] den Antipoden,

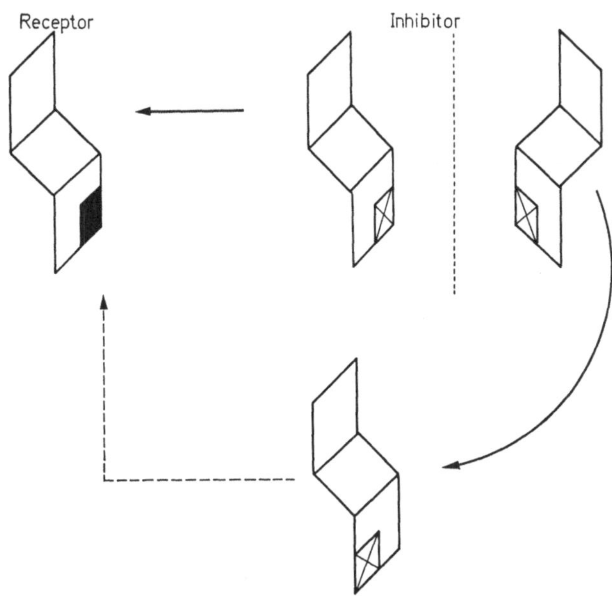

Abb. 2. Schema der Beziehung eines Receptors zu einer molekularasymmetrischen Verbindung und deren Spiegelbild

das (+)-Colchicin, hergestellt. Diese Verbindung wurde von uns auf ihre mitosehemmende Wirkung geprüft [6]; sie zeigte praktisch keine Wirksamkeit (Tab. 1). Diese Unwirksamkeit als Ausdruck einer absoluten stereochemischen Spezifität ist nicht überraschend, da zahlreiche andere Beispiele dieser Art bekannt sind.

Ein Problem ergibt sich erst aus der Gegenüberstellung mit der Wirksamkeit des Desacetylamino-colchicins [5]. In dieser Verbindung ist die $NH-CO-CH_3$-Gruppe des Colchicins durch Wasserstoff ersetzt, und damit ist das asymmetrische C-Atom symmetrisch geworden. Die Verbindung ist im sichtbaren Licht optisch inaktiv. Ihre Wirksamkeit steht in Widerspruch zu pharmakologischen Erfahrungen mit anderen Verbindungen; hiernach soll eine Verbindung ohne Asymmetriezentrum dem schwächer wirksamen Antipoden einer analogen Verbindung mit einem Asymmetriezentrum entsprechen [*8*]. Im Falle des hier beschriebenen Colchicinderivates ist die Situation aber umgekehrt.

Betrachtet man ein Molekülmodell des Colchicins, so sieht man, daß die Molekel nicht eben ist, sondern daß der aromatische Ring und der Tropolonring gegeneinander verdreht sind. Bei der Ungleichheit der Ringe existiert daher eine Molekularasymmetrie, die zu weiterer optischer Aktivität Anlaß gibt. Wir konnten feststellen, daß aus Colchicin hergestelltes Desacetylaminocolchicin zwar im sichtbaren Bereich des Lichtes nicht optisch aktiv ist, jedoch im Ultravioletten, bei 250 mμ, eine deutliche optische Aktivität besitzt. Die durch die Behinderung der freien Drehbarkeit gegebene Molekularasymmetrie bedingt das Auftreten hinlänglich stabiler optischer Antipoden. Das von SCHREIBER et al. [*9*] synthetisch dargestellte Desacetylaminocolchicin ist das Racemat beider Antipoden, während die aus dem natürlichen Colchicin hergestellte Form einen optisch aktiven Antipoden darstellt. Das natürliche Colchicin ist nicht einer von nur zwei möglichen Antipoden, sondern einer von vieren, die sich aus dem Vorhandensein molekularer Asymmetrie neben einem asymmetrischen C-Atom ergeben. In Abb. 2 ist schematisch wiedergegeben, wie eine Molekularasymmetrie sich bei der Wechselwirkung zwischen Rezeptor und den beiden isomeren Inhibitoren auswirkt. Unsere Befunde zeigen, daß für die antimitotische Wirksamkeit außer den notwendigen Strukturelementen eine bestimmte räumliche Form der Molekel gegeben sein muß. Außer der Struktur bestimmen die Konfiguration und bei Verbindungen mit freier Drehbarkeit die Konformation über diese biologische Wirkung.

Der eine von uns (TH. J. F.) dankt dem National Cancer Institute des Public Health Service, USA., sowie der Alexander von Humboldt-Stiftung für ein Forschungsstipendium.

Literatur

1. CORRODI, H. u. E. HARDEGGER: Herstellung des racemischen Colchicins und des unnatürlichen (+)-Colchicins. Helvet. chim. acta **40**, 193 (1957).
2. GRISEBACH, H.: Chemie und Biochemie der α-Liponsäure. Angew. Chem. **68**, 554 (1956).
3. LETTRÉ, H.: Über Mitosegifte. Erg. Physiol. **46**, 379–452 (1950).
4. — Zur Wirkung von Thioctsäure auf den Mäuse-Ascites-Tumor. Naturwissenschaften **45**, 217 (1958).
5. — TH. J. FITZGERALD u. W. SIEBS: Desacetylaminocolchicin und -isocolchicin. Naturwissenschaften **53**, 132 (1966).
6. — u. R. LETTRÉ: Zur antimitotischen Wirksamkeit der optischen Antipoden des Colchicins und eines Colchicinderivates. Naturwissenschaften **53**, 180 (1966).
7. MAZIA, D.: Mitosis and the physiology of cell division. In: J. Brachet and A. Mirsky. (Edit.): The Cell, Vol. III, p. 77. New York: Academic Press 1961.

8. Schaumann, O.: Zur Pharmakologie der optischen Isomeren des 3,4-Dioxy-nor-
ephedrins. In: Medizin und Chemie, Vol. III, S. 383 ff. Leverkusen: „Bayer"
1936.
9. Schreiber, J., W. Leimgruber, M. Pesaro, P. Schudel, T. Threlfall u.
A. Eschenmoser: Synthese des Colchicins. Helvet. chim. acta **44**, 540 (1960).
10. Shelanski, M. L. and E. W. Taylor: Isolation of a protein subunit from
microtubules. J. Cell Biology **34**, 549 (1967).

Zum Aufbau des Interphasechromosoms

Von

R. Lettré*

Die Ursache des zuweilen negativen Ausfalls der Feulgen-Reaktion an bestimmten Chromosomenabschnitten, in Abhängigkeit von dem Funktionszustand des betreffenden Bezirkes, der Fixierung und Vorbehandlung der Präparate und zuweilen auch der Dauer der Hydrolyse, hat uns im Rahmen eigener Untersuchungen seit längerer Zeit beschäftigt. Als Beispiele für Feulgen-negative Chromatinstrukturen seien genannt: die Chromosomen der Oogonien und des Synkarions (Agrell [1, 2]), die bei niedrigen Temperaturen auftretende sogenannte „Kältechromasie", die von Darlington und LaCour [8] für definierte Chromosomenbezirke bei Pflanzen beschrieben wurde, und schließlich die meist fehlende Anfärbbarkeit der nukleolenbildenden Chromosomenabschnitte während der Interphase und der Mitose, in der sie als die sogenannten Sekundärkonstriktionen in Erscheinung treten. Unsere Vermutungen gingen dahin, daß sich bei der Fixierung auf diesen Abschnitten ein – von der Funktion des betreffenden Abschnittes abhängiges – Präzipitat niederschlagen könnte, das die für eine positive Feulgen-Reaktion notwendige Angreifbarkeit der DNS-Strukturen durch die Hydrolyse behindern könnte. Als Bestandteile des die DNS begleitenden Materials sind mit Sicherheit Proteine und Ribonucleinsäure bekannt; unser Interesse galt seit langem der Rolle, welche Lipoide in diesem Zusammenhang spielen könnten.

Der Lipoidgehalt der Zellmasse beträgt im Durchschnitt 30% (Macheboeuf [15]); er ist in verschiedenen Geweben unterschiedlich hoch, ebenso differiert er in bezug auf die Relation zwischen Kernen und Cytoplasma. Von Stoneburg [19] wurden Lipoide, u. a. Cholesterin, in isolierten Kernen nachgewiesen; es blieb jedoch offen, ob sie im Kernsaft oder in den Chromatinstrukturen zu lokalsieren seien. So ist zu verstehen, daß Claude [7] zwar Lipoide als einen Bestandteil der Nukleolen anführt,

---

* Die Untersuchungen, über welche hier berichtet wird, wurden gemeinsam mit Dr. N. Paweletz und Dr. Dr. W. Siebs durchgeführt, denen ich für vielfältige Hilfe zu danken habe.

bei den Chromosomen selbst jedoch Lipoide nicht erwähnt. Die Befunde und Vorstellungen von CLAUDE erscheinen aber auch für das Chromatin von Bedeutung, so daß sie später noch ausführlicher erwähnt werden sollen.

1959 fanden CHAYEN u. Mitarb. [6], daß Lipoide auch einen Bestandteil der Chromosomen darstellen; sie konnten bei der Aufarbeitung des isolierten Nukleohistons einen Lipoidgehalt von 23% des Trockengewichtes feststellen. Wie wenig bekannt diese Befunde sind, läßt sich vielleicht daraus entnehmen, daß der in dem Handbuch ,,The Cell'' von MIRSKY and OSAWA [16] geschriebene Beitrag über den Interphasekern Lipoide überhaupt nicht erwähnt. Der Grund ist wohl darin zu suchen, daß diese Lipoide sich bei den konventionellen histochemischen Methoden meist dem Nachweis entziehen, und daß ein sehr erheblicher Anteil der Lipoide nur durch sehr drastische Methoden freigesetzt und dem Nachweis zugänglich gemacht werden kann.

1965 konnten LETTRÉ, SIEBS und PAWELETZ [14] berichten, daß sich sowohl im Chromatingerüst der Interphasekerne als auch innerhalb der Nukleolen eine Lipoproteinkomponente histochemisch nachweisen läßt: die Darstellung gelang mit $KMnO_4$, dessen Eigenschaft, bevorzugt Lipoproteine zu fixieren, von der Elektronenmikroskopie her bekannt ist. Für die gleichen Strukturen war eine bevorzugte Affinität des Sudan Schwarz B feststellbar, wenn nach der Methode von BERENBAUM [4] gefärbt wurde, d. h. wenn durch Einwirkung von 40° warmem Aceton die Lipoide demaskiert wurden. Elektronenmikroskopisch ließen sich nach Fixierung mit OsO_4, anschließender Demaskierung der Lipoide durch Pyridin und Versilberung nach der Methode von GONZALEZ-RAMIREZ [12] die feinsten Chromatinstrukturen indirekt darstellen: den nicht unmittelbar versilberten fädigen Strukturen fanden sich winzige tropfenförmige Silberniederschläge angelagert, welche die teilweise als feine Schrauben erkennbaren Chromatinstrukturen nachzeichneten (PAWELETZ, SIEBS u. LETTRÉ [18]). Die Fadenstrukturen, welche stellenweise als sich aufspaltende Doppelstränge sichtbar waren, zeigten im einzelnen Faden einen Durchmesser von ca. 50 Å, was der Größenordnung einer Elementarfibrille entspricht.

Auf unsere Bitte hin führte Herr Dr. BEHEIM [3] in unserem Institut eine Aufarbeitung von isoliertem Nukleoprotein mit einer Modifikation der von CHAYEN u. Mitarb. [6] beschriebenen Methode durch. Er konnte die Befunde von CHAYEN u. Mitarb. bestätigen und konnte zusätzlich nach mehrstündiger Hydrolyse mit Bariumhydroxyd und anschließend mit Salzsäure in dem mit Alkohol-Äther und Chloroform extrahierten Material chromatographisch Cholesterin nachweisen.

Daß es strukturgebundene Lipoide gibt, welche nur durch Zerstörung (CLAUDE [7] ,,severe disrupting'') der Strukturen feststellbar gemacht

werden können, wurde bereits von CLAUDE für Mitochondrien (Phosphor-
lipoidgehalt 25–30%) und Mikrosomen (40%) festgestellt. CLAUDE sieht
daher Lipoide als integrierende Bestandteile stoffwechselaktiver Strukturen innerhalb der Zelle an, die also nicht nur die Aufgabe haben, eine
Trennung verschiedener Phasen innerhalb der Zelle aufrecht zu erhalten,
sondern vermutlich enzymatische Reaktionen steuern. Die Befunde mit
dem Steroidhormon Ecdyson werden von KARLSON [13] so gedeutet, daß
Ecdyson sich unmittelbar als Derepressor oder Co-Derepressor derjenigen
Region des Chromosoms anlagert, in der daraufhin eine Puffbildung
erfolgt. Obwohl diese Auffassung noch nicht allgemein akzeptiert ist,
ließe sie sich gut im Sinne einer Wechselwirkung mit strukturgebundenen
Lipoiden des Chromatins verstehen.

Alle unsere bisherigen Versuche waren mit einer Demaskierung der
Lipoide fixierter Zellen durchgeführt worden, und wir suchten nun nach
einer Möglichkeit, eine Einwirkung auf intranukleäre Lipoide an lebenden
Zellen durchführen zu können. Wir hofften, evtl. die Feulgen-Reaktion
dadurch beeinflussen zu können.

Wir hatten in klinischen Berichten (u. a. NITZ-LITZOW [17]; ENGEL-
HARDT [9]; ZELLER, SCHÖN u. ALADAG [20]) über die Wirkung eines
Medikamentes SP54 gelesen, dem man die Fähigkeit einer Breitband-
lipolyse zuschreibt. Die Substanz stellt ein Heparinoid dar, einen Pentosan-
polysulfosäureester, der als Polyanion wirkt. Laboratoriumsunter-
suchungen von GILLERT [11] zeigten eine Beeinflussung des Verhaltens
von Lipoproteinen bei der Immunoelektrophorese oder bei der Immuno-
präzipitationsmethode in Agar.

Wir untersuchten die Wirkung der Substanz auf in vitro gezüchtete
normale Zellen (mesenchymale Hühnerfibroblasten) und maligne Zellen
(menschliche Carcinomzellen, Stamm HeLa). Den 24 resp. 48 Std vorher
angesetzten Kulturen wurde in einer Beobachtungskammer die Substanz
zugesetzt, und sie wurden bei verschiedener Konzentration der Substanz
kurzfristig oder auch über mehrere Stunden beobachtet. Die Auswertung
von Serien solcher Präparate erfolgte nach Fixierung und Färbung.

Wir möchten, um jedem Mißverständnis vorzubeugen, betonen, daß
wir erst mit einer Konzentration der Substanz, welche bereits vielfach die
klinisch angewandte Konzentration übersteigt, Wirkungen in der von uns
gewählten Versuchsanordnung sahen. Bei einer völlig aus dem Rahmen
sonstiger Versuche fallenden Substanzkonzentration, nämlich einer Endkonzentration von ca. 65 mg/ml sahen wir endlich so drastische Veränderungen, wie man von einem Eingriff in die Verteilung der Zellipoide
erwarten zu können glaubt. Die Schäden waren so schwerwiegend, daß
nach allen unseren bisherigen Erfahrungen an keine Erholung der
geschädigten Zellen zu denken war. Die zunächst leichten Veränderungen
an der Zelloberfläche waren für uns nicht überraschend, da wir vergleich-

bare Phänomene gelegentlich bei der Austestung von Steroiden gesehen hatten. Auffallend war jedoch die fast schlagartig einsetzende Hemmung der Mitosen, die offenbar auf eine Störung des Chromatins zurückzuführen ist, und auf die im Rahmen dieser Veröffentlichung nicht näher eingegangen werden soll. Sie lief einer entsprechenden Veränderung des Chromatins in den Interphasekernen parallel. Da gleichzeitig mit diesen Phänomenen die Beobachtung der lebenden Zellen im Phasenkontrastmikroskop durch eine leichte Trübung behindert wurde, haben wir diese Veränderung an den Chromatinstrukturen hauptsächlich an fixierten und gefärbten Präparaten studiert. Abb. 1a und 1b zeigen jeweils Ausschnitte von Kontrollkulturen mesenchymaler Hühnerfibroblasten; Abb. 1c und 1d Abbildungen aus Kulturen, welche 30 min unter der Einwirkung von ca. 65 mg/ml SP54 gestanden hatten. In unserer über fast drei Jahrzehnte gehenden Erfahrung mit Zellen in der Gewebekultur haben wir niemals eine Erholung einer derartig schwer geschädigten Kultur erlebt. Besonders auffällig ist die starke Kondensation des Chromatins und die anscheinende Lückenhaftigkeit der Kernmembran, welche sich allerdings in elektronenmikroskopischen Aufnahmen an vielen Kernen nicht bestätigen ließ.

Wider alles Erwarten erwiesen sich jedoch die Störungen noch nach 30 min dauernder Einwirkung der Substanz als reversibel. Bereits 30 min nach Auswaschen der Versuchslösung, Spülen der Kulturen mit Salzlösung und frischer Fütterung hatten sich die Zellen zum größten Teil wieder erholt (s. Abb. 1e und 1f.). Die Mehrzahl der Kerne zeigt eine normal feine Struktur, nur vereinzelt ist die Chromatinzeichnung noch etwas vergröbert. Prophasen von annähernd normalem Aussehen sind vorhanden, die späteren Mitosestadien weisen dagegen noch Anomalien auf. Das Cytoplasma zeigt teilweise eine mehr oder weniger starke Granulierung und Vakuolisierung. Die Zelloberfläche hat begonnen, sich zu glätten, die Form der Zellen beginnt sich zu normalisieren. Nur ganz vereinzelte Zellen gehen zugrunde.

Um festzustellen, ob die Schädigung in der Tat auf eine Mobilisierung von Lipoiden innerhalb der Zelle und vor allem innerhalb des Zellkernes zurückzuführen sei, färbten wir Versuchs- und Kontrollkulturen nach der von BERENBAUM [4] angegebenen Methode für die Darstellung maskierter Lipoide. Abb. 2a zeigt eine Zelle aus einer Kontrollkultur: das Cytoplasma läßt eine fein strukturierte Zeichnung erkennen, der Kern erscheint blasser als das Cytoplasma, die Nukleolen sind intensiv angefärbt und lassen andeutungsweise eine Strukturierung erkennen, die unter dem angefärbten, lipoidhaltigen, sie umhüllenden Material verborgen ist. Abb. 2b zeigt Zellen der gleichen Serie von Kulturen nach 30 min dauernder Behandlung mit SP54. Hier sind die Kerne etwas stärker getönt als das Cytoplasma, es ist jedoch keinerlei Strukturierung im Kern zu erkennen. Die Nukleolen sind deutlich blasser als in den Kontrollen. Man hat den Eindruck, daß durch die für demaskierte Lipoide charakteristische Färbung eine feinst verteilte Substanz dargestellt wird, welche die Strukturen „verschleiert". Nach der Erholung (30 min), finden sich Bilder, welche den Kontrollen bereits weitgehend ähnlich geworden sind: die Nukleolen sind dunkel und dicht, anscheinend meist etwas dunkler und kleiner als in den Kontrollkulturen; die Kerne haben sich weitgehend

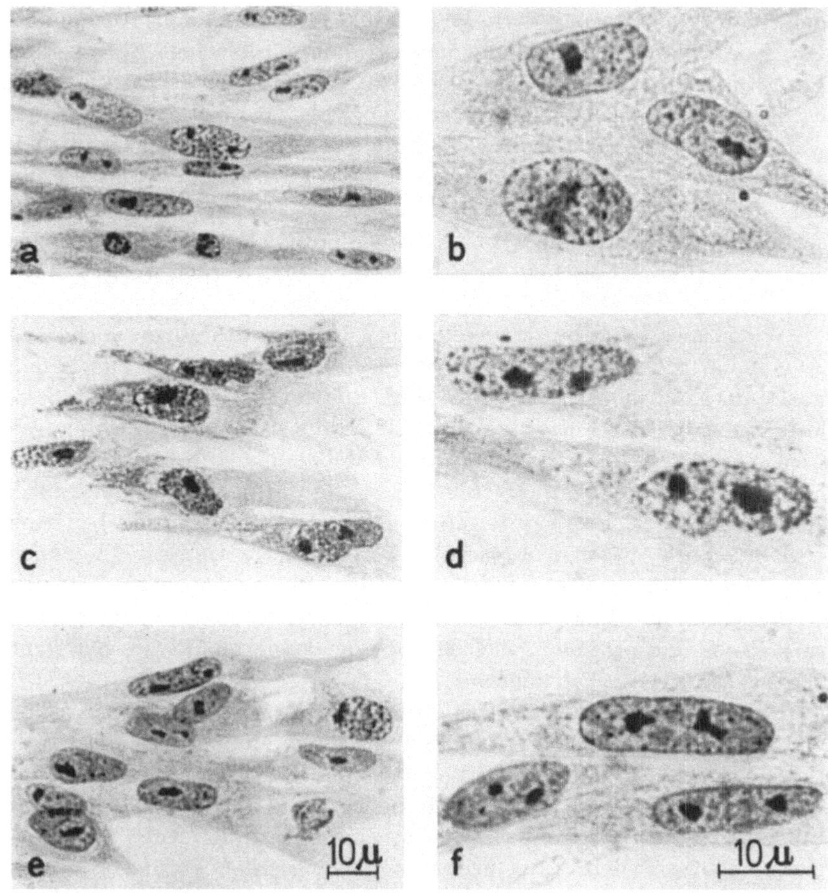

Abb. 1a–f. Ausschnitte aus Kulturen von Hühnerfibroblasten der gleichen Versuchsserie, ca. 24 Std in vitro gezüchtet. a und b Kontrollkultur, Zugabe physiologischer Salzlösung für 30–60 min; c und d Versuchskultur, Zugabe von SP54 für 30 min (Endkonzentration ca. 65 mg/ml); e und f Versuchskultur, Zugabe von SP54 wie bei c und d; Auswaschen und frische Fütterung; gesamte Erholungsphase 30 min. Fixierung nach Serra; Färbung Hämalaun

aufgehellt; im Cytoplasma fällt vor allem eine tropfige Ablagerung von Lipoiden auf, die in Kontrollkulturen nur selten zu sehen ist.

Diese Befunde sprechen dafür, daß hier in der Tat eine Einwirkung auf die intrazellulären und vor allem intranukleären Lipoide stattgefunden hat, welche offenbar für die im Kern sichtbar werdenden Kondensationseffekte an den Chromosomen verantwortlich zu machen ist. In der Erholungsphase läuft anscheinend die Normalisierung der Verteilung der Lipoide der Normalisierung des Kondensationszustandes der Chromosomen parallel.

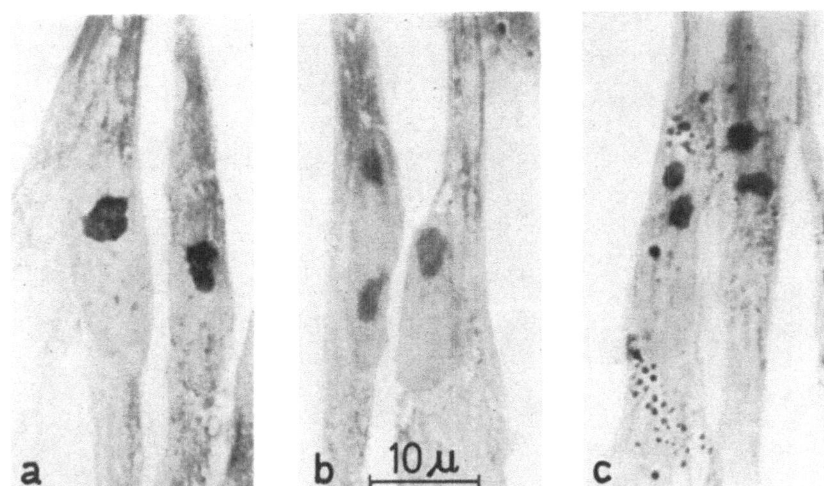

Abb. 2a–c. Ausschnitte aus Kulturen von Hühnerfibroblasten der gleichen Versuchsserie, ca. 24 Std in vitro gezüchtet. a Kontrollkultur, Zugabe physiologischer Salzlösung für 30–60 min; b Versuchskultur, Zugabe von SP 54 für 30 min (Endkonzentration ca. 65 mg/ml); c Versuchskultur, Zugabe von SP 54 wie bei b; Auswaschen und frische Fütterung; gesamte Erholungsphase 30 min. Fixierung Formalin; Färbung nach BERENBAUM [4]

Ob die beobachtete Erholung eine restitutio ad integrum darstellt, oder ob spätere Zellteilungen noch Folgeschäden an den Chromosomen erkennbar machen werden, läßt sich zur Zeit noch nicht sagen, da eine entsprechend lange Weiterzüchtung der behandelten Kulturen bisher noch nicht durchgeführt wurde.

Zum Abschluß möchten wir noch auf eine kürzlich erschienene Arbeit von FEIT u. OEHLERT [10] hinweisen, welche vielleicht mit dem Lipoidgehalt des Chromatins in Beziehung steht. Die Autoren verfolgten den Verbleib von mit ³H markiertem 3,4-Benzpyren an in vitro gezüchteten Leukocyten. Bereits 2 Std nach Zugabe des Benzpyrens fand sich eine Markierung bei 100% der Interphasekerne und ca. 50% der Mitosen. Die

der Arbeit von FEIT u. OEHLERT [10] entnommene Abb. 3 zeigt die
Markierung einer frühen Prophase (3a), einer späteren Prophase und
eines Interphasekernes (3b), und schließlich die Markierung von Meta-
phasechromosomen (3c). FEIT u. OEHLERT konnten an den Chromosomen
keine spezifische Lokalisation des Benzpyrens erkennen; sie diskutieren
die Möglichkeit einer Einlagerung des Benzpyrens in die Chromatin-
struktur in dem von BOYLAND [5] vorgeschlagenen Sinne, und betonen
ausdrücklich, daß die bereits nach 2 Std feststellbare Markierung der
Mitosechromosomen einen Zusammenhang des Einbaus mit der Chromo-
somenreduplikation ausschließt, da die G_2-Phase dieser Zellen $4^1/_2$ Std
beträgt.

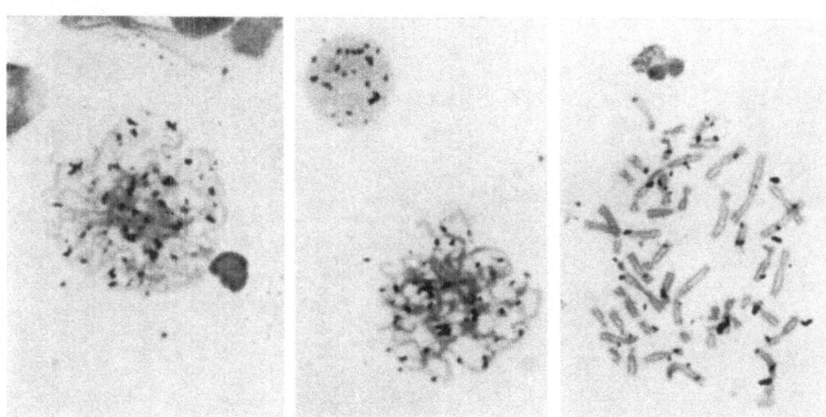

Abb. 3a–c. Autoradiogramme mit ^{3}H-3, 4-Benzpyren markierter menschlicher Blutzellen, 2 Std nach Inkubation. a Markierung des Kernchromatins in früher Prophase; b Chromosomenmarkierung in später Prophase, markierter Interphasekern;
c Chromosomenmarkierung in Metaphase. (Aus einer Arbeit von FEIT u. OEH-
LERT [10])

Es erscheint nicht unwahrscheinlich, daß die Einlagerung des Benzpyrens im Zusammenhang mit der strukturgebundenen Lipoidkompo-
nente der Chromosomen stehen könnte, und erst in der S-Phase, während
der Umstrukturierung im Verlaufe des Reduplikationsprozesses, eine
direkte Störung im Aufbau der DNS, eine Mutation, auslösen würde.

Literatur

1. AGRELL, I.: Cytochemical indication of deoxyribonucleic acid in the pronucleus
   of the mature sea urchin egg. Ark. Zool. **11**, 457–459 (1958).
2. — The structure of the chromatin of the pronucleus and the syncarion of the sea
   urchin egg. Ark. Zool. **12**, 95–98 (1958).
3. BEHEIM, P.: Publikation in Vorbereitung.

4. BERENBAUM, M. C.: The histochemistry of bound lipids. Quart. J. micr. Sci. **99**, 231–242 (1958).
5. BOYLAND, E. and B. GREEN: The interaction of polycyclic hydrocarbons and nucleic acids. Brit. J. Cancer **16**, 507–517 (1962).
6. CHAYEN, J., R. CHAYEN, G. C. CUNNINGHAM, and L. BITENSKY: Bound lipids and their significance in cell biology. Path.-Biol. **9**, 925–926 (1961).
7. CLAUDE, A.: Proteins, lipids and nucleic acids in cell structures and functions. In: Adv. in Protein Chem. **5**, 423–440 (1949).
8. DARLINGTON, C. D. and L. LaCour: Nucleic acid starvation of chromosomes in Trillium. J. Genet. **40**, 185–213 (1940).
9. ENGELHARDT, A.: SP54 – ein Polysaccharidsulfoester zur Anregung der Fibrinolyse. Fortschr. Med. **81**, 728–731 (1963).
10. FEIT, J. u. W. OEHLERT: Autoradiographischer Nachweis von ^{3}H-3,4-Benzpyren in Chromosomen menschlicher Blutzellen. Z. Krebsforsch. **69**, 370–372 (1967).
11. GILLERT, K. E.: Zusatz von Mucopolysacchariden und anderen Polyanionen bei Gelpräpipitationsreaktionen. In Peeters (Edit.): Protides of the Biological Fluid Amsterdam: Elsevier 1964.
12. GONZALEZ-RAMIREZ, J.: Nucleolar physiology. III Considerations about the meaning of nucleolar silver impregnations in cultured HeLa cells. Bol. Inst. Estud. méd. biol. (Mex.) **19**, 195–206 (1961).
13. KARLSON, P.: Morphogenese und Metamorphose der Insekten. In: Induktion und Morphogenese (Mosbacher Colloquium 1962). Berlin-Göttingen-Heidelberg: Springer 1963.
14. LETTRÉ, R., W. SIEBS, and N. PAWELETZ: Morphological observations on the nucleolus of cells in tissue culture, with special regard to its composition. Nat. Cancer Inst. Monogr. **23**, 107–123 (1966).
15. MACHEBOEUF, M.: États des lipides dans la matière vivante. Actualités Scientifiques et Industrielles. Paris: Hermann et Cie 1936.
16. MIRSKY, A. E. and S. OSAWA: The Interphase Nucleus. In: J. BRACHET and A. MIRSKY (Edit.): The Cell, Vol. II, p. 677. New York: Academic Press 1961.
17. NITZ-LITZOW, D.: Klinisch-chemische Untersuchungen zur Lipolyse mit einem neuen Heparinoid. Ärztl. Forsch. **15**, 33–38 (1961).
18. PAWELETZ, N., W. SIEBS u. R. LETTRÉ: Untersuchungen zur Argentaffinreaktion des Nukleolus. Z. Zellforsch. **76**, 577–605 (1967).
19. STONEBURG, C. A.: Lipids of the cell nuclei. J. biol. Chem. **129**, 189–196 (1939).
20. ZELLER, W., H. SCHÖN u. I. ALADAG: Untersuchungen über die Behandlung der hyperglykämischen Atherosklerose mit SP54. Med. Welt **15**, 2231–2238 (1964).

Reaggregation getrennter Tumorzellen

Von

A. Schleich

Die Versuche, maligne Gewebe im Reagensglas zu züchten, sind
annähernd so alt und so vielfältig wie die Technik der Gewebekultur
überhaupt, und die sich bietenden experimentellen Möglichkeiten
wachsen mit der Raffinesse der technischen Durchführung. Wir haben
dabei den großen Vorteil, die lebende Tumorzelle außerhalb des Organismus der chemischen oder physikalischen Beeinflussung und der optischen
Beobachtung zugänglich machen zu können. Dem steht natürlich auch
hier, wie bei jeder Kultur in vitro, der Nachteil eines mehr oder minder
unphysiologischen Milieus und die dadurch bewirkte selektive Veränderung der Zellpopulation gegenüber. Bei den ersten Tumorzüchtungen in
vitro explantierte man kleinere Gewebefragmente ins Koagulum auf Glas
oder Glimmer [2], später versuchte man es mit Zugabe von gesundem
Gewebe als Stütz- oder Nährsubstanz. Trowell [6] in England züchtete
Tumorgewebe in größeren Fragmenten auf einem feinen Drahtnetz,
H. Fell [1] auf Linsenpapier. Leighton [3] in den USA benutzt eine
Matrix aus Schwamm; Etienne Wolff [7] und seine Mitarbeiter in Paris
züchten mit Erfolg menschliche Tumoren auf Mesonephros von Hühner-
embryonen. Das sind nur einige Techniken unter einer großen Anzahl.
Alle diese Bemühungen haben eine Annäherung an die im Organismus
herrschenden Verhältnisse zum Ziel und sind vorwiegend nach morphologischen Gesichtspunkten ausgerichtet. Die Proliferation, d. h. die Vermehrung der Zellen, geht dabei nicht auf Kosten der Differenzierung,
wie das z. B. bei den Tumorzellstämmen der Fall ist, die in Dauerzüchtung
als einschichtige Zellrasen für biochemische und virologische Studien in
den Laboratorien der ganzen Welt gehalten werden.

Wenn bei einem Tumor in vitro noch seine ursprüngliche Zellpopulation weitgehend erhalten bleiben soll, dann muß ihm Gelegenheit
gegeben sein, seine dreidimensionale Struktur zu wahren. Dabei können
im Zentralstück der Primär-Kultur Ernährungsschwierigkeiten auftreten,
und die daraus resultierenden Produkte des Zellzerfalls werden zur Gefahr
für die übrigen Zellen. Andererseits finden wir Differenzierung und
Funktion nur selten in der dem stimulierenden Nährmedium zunächst

liegenden Wachstumszone. So spielt sich auch in der klassischen Gewebe-
Kultur der Proliferationsprozeß in der Randzone ab, und mit dem Ein-
setzen der mitotischen Tätigkeit ist die Differenzierung blockiert. Nach
einigen Passagen nimmt sehr häufig das Bindegewebe überhand auf
Kosten der langsam verschwindenden mehr oder minder differenzierten
Tumorzellen. Dieses Phänomen der Umwandlung zu uncharakteristischen
Bindegewebekulturen begegnet uns bei einem großen Prozentsatz explan-
tierter Tumoren.

Die häufige Erfahrung, daß das Metastasengewebe in vitro besser
wächst als der Primärtumor, ließe auf eine progressive Dedifferenzierung
der in vivo abgewanderten Tumorzellen schließen, und man sollte deshalb
z. B. von den Zellen eines Ascites oder eines Pleuraexsudats, die im
weiten Sinne als Metastase anzusehen sind, keine besonderen histo-
genetischen Potenzen mehr erwarten. Unsere Ergebnisse bewiesen jedoch
das Gegenteil [5]. Die dazu verwendeten Ascites- und Pleuraexsudate
wurden uns freundlicherweise von Herrn Prof. KÄRCHER aus der Strahlen-
klinik zur Verfügung gestellt. An der praktischen Durchführung unserer
Versuche waren Frau M. FRICK und Herr A. MAYER beteiligt.

Wir bauten unsere Experimente auf einer Züchtungsmethode auf, die
MOSCONA [4] in den USA in den 50er Jahren entwickelt hatte. Er disso-
ziierte embryonales Organ-Gewebe mit Trypsin zu Einzelzellen, brachte
diese Suspension in einem Brutkasten in mäßige Schüttelbewegung und
erreichte damit innerhalb 48 Std eine histologisch einwandfreie Reaggregation der einzelnen dissoziierten, embryonalen Organe. Diese
Technik schien uns bei unseren bereits in Suspension vorhandenen
Ascitestumoren sinnvoll. Unser Arbeitsgerät ist ein New Brunswick-
Gyrotory Shaker in Form einer Truhe, in der auf einer, in elliptische
Rotation versetzten Platte, die Erlenmeyerkolben mit dem Zellmaterial
festgeklammert sind. Die Körperflüssigkeiten wurden sofort nach der
Punktion zentrifugiert, im Bedarfsfall von den Erythrocyten befreit und
kurz trypsiniert. Je 5 ml Nährlösung (40% menschl. Placentaserum, 40%
Hanks Salzlösung, 20% Hühner-Embryonalextrakt) enthielten ca. 5 bis
6 Millionen Zellen. Die Temperatur im Shaker war 37 °C bei 65 Rota-
tionen/min.

Bei den Tumorzellen dauert die Reaggregation im Durchschnitt 2 bis
3 Wochen. Die Aggregate bilden während der ersten Woche ein wirres,
anscheinend vom Zufall diktiertes Konglomerat. Bei überwiegend
epithelialen Tumoren hängt das Zustandekommen eines Aggregats vom
Vorhandensein einer bindegewebigen Komponente ab. In der zweiten
Woche beginnt sich die Struktur auszubilden. Eine kapselartige Umran-
dung entsteht, und im Innern des Aggregats kommt es zur Differenzierung. Deutlichere Ansätze zu mehr oder minder geordneten Strukturen
werden erkennbar. HE-, Azan- und PAS-Färbungen demonstrieren das

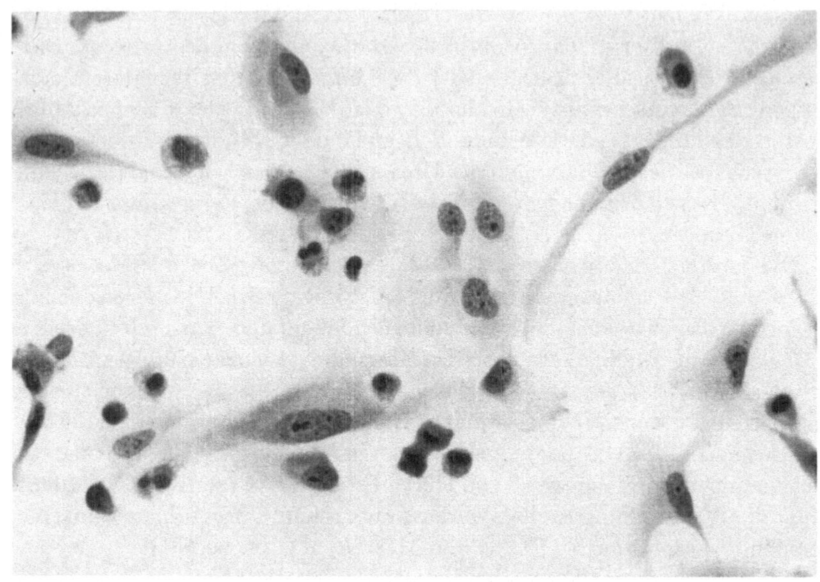

Abb. 1 a

Abb. 1 b   Abb. 1 c

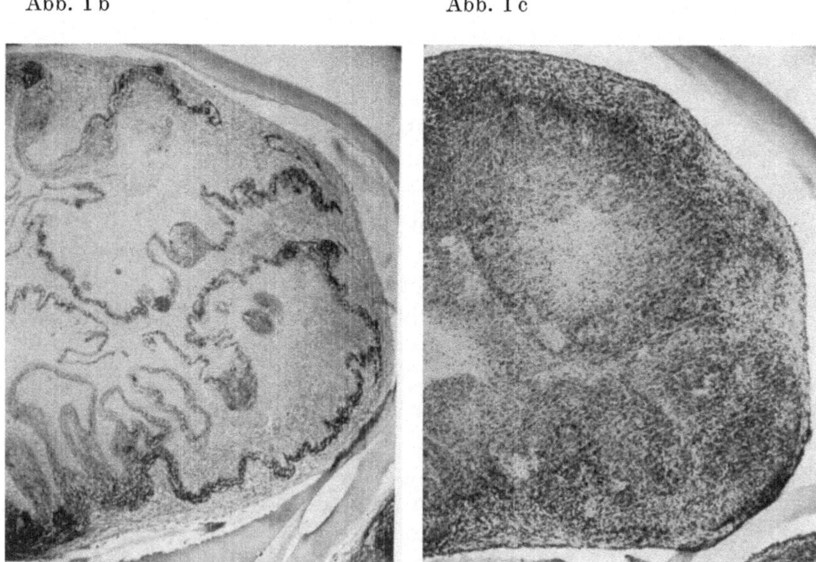

Abb. 1. Ascites, Ovarial-Carcinom. a Einzelzellen, 6 Std nach Punktion. HE-Färbung. b, c Schnittserie eines Aggregats, 33 Tage im Shaker. b Färbung: PAS. c Färbung: HE

Vorhandensein sowohl mesenchymaler als auch epithelialer Komponenten. Die Schleimbildung beweist, daß es sich um funktionell intaktes Gewebe handelt (Abb. 1 a–c).

Auf diesen Befunden wollen wir unsere weiteren Versuche aufbauen. Wir wissen nun, daß Ascitestumoren und dissoziierte Zellen fester Tumoren histogenetische Potenzen behalten. Wir wissen auch, daß eine sinnvolle Aggregation nur in Gegenwart von Zellen mesenchymalen Ursprungs stattfindet. Wir wissen drittens, daß alle diese Aggregationen nur in Gegenwart von menschlichem Placentaserum im Nährmedium über Zeiträume möglich sind, die über 48 Std hinausführen. Rund fünfzig Exsudate bei Mamma- und Ovarialtumoren und bei fortgeschrittenen Melanomen haben wir bis heute mit dieser Technik zur Reaggregation gebracht. Neue Versuche mit soliden Primärexplantaten sind im Gang. Ein dankbares Studienobjekt bietet auch der Laborstamm des menschlichen Cervixcarcinoms HeLa (GEY). Diese in Gewebekultur in einschichtiger Membran wachsenden Tumorzellen waren in Reinkultur nicht zur Aggregation über einen längeren Zeitraum zu bewegen. Doch jede Zugabe von Mesenchymzellen, ob von Hühnchen, Ratte oder Mensch, befähigte die Zellen zur Aggregation.

Es bieten sich mit dieser Aggregationsmethode reizvolle Experimentierobjekte, beginnend mit dem Studium des gesamten Komplexes der Dynamik der Aggregation über Invasion, Infiltration und Zellinteraktion bis hin zur Beeinflussung der Aggregation durch oberflächenwirksame Substanzen und Cytostatika.

Literatur

1. FELL, H. B.: Recent advances in organ culture. Sci. Progr. **41**, 212–231 (1953).
2. GEY, G. O., W. D. COFFMAN, and M. T. KUBICEK: Tissue culture studies of the proliferative capacity of cervical carcinoma and normal epithelium. Cancer Res. **12**, 264–265 (1952).
3. LEIGHTON, J., I. KLINE, M. BELKIN, and Z. TETENBAUM: Studies on human cancer using sponge matrix tissue culture. J. nat. Cancer Inst. **16**, 1353–1373 (1956).
4. MOSCONA, A. A.: Rotation-mediated histogenetic aggregation of dissociated cells. Exp. Cell Res. **22**, 455–475 (1961).
5. SCHLEICH, A.: Studies on aggregation of human ascites tumor cells. Europ. J. Cancer **3**, 243–246 (1967).
6. TROWELL, O. A.: The culture of mature organs in a synthetic medium. Exp. Cell Res. **16**, 118–147 (1959).
7. WOLFF, E. et E. WOLFF: Les résultats d'une nouvelle méthode de culture de cellules cancéreuses „in vitro". Rev. Franç. études clin. et biol. **3**, 945–951 (1958).

Cytometrische Methoden und ihre Bedeutung für therapeutische und prognostische Fragen der Cancerologie*

Von

H. G. Schiemer

Auf vielen Gebieten der Krebsforschung sind in den letzten Jahren erfolgversprechende Untersuchungsmethoden neu entwickelt worden; über zwei Methoden möchte ich im folgenden berichten.

Zunächst sei es erlaubt, auf einige bio- und cytochemische sowie histologische Probleme einzugehen, dann kurz unsere cytometrischen Verfahren zu skizzieren. Es handelt sich dabei vor allem um die Interferenzmikroskopie und UV-Cytophotometrie, die ich zunächst im Pathologischen Institut in Frankfurt a. M. mit Herrn Professor W. Sandritter (s. Schiemer [40]), dann unter Herrn Professor W. Rotter (s. Schiemer [42]) und seit 1966 in Heidelberg so weit fortentwickeln konnte, daß es jetzt möglich ist, in Sekunden oder Minuten Resultate zu erhalten. Im weiteren folgen Ergebnisse von Untersuchungen an normalen tierischen und menschlichen Zellen im Vergleich zu Tumorzellen, wobei auf die beachtliche Tatsache hingewiesen werden sollte, daß man heutzutage cytometrisch Substanzmengen bis zu 1 billionstel Gramm exakt bestimmen kann. Eine neue objektive Beschreibung des Tumorzellwachstums wird erörtert. Daran knüpfen erste strahlen- und chemotherapeutische sowie prognostische Überlegungen an.

Bio- und cytochemische sowie cytologische Probleme

Seinerzeit wurden erhebliche Hoffnungen auf die Biochemie der bösartigen Tumoren gesetzt, z. B. Untersuchungen von Kögl [23] in der Art, daß es möglich sei, grundsätzliche Abweichungen zwischen normalem Gewebe und Tumorgewebe zu erarbeiten. Aber gerade diesen Bemühungen war kein großer Erfolg beschieden (s. dazu Behrens et al. [1, 2], Dittmar [11, 12], Warburg u. Christian [49]). Dagegen sind auf

---

* Mit Unterstützung durch die Deutsche Forschungsgemeinschaft und die Strebelstiftung Mannheim.

anderen Teilgebieten der Biochemie, z. B. der Enzymforschung (z. B. WARBURG [47, 48]), der Nucleinsäure-Forschung (CRICK-WATSON [9], MESELSON u. STAHL [33], BRACHET [4], usw.; s. auch Literatur bei HARBERS, DOMAGK u. MÜLLER [17]) ganz erhebliche Erfolge erzielt worden. Man hat in den Nucleinsäuren die Träger der genetischen Informationen erkannt. Die Erfassung von Menge und Konzentration an Nucleinsäure innerhalb einer Zelle (im Cytoplasma und im Nucleolus RNS; im Kern vor allem DNS) ist daher von erheblicher Bedeutung. Die Untersuchungen von CASPERSSON [5, 6, 7] haben uns die Methoden zur quantitativen physikalischen Bestimmung der Nucleinsäure aufgezeichnet. Die Nucleinsäuren sind in Carcinomzellen oft in absoluter Menge, aber auch in der Konzentration vermehrt. Dies stellt jedoch keine Regel dar. Doch ungeachtet des Letzteren müssen auch schon unterschiedliche DNS-Substanzen gefordert werden, wenn man das Carcinomgewebe histologisch betrachtet, oder wenn man z. B. aus den umfangreichen Chromosomen-Untersuchungen von MAKINO [30], MAKINO u. KANO [31] die logische Konsequenz zieht.

Diese fanden bei malignen Tumoren gehäuft bestimmte Chromosomen-vorkommen, meist war auch die Chromosomenzahl vermehrt. Man diskutiert seitdem das Problem der Stammlinie eines Tumors. Die Vielfalt der morphologischen Details im malignen Tumor gegenüber dem Primärtumor – selbst der gleiche Typ im gleichen Organ von zwei Erkrankten erbringt unterschiedliche Befunde, und in den Metastasen finden sich oft große morphologische Verschiedenheiten – läßt uns heute nicht mehr an jene Unbedingtheit von Stammlinien glauben. Ein genaueres Urteil zu diesen Fragen ist aber nur durch sorgfältige Untersuchungen vieler Tumoren möglich. Nicht nur die NS, sondern auch die Gesamt-Eiweiß-menge und die Menge an einzelnen Substanz-Fraktionen innerhalb der Zelle sind von größtem Interesse. Man glaubt, dadurch den Steuer-mechanismus der RNS- und DNS-Synthese besser erfassen und über die Leistung der Zelle besser aussagen zu können. So ist bis heute immer noch unklar, was die eigentliche Ursache ist, die zum Start der DNS-Synthese führt und die Voraussetzung dafür bildet.

Cytometrische Untersuchungsmethoden

Zwei Verfahren, nämlich die Interferenzmikroskopie und die Cyto-photometrie, haben sich in den letzten 10 Jahren als besonders geeignet erwiesen, die Bedingungen von normalem und pathologischem Wachstum zu studieren. Nur kurz sollen die beiden Methoden dem Wesen nach erklärt werden:

1. Bei der Interferenzmikroskopie (JAMIN [20], LEBEDEFF [24] und JAMIN-MACH [19], ZEHNDER [50]) bestimmt man den Phasen-, optischen

280*

TN 025* TK 055* TC 088* SIN

1+	.	.	.	.	.	.	.	.	.	.	.	.	.	.	.	.	.	.	.	.	.	.	.	.	.	85	.	.	.	.	.	.	.	.	.	.	.	.
2+	.	.	.	.	.	.	.	.	.	.	.	.	.	.	.	.	.	.	.	.	.	.	.	.	.	.	.	.	.	.	.	.	.	.	.	.	.	.
3+	.	.	.	.	.	.	.	.	.	.	.	.	.	.	.	.	.	.	.	.	.	.	86	.	86	82	85	.	.	.	.	.	.	.	.	.	.	.
4+	.	.	.	.	.	.	.	.	.	.	.	.	.	.	.	.	.	.	.	.	.	86	84	82	87	85	84	85	.	.	.	.	.	.	.	.	.	.
5+	.	.	.	.	.	.	.	.	.	.	.	.	.	.	.	.	.	.	.	.	87	.	86	87	83	84	75	78	80	83	79	.	.	.	.	.	.	.
6+	.	.	.	.	.	.	.	.	.	.	.	.	.	.	.	.	.	.	.	86	.	85	83	83	80	80	73	73	75	75	79	79	.	.	.	.	.	.
7+	.	.	.	.	.	.	.	.	.	.	.	.	.	.	.	.	.	.	85	79	81	78	74	73	70	69	65	74	76	.	.	.	.	.	.	.	.	.
8+	.	.	.	.	.	.	.	.	.	.	.	.	.	.	.	87	.	82	76	72	75	71	70	65	63	63	67	65	80	82	84	.	.	.	.	.	.	.
9+	.	.	.	.	.	.	.	.	.	.	.	.	.	.	82	79	76	72	69	66	65	66	60	61	65	72	68	77	85	.	.	.	.	.	.	.	.	.
0+	.	.	.	.	.	.	.	.	.	.	.	.	.	.	83	79	77	69	68	67	67	64	62	59	62	64	66	72	76	85	.	.	.	.	.	.	.	.
1+	.	.	.	.	.	.	.	.	.	.	.	.	.	87	81	75	75	71	68	65	73	63	65	68	66	65	67	76	84	.	.	.	.	.	.	.	.	.
2+	.	.	.	.	.	.	.	.	.	.	.	.	.	86	82	74	72	68	70	70	65	69	62	67	75	69	80	.	.	.	.	.	.	.	.	.	.	.
3+	.	.	.	.	.	.	.	.	.	.	.	.	.	84	75	78	74	75	70	71	73	67	68	66	71	78	78	83	.	.	.	.	.	.	.	.	.	.
4+	.	.	.	.	.	.	.	.	.	.	.	.	87	82	79	70	69	77	71	69	74	68	70	72	66	74	70	78	86	.	.	.	.	.	.	.	.	.
5+	.	.	.	.	.	.	.	.	.	.	.	.	87	80	74	71	69	69	65	66	65	64	67	70	68	63	71	68	77	81	.	.	.	.	.	.	.	.
6+	.	.	.	.	.	.	.	.	86	83	78	76	69	74	66	68	62	65	66	64	67	66	64	63	69	74	78	84	81	.	.	.	.	.	.	.	.	.
7+	.	.	.	.	.	.	.	.	85	76	75	70	63	69	62	66	59	62	61	68	66	64	62	65	67	70	73	78	.	.	.	.	.	.	.	.	.	.
8+	.	.	.	.	.	.	.	.	77	73	67	59	61	60	62	63	61	63	65	65	63	68	63	62	66	74	77	73	.	.	.	.	.	.	.	.	.	.
9+	.	.	.	.	.	.	86	.	69	78	61	50	54	53	53	56	49	60	61	61	62	62	62	64	65	71	74	75	82	82	86	.	.	.	.	.	.	.
0+	.	.	.	.	.	87	.	76	66	54	49	46	44	48	48	52	54	58	58	58	58	63	65	67	67	76	83	81	81	.	.	.	.	.	.	.	.	.
1+	.	.	.	.	86	.	.	73	57	52	50	44	43	39	41	42	41	49	52	56	57	62	59	60	70	73	73	86	83	.	.	.	.	.	.	.	.	.
2+	.	.	.	.	86	79	68	64	51	44	48	45	39	35	38	41	44	42	40	50	53	58	62	63	61	68	76	82	84	85	.	.	.	.	.	.	.	.
3+	.	.	.	.	85	74	73	53	46	42	42	37	33	34	37	36	38	37	39	45	49	55	61	59	64	73	78	83	.	.	.	.	.	.	.	.	.	.
4+	.	.	.	.	81	77	59	41	42	40	40	35	33	32	36	36	36	35	38	39	48	65	66	68	66	74	79	79	84	77	.	.	.	.	.	.	.	.
5+	.	.	.	86	78	66	56	45	42	42	40	34	33	38	35	34	36	38	41	40	56	57	66	64	67	78	82	87	84	.	.	.	.	.	.	.	.	.
6+	.	.	.	82	75	62	49	45	44	42	40	36	30	35	39	33	31	37	39	40	49	59	68	63	73	79	86	84	.	.	.	.	.	.	.	.	.	.
7+	.	.	86	76	71	55	52	46	41	40	40	25	33	31	34	33	38	40	42	42	49	62	64	69	81	.	.	.	.	.	.	.	.	.	.	.	.	.
8+	.	.	.	67	65	56	51	49	38	36	40	35	32	34	35	39	41	45	38	43	52	62	68	72	84	81	.	.	.	.	.	.	.	.	.	.	.	.
9+	.	84	81	69	64	59	49	44	42	42	41	34	36	36	34	38	38	42	48	48	59	70	70	81	87	.	.	.	.	.	.	.	.	.	.	.	.	.
0+	.	81	74	70	67	53	48	46	39	38	39	37	38	38	37	37	35	44	49	52	66	65	75	87	87	.	.	.	.	.	.	.	.	.	.	.	.	.
1+	.	82	68	68	61	53	48	44	42	40	35	35	37	39	37	37	44	48	52	57	62	81	.	85	.	.	.	.	.	.	.	.	.	.	.	.	.	.
2+	.	78	74	67	66	57	55	46	46	44	43	38	35	36	41	44	43	45	50	56	61	65	77	77	.	.	.	.	.	.	.	.	.	.	.	.	.	.
3+	.	84	83	75	69	62	67	60	54	51	45	43	43	41	41	43	45	48	49	55	61	62	70	72	82	85	87	86	.	.	.	.	.	.	.	.	.	.
4+	.	.	79	69	70	67	66	58	56	52	47	48	42	45	48	49	51	53	53	59	66	72	74	79	.	81	.	.	.	.	.	.	.	.	.	.	.	.
5+	.	.	80	71	63	69	62	61	59	54	49	54	47	55	51	54	53	62	63	69	74	76	82	.	84	.	.	.	.	.	.	.	.	.	.	.	.	.
6+	.	.	80	72	76	66	62	62	58	63	49	59	58	62	59	61	67	69	69	74	75	80	78	.	.	87	.	.	.	.	.	.	.	.	.	.	.	.
7+	.	86	77	71	71	69	75	67	63	65	59	58	63	66	73	77	71	79	76	.	80	84	.	.	86	.	.	.	.	.	.	.	.	.	.	.	.	.
8+	.	.	80	74	76	71	68	76	69	58	75	66	77	70	70	75	79	83	73	82	85	84	87	84	.	.	.	.	.	.	.	.	.	.	.	.	.	.
9+	.	79	.	75	77	73	77	72	66	72	73	80	80	73	83	77	.	86	83	.	86	87	.	.	.	.	.	.	.	.	.	.	.	.	.	.	.	.
0+	84	.	.	82	77	73	75	77	74	75	75	82	83	83	82	84	84	86	83	.	.	.	.	.	.	.	.	.	.	.	.	.	.	.	.	.	.	.
1+	.	85	82	77	74	79	76	78	78	79	83	81	86	.	87	86	.	82	.	87	86	86	86	.	.	.	.	.	.	.	.	.	85	.	.	.	87	.
2+	.	84	80	78	82	81	80	86	85	.	86	.	87	.	.	.	.	.	.	.	.	.	.	.	.	.	.	.	.	86	83	84	.	86	.	.	.	.
3+	.	85	85	84	83	.	87	.	86	.	85	.	.	.	.	.	.	86	.	.	.	.	.	87	87	85	85	.	.	.	85	.	.	.	.	.	.	.
4+	.	.	.	.	.	.	.	.	.	.	.	.	.	.	.	.	.	.	.	.	.	.	.	.	.	.	.	.	.	.	.	.	.	.	.	.	.	.

FN 003*	FK 040*	FC 050*	TN 025*	TK 055*	TC 080*	SH 010*	AP 041*	HU 010*	AL 0423*	NR	MB	19951*
1*	*	*										
2*	*	*										
3*	*	*										
4*	*	*										
5*	*	*										
6*	6*	*										
7*	8*	6*										
8*	10*	14*										
9*	13*	24*										
10*	14*	37*										
11*	13*	51*										
12*	11*	64*										
13*	13*	75*										
14*	14*	88*										
15*	15*	102*										
16*	17*	117*										
17*	19*	134*										
18*	20*	153*										
19*	20*	173*										
20*	19*	193*										
21*	20*	212*										
22*	22*	232*										
23*	22*	254*										
24*	23*	276*										
25*	22*	299*										
26*	22*	321*										
27*	21*	343*										
28*	21*	364*										
29*	20*	385*										
30*	21*	405*										
31*	19*	426*										
32*	23*	445*										
33*	21*	468*										
34*	22*	489*										
35*	19*	511*										
36*	18*	530*										
37*	17*	548*										
38*	14*	565*										
39*	8*	579*										
40*	7*	587*										
41*	7*	594*										
42*	*	601*										

MB   19951*   100*   *   *   425*   2060*   683*   6010*

Tab. 1a zeigt den Maschinenausdruck einer berechneten Carcinomzelle (Mammacarcinom). Der obere Teil der Abbildung stellt die Zelle dar. Der Ausdruck wurde mit Hilfe des Niveaudiagramm-Systems des MCZ-Programms erstellt. Die Umgebung der Zelle erscheint als Leerfeld, indem die Niveaubegrenzung bei 88% Transmission eingestellt wurde. Das Cytoplasma ist durch geradstehende %-Transmissionszahlen, der Kern durch schrägstehende halbfette %-Zahlen wiedergegeben. Bis zu 4 Ausläufer nach links oder rechts oder nach oben oder unten können von dem Programm unterschieden werden. Jede Fremdzelle am Rande der Zelle wird eliminiert, sofern das Programm die zentrale Zelle getrennt von den anderen Objektdetails findet. Innerhalb des Cytoplasmas können bis zu 4 Kerne erkannt werden, innerhalb jedes Kernes wiederum bis zu 4 kleinere Objekte (z. B. Nucleoli) unterschieden werden.

In 1b des Maschinenausdrucks werden in der ersten Zeile die notwendigen Berechnungsparameter angegeben. FN, FK und FC bedeuten die Minimalflächen für Nucleolus, Kern und Cytoplasma; TN, TK und TC die %-Transmissionswertgrenze; SH: Schrittweite, AP: Anzahl der einzelnen Meßpunkte pro Zeile, HU: Hubweite, AL: Anzahl der gemessenen Linien. NB 19951 ist die Kennzeichnung des Meßobjektes.

Die drei folgenden Zahlenkolonnen stellen einmal die Numerierung der Zeilenlinie in der ersten Kolonne dar; in der zweiten Kolonne findet sich die Anzahl der aufzusummierenden Meßwerte für das Cytoplasma; in der dritten Kolonne sind die Summenwerte abzulesen. Am Schluß der Zeile wird sowohl auf Schreibmaschine als auch auf Lochstreifen das Ergebnis der Berechnung ausgedruckt. Hier wurde bei der Zelle MB 19951 ein Kern mit einer mittleren Transmission von 42,5% bei einer Fläche von $206\mu^2$ und ein Cytoplasma mit mittlerer Transmission von 68,3% bei einer Gesamtzellfläche von $601,0\mu^2$ gefunden. Weiteres siehe Text

Weglängen- oder optischen Gang-Unterschied zwischen Objekt und Referenzstrahlen mit einem Kompensator. Berücksichtigt man das spezifische Refraktionsvermögen (χ), z. B. für Eiweiß, so kann durch eine Gangunterschiedsmessung über dem Zellkern (innerhalb des mikroskopischen Gesichtsfeldes) und indem zugleich auch dessen Fläche berücksichtigt wird, die Trockenmasse des Kernes ermittelt werden (SCHIEMER [41]; s. a. DAVIES u. DEELEY [10]).

Die so bestimmten Substanzmengen liegen bei normalen Zellen pro Kern etwa zwischen $20\text{--}80 \times 10^{-12}$ g. Desgleichen verfährt man bei der Untersuchung des Cytoplasmas.

2. Die Cytometrie ist besonders durch das Gerät von Barr & Stroud und ein weiteres von der Firma Carl Zeiß bekannt geworden. Wir haben uns in letzter Zeit aus methodischen Gründen vor allem mit der UV-Photometrie befaßt. Durch diese ist es möglich, die Nucleinsäuren ohne färberischen Eingriff im Bereich der spezifischen Absorption bei der Wellenlänge 263 nm quantitativ zu bestimmen.

Ich habe die langwierige Registrierung durch den Schnellmeßzusatz der Firma Carl Zeiß auf ein Minimum reduzieren können. Mit Hilfe eines Magnetbandspeichers* lassen sich die Meßdaten während der Registrierung festhalten und anschließend von einem Computer analysieren. Es entstehen Zahlenfelder, die %-Transmissionswerte bedeuten (s. Tab. 1). Die Zellumgebung wird durch Leertastenanschläge, das Cytoplasma durch schwarze, der Zellkern durch rote Zahlen veranschaulicht. Dieses Niveaudiagramm dient der Kontrolle; anschließend wird in wenigen Minuten die mittlere Transmission der jeweiligen Zellareale und deren genaue Fläche in μ^2 angegeben. Diese Daten werden der größeren Schnelligkeit wegen und wegen des Umfanges des benutzten statistischen Programmes im Deutschen Rechenzentrum in Darmstadt weiterverarbeitet.

Zur Auswertung muß folgendes vermerkt werden:

Der wahre Wert solcher Untersuchungen hängt heute und in Zukunft von der schnellen und umfangreichen statistischen Auswertung ab. Früher mußte ich mit vielen Hilfskräften lange Zahlenkolonnen monatelang durcharbeiten. Heute kann man dafür die elektronischen Datenverarbeitungsanlagen einsetzen. Mit unseren Zellanalyse-Programmen werden nicht nur die Einzelwerte von Trockengewicht, Volumen, DNS-Menge usw., sondern auch die jeweiligen Mittelwerte mit den dazugehörigen Sigmawerten berechnet und ausgegeben. Es werden ferner Regressionsanalysen vorgenommen und Verteilungshistogramme aufgestellt und in Sekundenschnelle ausgedruckt.

---

* Es handelt sich um eine Entwicklung der Firmen Assmann und Kienzle, benutzt wird dabei u. a. ein sog. endloses Magnetband.

Vergleichende cytometrische Untersuchungen

Wir sind also in der Lage, kurzzeitig die Zelle auf ihren Substanz-
gehalt zu untersuchen. Wir werden in einem Kollektiv kleine, normale
mit reduzierter und solche mit gesteigerter Funktion oder zugrunde
gehende Zellen finden. Substanz- und Wassergehalt sind entsprechend
verändert. Diesen „Normzellen" stehen die Tumorzellen gegenüber.

Für die experimentelle Krebsforschung ist eine vergleichende
Pathologie von besonderer Bedeutung. Viele Organveränderungen sind
bei den einzelnen Tierspecies häufig, bei anderen wiederum nicht. Bei den
weiblichen Mammaliern darf der Hormonstoffwechsel nicht übersehen
werden. Schon beim Menschen (SCHIEMER [43]) werden menstruations-
cyclusabhängige Organveränderungen festgestellt (bei der Ratte z. B.
beträgt der Cyclus nur etwa 4–6 Tage). Die Einflüsse gesteigerter Organ-
und Zell-Leistungen (z. B. bei lokalen oder generalisierten Entzündungen)
müssen berücksichtigt werden. Das Alter von tierischen oder menschlichen Probanden ist stets zu beachten. Mehr erkennt man durch die
Verteilungskurven (Abb. 1). In den Trockengewichtshistogrammen sind
die Ergebnisse einiger tierischer und menschlicher Zelluntersuchungen
zusammengetragen. In der oberen Hälfte der Abb. 1 sind vor allem die
haploiden und diploiden tierischen Zellen einander gegenübergestellt. Bei
dem menschlichen Untersuchungsgut werden normale Zellen und Tumorzellen miteinander verglichen. Entsprechend der Zellklasseneinteilung
von COWDRY [8] finden sich auch entsprechende Anordnungen, die man
an der Kern/Plasma-Gruppierung erkennt. Bei Carcinomzellen sind
häufig die Kern- und Cytoplasmadiagramme ineinander verschoben.
Beim Vergleich von normalen und Tumorzellen erkennt man insbesondere
die Reduktion der Cytoplasmastruktur. Die Tumorzellen kann man
formal von der I. und II. Klasse der COWDRYschen Einteilung nur durch
ihre Histogramme sicher unterscheiden.

Eine alleinige Bestimmung der Mittelwerte von Trockengewicht,
Volumen- oder %-Trockengewicht ergibt keine eindeutigen charakteristischen Hinweise auf Malignität. Wir beobachten, daß auch Carcinomzellen Mittelwerte im Bereiche von normalen Zellen besitzen. Ebenfalls gilt das für Bestimmungen der Nucleinsäuren; Zellen maligner
Tumoren können im Mittel normale NS-Werte aufweisen.

Strahlentherapeutische Überlegungen

Lange Zeit hatte man gehofft, durch Erkennen einer sog. Stammlinie
auf den voraussichtlichen DNS-Gehalt und auf die Eigenart des Tumors
schließen zu können. Man sah in dieser Konstanz auch einen Ansatzpunkt,
strahlentherapeutisch wirksam zu werden. Diese Konstanz ist aber nur
in seltenen Fällen vorhanden.

H. G. Schiemer

Tier
Mensch
%
40
20
0
Forellen-u.Saibling-Spermien
n=44; Tr.=4,24·10⁻¹²g
Erythrocyten(Zellkerne)
n=34; Tr.=8,36·10⁻¹²g
Krötenerythrocyten
(Zellkerne)
(Bufo viridans)
n=35; Tr.=18,07·10⁻¹²g
Froscherythrocyten
(Zellkerne)
(Rana temporaria)
n=32; Tr.=7,17·10⁻¹²g
Kaninchenspermien
n=44; Tr.=6,75·10⁻¹²g
Erythrocyten(Zellkerne)
n=28; Tr.=13,28·10⁻¹²g
Rattenspermien
n=31; Tr.=6,04·10⁻¹²g
Thymus(Zellkerne)
n=75; Tr.=11,24·10⁻¹²g
Spermien
Thymocyten(Zellkerne)
UHLIG, 1958
Leber
55 J.
GÜNTHER, 1965
Aortenendothelien
26 J.
SCHIEMER, STAHR, 1964
Plattenepithelien
der Mundschleimhaut
ZAHN, 1965
Kleinzelliges Karzinom
POLLAK, 1958
Mamma-Ca, solide, teils
undifferenziert, scirrhös
E 12617/66; 72 J.
Mamma-Ca, solide, undif-
ferenziert, scirrhös
E 13072/66; 73 J.
0   5   10   50   100   500   1000·10⁻¹²g

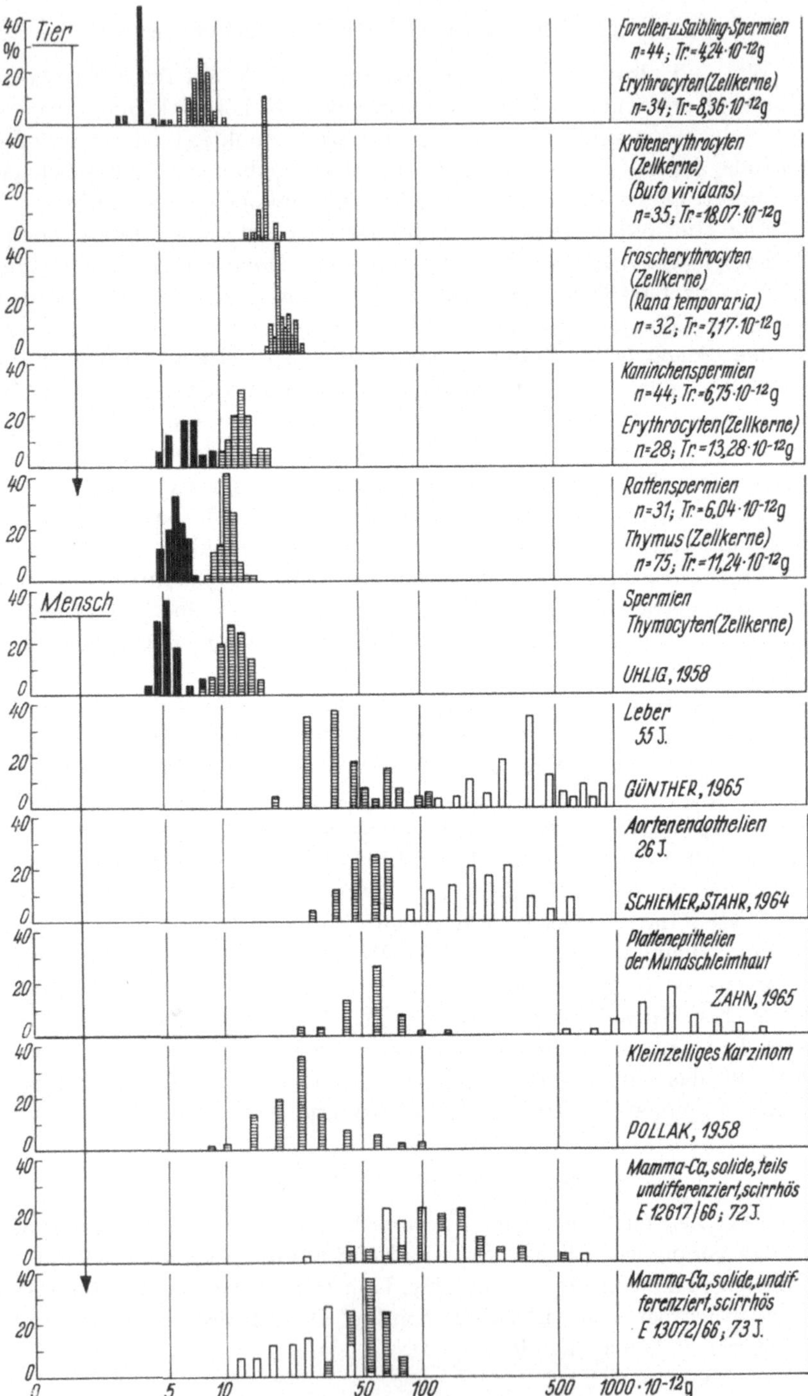

Die Treffer-theoretischen Überlegungen ergeben einen direkten therapeutischen Einsatz für nur 20% der Fälle, der andere Prozentsatz der Strahlung wird durch Alkylierungs-Effekte (durch Bildung von H_2O_2) im Zellgewebe wirksam (MAURER [32], RAJEWSKY [37]). Durch eine Röntgenbestrahlung wird DNS auf Grund ihrer (partiellen) Singularität molekular irreversibel geschädigt. Aber auch die RNS wird durch Röntgenstrahlen verändert. Eine strahlentherapeutische Voraussetzung ist eine hohe Konzentration an Nucleinsäure (RNS und auch DNS) gegenüber den normalen Zellen. Nun sind bei weitem nicht alle Carcinomzellen mit hoher Nucleinsäurekonzentration behaftet. Auch innerhalb eines Zellkollektivs können weite Streuungen vorkommen. Aus diesem Grunde dürften sich besonders die kleinen dichten, wenig streuenden nucleinsäurereichen Tumorzellen für eine Strahlenbehandlung eignen, wie wir das oft auch aus klinischen und autoptischen Berichten entnehmen.

Ein Beispiel zur Frage der morphologischen und auch objektiv faßbaren Verschiedenheit bei Primärtumor und Metastasen ist in Abb. 2 und Tab. 2 aufgezeigt. Die Carcinommetastase ist danach objektiv stärker verwildert als der Primärtumor. Ich möchte darüber hinaus mit diesen Befunden zu Überlegungen anregen, ob z. B. nur die in ihren Histogrammen eng gruppierten Carcinomzellkollektive optimal radiologisch zu behandeln sind.

Objektivierende Methoden zur Beobachtung des Zellwachstums

Die cytometrischen Untersuchungen lassen in gewisser Näherung (1. und 2. Grades) eine Aussage über die Syntheseleistungen der Zellen zu, hinsichtlich der Gesamtproteinmenge, hinsichtlich der RNS im Cytoplasma oder der DNS im Zellkern. Man benutzt dazu die Methode der Regressionsanalyse. Nehmen wir ein einfaches anschauliches Beispiel: Innerhalb einer Bevölkerung kann man Säuglinge, Kinder und Erwachsene unterscheiden. Da ein Kind in der Regel bei einer gewissen Größe auch ein bestimmtes Gewicht hat, desgleichen der Erwachsene, kann man schon aus den Gewichtsangaben auf das Alter irgendeiner Person schließen. Unser Beispiel übertragen auf die Zelle: Wir setzen voraus, daß – statistisch gesehen – die größere Zelle, die an Substanz

Legende zur Abb. 1 (siehe Seite 224).

Abb. 1. Histogramme der Trockengewichte von tierischen und menschlichen Zellen. Bei der oberen Gruppe sind vor allem die haploiden und diploiden Zelltypen berücksichtigt. Beim Menschen sind die verschiedenen Zellklassen-Einteilungen nach COWDRY zu erkennen, so z. B. Leberzellen und Plattenepithelien. Diesen Normalzellkollektiven stehen verschiedene Carcinomzelltypen gegenüber. Die Ineinanderschachtelung der Kern- und Cytoplasma-Diagramme der letzten 2 Carcinome sind für maligne Tumoren typisch

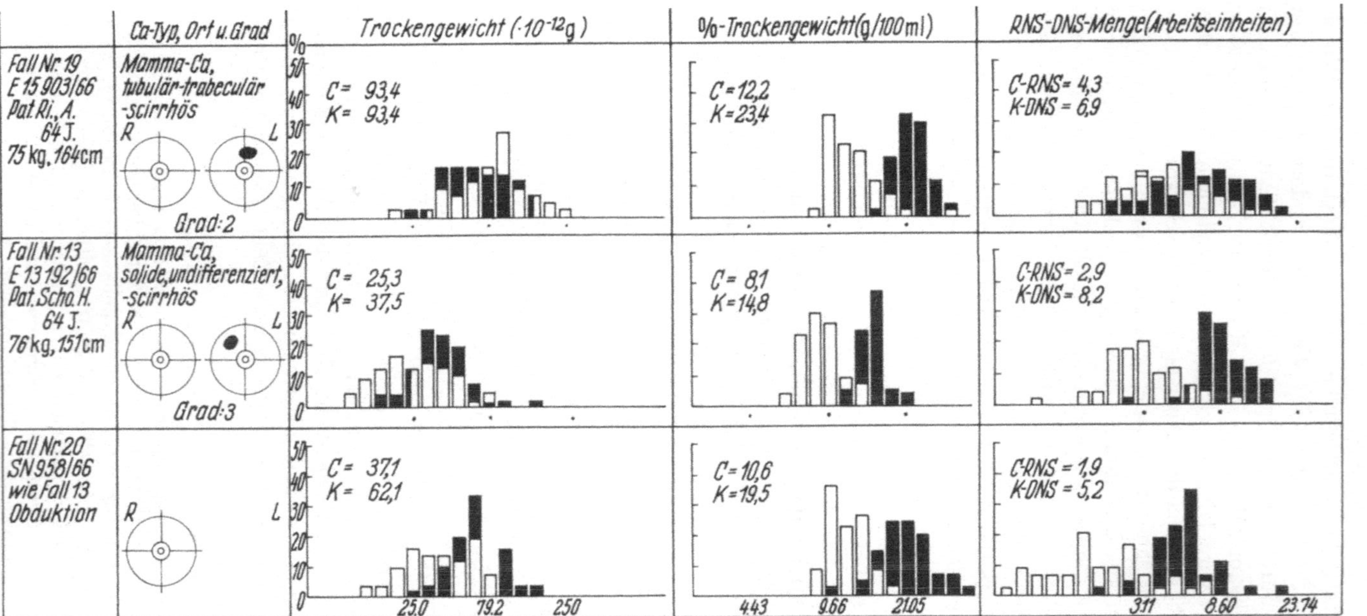

Abb. 2. Zusammenstellung einiger Ergebnisse unserer cytometrischen Untersuchungen von Mammacarcinomen. Es sind 3 Fälle dargestellt: Es handelt sich um Patientinnen, die inzwischen verstorben sind. Im 1. Fall wurde eine Bestrahlungstherapie vorgenommen. Im 2. Fall war sie beabsichtigt; die Patientin verstarb kurz vor Beginn der Therapie an einer fulminanten Lungenembolie bei paraneoplastischem Syndrom; der 3. Fall weist die cytometrischen Ergebnisse des Autopsiegutes auf. In der zweiten Spalte ist die Lokalisation der Mammatumoren zu erkennen und die Malignitäts-Graduierung nach HAAGENSEN. In der dritten und vierten Spalte sind Trocken-, %-Trockengewicht und Nucleinsäuremengen sowohl durch Histogramm als auch in den Mittelwerten angegeben. „C" bedeutet Cytoplasma, „K" Kern. Trockengewicht und %-Trockengewicht wurden durch interferenzmikroskopische Untersuchungen, die Nucleinsäuremengen durch cytophotometrische Untersuchungen erhalten. Weiteres siehe Text

reichere Zelle, auch die für das Zell-Leben ältere Zelle ist, gegenüber den deutlich kleineren und leichteren Zellen. Die Regressionsgerade gewinnt dadurch die Bedeutung eines Vektors, dessen Winkelsteilheit zugleich auch ein Maß der beschleunigten oder herabgesetzten Substanzsynthese ist.

Man wird zu diesen Überlegungen durch gewisse Befunde cytometrischer Untersuchungen geführt, z. B. durch eine Gegenüberstellung von Tr. und Volumen von Leberzellen (Abb. 3). Im doppeltlogarithmischen

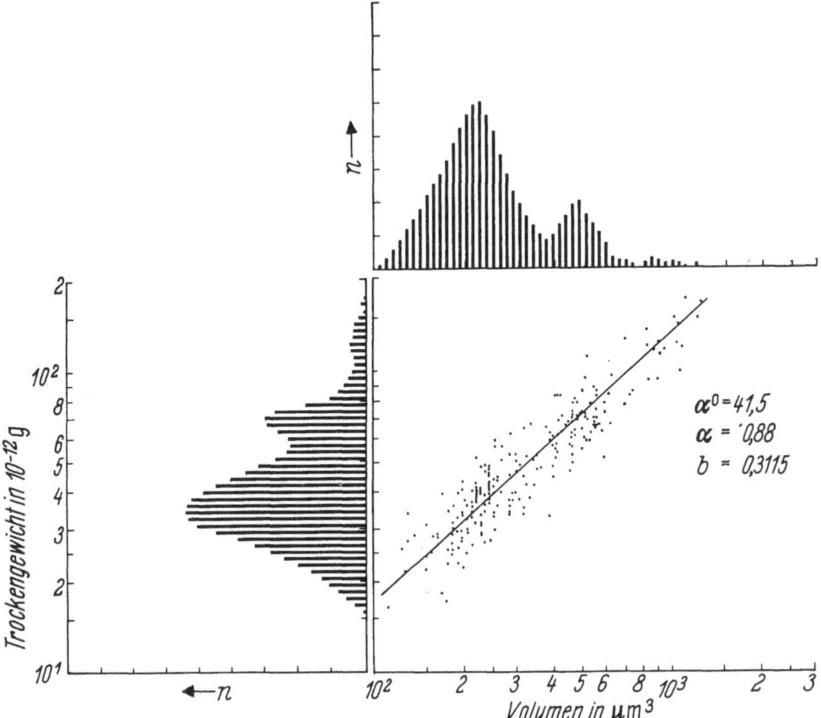

Abb. 3. Halblogarithmische Darstellung (modifiziert nach SCHIEMER, 1965) von Volumen und Trockengewichtsverteilung in doppeltlogarithmischer Form. Es handelt sich um eine allometrische (Regressions-)Analyse eines Kollektivs von Leberzellkernen (225 normale menschliche Leberzellen). Es sind die Trockengewichtswerte links seitlich, in der oberen rechten Abteilung die Volumenwerte aufgetragen. In der doppeltlogarithmischen Darstellung rechts unten ist die Korrelation zwischen Volumen und dem jeweiligen Trockengewicht der einzelnen Kerne graphisch dargestellt. Die „Punktwolken" zeigen 2 Schwerpunkte, die mit den jeweiligen diploiden und tetraploiden Gipfeln von Volumen und Trockengewicht übereinstimmen. Es ergibt sich daraus eine Regressionsgerade, deren Anstiegswinkel (α) ein Maß für die Syntheseleistung ist. Man gibt im allgemeinen die Tangenswerte an. „b" beinhaltet den Abschnitt auf der X- oder Y-Achse. Es handelt sich hier um den somatischen Wachstumsfaktor oder initialen Wachstumsindex. „b" könnte etwas über den Zellinformationsgehalt aussagen. Weiteres siehe Text

Raster ergibt sich dann eine enge Gruppierung um eine Regressionsgerade. Auch die sicher tetraploiden Zellkerne setzen sich in der gleichen Richtung geordnet fort. Es handelt sich also um ein biologisches Prinzip. Wir kennen derartige Untersuchungen schon durch SNELL [*39*], DUBOIS [*14, 15*], KLATT [*22*], NEEDHAM [*35*], LINZBACH [*27*], SANDRITTER et al. [*38*]. Ob es um Vergleiche zwischen Gehirngewicht und Körpergewicht, zwischen biochemisch faßbaren Größen und dem Gesamtgewicht des bezogenen Objektes ging, es erwies sich immer, daß die Korrelation eines Teiles des Ganzen zum Ganzen bei biologischen Objekten gesetzmäßige Befundverteilungen ergibt, die besonders gut in geometrisch unterteilten

Tabelle 2. *Allometrische Daten der Nucleinsäure/Volumen-Korrelation (Regressionsanalyse) von 3 cytophotometrisch untersuchten Mammacarcinomen. Es handelt sich um die gleichen Fälle wie in Abb. 2.*

Beim 1. Fall, der 64jährigen Frau, fallen die erhöhten α-Werte auf, die für eine gesteigerte Nucleinsäuresynthese sprechen. Demgegenüber scheint der Informationsgehalt niedrig zu sein, was aus den niedrigen Werten für „b" zu entnehmen ist. Die allometrischen Untersuchungen im 2. Fall, der 64jährigen Frau, zeigen im Primärtumor für Protoplasma einen hohen „Informationsgehalt" mit gesteigerter Syntheseleistung. Diese Syntheseleistung findet sich auch für das untersuchte Zellkollektiv der Knochenmetastase bei der Obduktion (zwei Monate später), jedoch ist jetzt der „Informationsgehalt" des Cytoplasmas außerordentlich niedrig

	Kern (DNS)	Cytoplasma (RNS)	Bemerkungen:
Fall E 15903/66 64 Jahre ♀ tubuläres, scirrhös gewachsenes Mamma-Ca.	$\alpha = 0,8781$ $b = 0,0253$	$\alpha = 1,1606$ $b = 0,0021*$	Ausgedehnte Metastasierung, seit 1 Monat ziehende Schmerzen. Relat. wasserarme Zellen (% Tr_k 23,4, % Tr_c 12,2) Tr_k/DNS = 13,5:1
Fall E 13192/66 64 Jahre ♀ Solides, undifferenziertes scirrhös gewachsenes Mamma-Ca.	$\alpha = 0,7593$ $b = 0,1910$	$\alpha = 1,0344$ $b = 0,9888$	Tumor seit 5 Monaten getastet, Lymphknoten-Metastasen; Zell-Wassergehalt im Bereich der Norm (% Tr_k 14,8; % Tr_c 5,8) Tr_k/ DNS = 4,5:1
Fall SN 958/66 64 Jahre ♀ (E 13192/66) Autopsie 2 Monate später! Solides, teils stark verwildertes Ca.	$\alpha = 0,7258$ $b = 0,3061$	$\alpha = 1,0858$ $b = 0,0123*$	Generalisierte Metastasierung, relat. wasserarme Zellen (% Tr_k 19,1; % Tr_c 10,6) Tr_k/DNS 12:1

* Informationsarmes Cytoplasma!

Papieren graphisch dargestellt werden können. Man unterscheidet einen sog. Wachstumsexponenten ‚α' (auch Wachstumskonstante) und den initialen Wachstumsindex ‚b'. Vereinfacht gesagt, bedeutet ‚α' einen Gradienten der Syntheseleistung ($1,0$ = volumenbezogene Substanzvermehrung; $0,66$ = oberflächenbezogene Substanz- oder Stoffwechselleistung). ‚b' könnte etwas mit der Differenziertheit der biologischen Leistung („Mitgift") zu tun haben, z. B. Cytoplasmainformation, wie in Tab. 2 erkennbar.

Wir besitzen somit Methoden, die die Zell-Leistung quantitativ und qualitativ erfassen. Diese Feststellung ist von besonderer Bedeutung für die Beurteilung der Wirksamkeit vor allem chemotherapeutischer Maßnahmen.

Chemotherapeutische Überlegungen

Man kann eine folgende Zusammenstellung verschiedener tumorwirksamer Hemmstoffe vornehmen (siehe dazu auch LETTRÉ [25], GASTPAR u. HERRMANN [16], MEYTHALER [34], PÜTTER [36]):

a) alkylierende Agentien,
b) Antimetabolite (Antiwirkstoffe),
c) Mitosegifte,
d) Antibiotika,
e) Hormone.

Die Zusammenstellung erhebt keinen Anspruch auf Vollständigkeit. Für die *alkylierenden* Substanzen gilt im Grunde das gleiche, wie es oben für die Strahlentherapie gesagt wurde.

Folgendes sei noch hinsichtlich der die Strahlensensibilität aufhebenden Wirkung schwefelhaltiger organischer Verbindungen erwähnt. Soviel aus der uns zugänglichen Literatur zu ersehen ist, könnte hier eine Chemotherapie der Bestrahlung überlegen sein. Letzteres gilt unter Umständen besonders für Krebsfälle, bei denen wir mit cytometrischen Untersuchungen z. B. im Zellkern viel Trockensubstanz, aber prozentual wenig Nucleinsäure nachgewiesen haben.

Die Wirkung von *Antimetaboliten* konnten wir selbst an regenerierenden, teilektomierten Rattenlebern studieren. Unter Methotrexat weist insbesondere die Substanzsynthese im Zellkern eine Hemmung auf gegenüber den normal regenerierenden Leberzellen (SCHIEMER et al. [45]).

Die *Mitosegifte*, im Zusammenhang mit cytometrischen Untersuchungen gesehen, lassen die größte Wirksamkeit bei schnell DNS-synthetisierenden Zellen erwarten. Das sind vor allem Tumorzellen mit sehr kurzen Interphasezeiten, also kleinzellige Tumoren. Diese bilden meist auch wenig Cytoplasmastrukturen aus.

Über die Wirkung von *Antibiotika* läßt sich hier wenig aussagen, da wir auf diesem Gebiete noch keine Erfahrungen sammeln konnten.

Die Einführung der *Tumorbehandlung mit Hormonen* verdanken wir vor allem den Arbeiten von BIELSCHOWSKY et al. [*3*], HUGGINS [*18*] und LOESER [*28*]. Durch unsere menstruationscyclusabhängigen Untersuchungen an Mundschleimhautepithelien konnten wir bereits zeigen, wie sehr hormonelle Einflüsse am Kern und Cytoplasma hinsichtlich des Substanz- und Wassergehaltes wirksam sind.

Prognostische Überlegungen

An einigen Fällen von Plasmocytomerkrankungen, die wir durch Autopsie genauer untersuchen konnten, läßt sich paradigmatisch das Problem deutlich machen. In Tab. 3 sind die interferenzmikroskopischen Ergebnisse zusammengestellt. Außerdem sind einige normale Vergleichswerte angeführt. Kerntrockengewicht und Volumenwerte sind gegenüber normalen Werten durchweg höher. Gegenüber der Norm sind andererseits die Trockengewichte und Volumina für Cytoplasma deutlich erniedrigt. Die Fälle 3 (70jährige Frau), 4 (65jährige Frau), 6 (44jährige Frau) zeichnen sich durch eine kurze Krankheitsdauer aus. In der dazugehörigen allometrischen Untersuchung finden wir Hinweise auf eine erhöhte Syntheseleistung in Kern und Cytoplasma. Zwei Fälle verstarben an den Folgen einer Paraproteinnephrose. Die hohen %-Tr.-Werte im Falle der 65jährigen Frau deuten auf eine Besonderheit hin: Es handelt sich um eine extreme Paraproteinose (s. JANSEN et al. [*21*]). In dem letzten in der Tabelle aufgeführten Falle wurde massiv mit Endoxan behandelt. Die hämorrhagische Diathese ist wohl vor allem darauf zurückzuführen. Man muß sich allerdings in diesem Zusammenhang fragen, zu welchen Ergebnissen eine cytometrische Untersuchung in einem Zeitpunkt vor Beginn der Chemotherapie geführt hätte. Die bei der Sektion erhobenen Befunde sprechen jetzt für ein langsames Myelomwachstum.

Es ist unsere Aufgabe, an weiteren Fällen zu prüfen, ob tatsächlich bei derartigen Kombinationen von cytometrischen Werten mit genügender Häufigkeit die Art des Krankheitsverlaufes vorausgesagt werden kann.

Auch scheinen mir für die Tumorbehandlung einige Ansatzpunkte gegeben zu sein, nämlich derart, daß das cytometrische Ergebnis bei manchen Myelomerkrankungen die Wahl der Therapie bestimmen könnte. Z. B. wäre in manchen Fällen zu versuchen, nur die Gammaglobulin-Synthese im Protoplasma der Myelomzellen durch Antimetaboliten zu hemmen, wenn wir mit unseren Untersuchungen eine derartige gesteigerte Proteinsynthese cytometrisch erfassen.

Tabelle 3. *Plasmocytomwerte und normale Vergleichswerte sind tabellarisch gegenüber-*
gestellt.

In der oberen Abteilung Normalwerte; in der unteren Abteilung erkennt man die
erhöhten Kerntrockengewichte einerseits und die erniedrigten Cytoplasmatrocken-
gewichte andererseits.
Auffällig ist Fall 4 (65jähr. Frau). Hier handelt es sich um eine außerordentlich
starke Eiweißsyntheseleistung der Plasmazellen, die zu einem Karpaltunnel-
Syndrom geführt haben. Die Patientin ist an den Folgen einer paraprotein-
ämischen Nephrose verstorben.

Weiteres siehe Text

a) normale Vergleichswerte
b) Plasmocytomfälle

a)	Trockengewicht in 10^{-12} g		Volumen in 10^{-12} cm³		%-Trockengew. in g/100 ml		
	Kern	Cytopl.	Kern	Cytopl.	Kern	Cytopl.	
Nasenpolyp (Schleimhaut)	15,5	91,3	121,0	1260,0	14,0	7,8	HÜBNER u. SCHIEMER 1962
Lebercirrhose (Knochenmark)	18,1	83,3	118,0	938,0	15,8	9,6	HÜBNER u. SCHIEMER 1962
Thymus (Zellkerne)	25,0		119,0		21,8		SCHIEMER 1967

b) Fall-Nr. Alter u. Geschlecht	Trockengewicht in 10^{-12} g		Volumen in 10^{-12} cm³		%-Trockengew. in g/100 ml		Eigene Untersuch. Krankheitsdauer
	Kern	Cytopl.	Kern	Cytopl.	Kern	Cytopl.	
1 SN 110/66 51 Jahre ♂	23,6	33,3	105,7	292,4	23,5	11,6	1 Jahr
2 SN 474/66 63 Jahre ♂	38,3	28,0	217,2	317,3	18,5	9,3	3 Jahre
3 SN 652/66 70 Jahre ♀	28,3	20,7	128,2	195,4	22,6	10,7	¹/₂ Jahr
4 SN 1104/66 65 Jahre ♀	34,7	34,7	145,6	241,1	24,6	14,5	¹/₂ Jahr
5 SN 1130/66 54 Jahre ♂	36,3	29,0	169,0	254,9	23,1	11,5	5 Jahre
6 SN 19/67 44 Jahre ♀	45,8	56,1	236,6	503,7	20,9	11,5	¹/₂ Jahr

Zusammenfassung und Ausblick

Die gegebene Übersicht möge folgendes gezeigt haben:

1. Es gibt heutzutage cytometrische (interferenzmikroskopische und cytophotometrische) Methoden, die es uns erlauben, innerhalb von Sekunden oder Minuten Substanzmengen (z. B. Trockensubstanz, DNS oder RNS) im Protoplasma, Zellkern und Kernkörperchen einer Zelle zu bestimmen.

2. Dies ließ sich nur durch den Einsatz moderner kybernetischer Auswerteverfahren erreichen. Mit Hilfe des eigenen Computers RPC 4000 und der elektronischen Datenverarbeitungsanlage IBM 7094 im Deutschen Rechenzentrum in Darmstadt können unsere cytometrischen Daten unter Umständen für einen Untersuchungsfall innerhalb weniger Stunden verarbeitet werden und im Ergebnis vorliegen. Nicht nur Einzelwerte, Mittelwerte und Standardabweichungen, sondern auch Histogramme und Regressionsanalysen werden im Maschinenausdruck dargestellt.

3. Durch die Regressionsanalyse (allometrische Wachstums-Untersuchungen) lassen sich über Syntheseleistungen der Zelle Informationen erhalten. Es zeigt sich, daß Kern und Cytoplasma oft unterschiedliche Wachstumsgradienten hinsichtlich Substanz und Nucleinsäure-Zunahme aufweisen. Bei Tumorzellen ist das besonders ausgeprägt.

Diese Resultate können zusätzlich – neben den Mittelwerten und Histogrammen für Substanzmenge und Konzentration sowie Nucleinsäuregehalt der jeweils untersuchten Zellkollektive – für diagnostische, therapeutische und prognostische Überlegungen herangezogen werden.

4. Die vorgetragenen Ergebnisse berechtigen uns, den eingeschlagenen Weg auch weiter zu verfolgen. Es gilt jedoch zunächst: daß uns nur das sorgfältige Registrieren aller Befundeinzelheiten weiterhelfen wird. Dieser Grundsatz wurde bereits vor Jahren (DOERR [13]) allgemein für das Krebsproblem formuliert. Gegenüber früher verfügen wir heute aber über weitergehende Methoden. Die notwendigen Analysen der gegenseitigen Abhängigkeiten oder das syndromhafte Zusammentreffen z. B. von klinischen, patho-anatomischen und cytometrischen Befunden wird auch in solchen Fällen durch die moderne Kybernetik erleichtert (SCHIEMER [44]; SCHIEMER, BLEYL u. ROSSNER [46]).

Literatur

1. BAUER, K. H.: Das Krebsproblem. Berlin-Göttingen-Heidelberg: Springer 2. Aufl. 1963.
2. BEHRENS, O. K., F. LIPMANN, M. COHN u. D. BURK: Das Krebsproblem. Zit. nach: K. H. BAUER (1963).
3. BIELSCHOWSKI, F., W. E. GRIESBACH, W. H. HALL, T. H. KENNEDY, and D. H. PURVES: Studies on experimental goitre: the transplantability of experimental thyroid tumors of the rat. Brit. J. Cancer 3, 541–546 (1959).

4. Brachet, I.: The biological role of ribonucleic acids. Amsterdam-London-New York: Elsevier 1960.

5. Caspersson, T.: Über den chemischen Aufbau der Strukturen des Zellkerns. Skand. Arch. Physiol. **73**, Suppl. **8** (1936).

6. — Studies on protein metabolism in the cells of epithelial tumors. Acta radiol. Suppl. **46** (1942).

7. — Cell growth and function. New York: N. W. Norton 1950.

8. Cowdry, E. V.: Ageing of individual cells. In: Cowdrys Problems of Ageing; Biological and Medical Aspects. S. 50–88. Baltimore: A. J. Lansing 1952.

9. Crick, F. H. C. and I. D. Watson: Molecular structure of nucleic acids. A structure for Desoxyribose Nucleic Acid. Nature **171**, 737–738 (1953).

10. Davies, H. G. and E. M. Deeley: An integrator for measuring the 'dry mass' of cells and isolated components. Exp. Cell Res. **11**, 169–185 (1956).

11. Dittmar: Über das Vorkommen von d-Glutaminsäure in Tumorproteinen. I. Z. Krebsforsch. **49**, 397–442 (1939).

12. — Über das Vorkommen von d-Glutaminsäure in Tumorproteinen. III. Z. Krebsforsch. **50**, 170–177 (1940).

13. Doerr, W.: Bösartige Geschwülste des Verdauungskanals. Internist **2**, 457–472 (1961).

14. Dubois, E.: Über die Abhängigkeit des Hirngewichtes von der Körpergröße, I. Bei den Säugetieren. Arch. Anthropol. **25**, 1–22 (1898).

15. — Über die Abhängigkeit des Hirngewichtes von der Körpergröße des Menschen. Arch. Anthropol. **25**, 423–441 (1898).

16. Gastpar, H. u. A. Herrmann: Anwendung von Cytostatica in der Hals-, Nasen-, Ohrenheilkunde. In: Therapie maligner Tumoren, Hämoblastome und Hämoblastosen. S. 666–709. Stuttgart: Enke 1966.

17. Harbers, E., G. Domagk u. W. Müller: Die Nukleinsäuren. Stuttgart: Thieme 1964.

18. Huggins, Ch.: Control of Cancers in man by endocrinological methods. Cancer Res. **17**, 467–472 (1957).

19. Jamin, J.: Description d'un nouvel appareil de recherches, fondé sur les interférences. C. R. Acad. Sci. **42**, 482–485 (1856).

20. — Sur un réfrateur différentiel pour la lumière polarisée. C. R. Acad. Sci. **67**, 814–816 (1868).

21. Jansen, H. H., H. G. Schiemer u. U. Bleyl: In Vorbereitung.

22. Klatt, B.: Zur Methodik vergleichender metrischer Untersuchungen, besonders des Herzgewichtes. Biol. Zbl. **39**, 406–430 (1919).

23. Kögl, F.: Zur Ätiologie der Tumoren. Klin. Wschr. **18**, 801–806 (1935).

24. Lebedeff, A. A.: L'interféromètre à polarisation et ses applications. Rev. Opt. **9**, 385–414 (1930).

25. Lettré, H.: Cytostatische Substanzen und ihre Wirkung. Grundlag. u. Praxis chem. Tumorbehandlung. Berlin-Göttingen-Heidelberg: Springer 1953.

26. — Zusammenfassung der experimentellen Arbeiten über antimitotische Therapie. Antibiot. et Chemother. **8**, 166–193 (1960).

27. Linzbach, A. J.: Quantitative Biologie und Morphologie des Wachstums einschl. Hypertrophie u. Riesenzellen. Handb. allg. Path., 6, I. S. 180 ff. (1955).

28. Loeser, A. A.: Mammary carcinoma response to inplantation of male hormone and progesteron. Lancet, II, 698–700 (1941).

29. Mach, L.: Über ein Interferenzrefractometer. Wiener Sitzgsber. **101**, Abth. IIa. (1892).

30. Makino, S.: The chromosomes cytology of the ascites tumors of rats, with special reference to the concept of stemline cell. In: Internat. review of cytology, IV, S. 25–84. New York: Academic Press 1967.

31. Makino, S. and Kano: Cytological studies of tumors. IX. Characteristic chromosome individuality of tumorstrain cells in ascites tumors of rats. J. nat. Cancer Ins. **13**, 1213 (1953).

32. Maurer, H. J.: Beitrag zur biologischen und biochemischen Wirkung ionisierender Strahlungen. I. Grundzüge der Chemie ionisierender Strahlungen. Strahlentherapie **106**, 491–504 (1958).

33. Meselson, M. and F. Stahl: The reduplication of DNA in Escherichia coli. Proc. nat. Acad. Sci. **44**, 671–682 (1958).

34. Meythaler, F.: Cytostatische Therapie der Hämoblastosen und Hämoblastome. In: Therapie maligner Tumoren, Hämoblastome und Hämoblastosen. S. 341 bis 428. Stuttgart: Enke 1966.

35. Needham, J.: Biochemistry and Morphogenesis. Cambridge: Univ. Press 1942, 1950.

36. Pütter, J.: Über die biochemischen Wirkungen von Cytostatica auf Tumorzellen. In: Therapie maligner Tumoren, Hämoblastome und Hämoblastosen. S. 80–146. Stuttgart: Enke 1966.

37. Rajewsky, B.: zit. nach: Maurer.

38. Sandritter, W., H. G. Schiemer, W. Alt u. E. Behrouzi: Histochemie von Sputumzellen. III. Interferenzmikroskopische Trockengewichtsbestimmungen. Frankfurt. Z. Path. **69**, 167–193 (1958).

39. Snell, O.: Die Abhängigkeit des Hirngewichtes von dem Körpergewicht und den geistigen Fähigkeiten. Arch. Psych. **23**, 436–445 (1891).

40. Schiemer, H. G.: Vergleichende Trockengewichtsbestimmungen an Kern und Zytoplasma verschiedener Karzinome. Verh. Dtsch. Ges. Path. **43**, 359–365 (1959).

41. — Prinzip und Erfahrungen mit dem Bakerschen Interferenzmikroskop. Acta histochem. **9**, 207–215 (1960).

42. — Pathologisches Wachstum. Acta histochem., Suppl. VI, 435–451 (1965).

43. — Neue Wege der Cytometrie auf dem Gebiete der Krebsforschung, der allgemeinen Biologie und Pathologie. Klin. Wschr. **45**, 393–399 (1967).

44. — Vergleichende histologische und zytometrische Untersuchungen an menschlichen Mammakarzinomen. – Ein Paradigma synoptischer Lösungsmethoden in der Kanzerologie. Habilitationsschrift (1967).

45. —, G. Günther u. D. Sina: Die Wirkung des Cytostaticum Methotrexat auf den Wassergehalt und das Trockengewicht von Kern und Cytoplasma der Leberzellen der Ratte bei der Regeneration und Teilhepatektomie. Frankfurt. Z. Path. **76**, 427–434 (1967).

46. —, U. Bleyl u. A. Rossner: Vergleichende Untersuchungen zwischen Sexchromatingehalt, zytometrischen und elektronenmikroskopischen Befunden an Mammakarzinomen. IV. Tg. Dtsch. Ges. Angew. Zytologie, Mannheim 1967.

47. Warburg, O.: Über die letzte Ursache und die entfernten Ursachen des Krebses. Würzburg: Triltsch 1966.

48. — Über die letzte Ursache und die entfernten Ursachen des Krebses. In: 17. Mosbacher Kolloquium v. 21.–23. 4. 1966. Berlin-Heidelberg-New York: Springer 1966.

49. — u. W. Christian: Gärungsfermente im Blutserum von Tumorratten. Biochem. Z. **314**, 399 (1943).

50. Zehnder, L.: Ein neuer Interferenzrefraktor. Z. Instrkd. **11**, 275–285 (1891).

Enzymatischer Abbau xenobiotischer Purinderivate

Von

D. WERNER

Die cytotoxische Wirkung einiger xenobiotischer Purinderivate, insbesondere die selektive Wirkung einiger Vertreter dieser Verbindungsklasse auf Tumorzellen in vitro [1], hat uns zu Untersuchungen über den enzymatischen Abbau dieser Verbindungen angeregt.

Von der Kenntnis dieses Abbauweges wurden Hinweise für einen Wirkungsmechanismus und eine Erklärung für das selektive cytotoxische Verhalten einiger Purinderivate erwartet.

Insbesondere wurden fünf Typen puryl-6-substituierter Amine untersucht: Puryl-6-substituierte primäre, sekundäre und tertiäre Amine, puryl-6-substituierte Aminosäuren und puryl-6-substituierte cyclische Imine.

Diese xenobiotischen Purinderivate wurden zunächst auf ihre Substratfähigkeit gegenüber Xanthinoxidase geprüft. Die substratfähigen Verbindungen wurden von dem Enzym in 2- bzw. 8-Stellung des Purinrings hydroxyliert. Der Substratnachweis mit spektrophotometrischen und radiochromatographischen Methoden, sowie der weitere Abbau der 2,8-dihydroxylierten xenobiotischen Purinderivate mit verschiedenen peroxidativen Systemen wurde bereits an anderer Stelle beschrieben [2].

Wir konnten nun zeigen, daß unser „in vitro“-Modell für den Abbau xenobiotischer Purinderivate repräsentativ für die tatsächlichen biologischen Vorgänge ist:

Die orale Verabreichung eines ^{14}C-markierten xenobiotischen Purinderivats, das Substrat für Xanthinoxidase ist, führt nach Chromatographie des Urins (Maus) zur gleichen Aktivitätsverteilung auf dem Chromatogramm, wie sie auch nach Chromatographie einer Inkubationsmischung von markierter Verbindung und Xanthinoxidase erhalten wird. Nach längerer Verabreichung treten neben dem Hauptmetaboliten (2,8-dihydroxyliertes Derivat) noch weitere Metabolite auf (Abb. 1). Ferner läßt sich in der Atemluft des Tieres markiertes Kohlendioxid nachweisen.

Füttert man das Tier gleichzeitig noch mit Allo-Purinol, einem Hemmstoff der Xanthinoxidase, so wird die markierte Purinverbindung nahezu unverändert ausgeschieden.

Zusammenfassend kann also gesagt werden, daß xenobiotische Purine, die Substrate für Xanthinoxidase sind, in vivo in zwei Schritten abgebaut werden: Zuerst werden über die monohydroxylierten Zwischenstufen die 2,8-dihydroxylierten Derivate gebildet. Letztere werden durch unspezifische Peroxidasen in kleinere Zwischenprodukte abgebaut, die

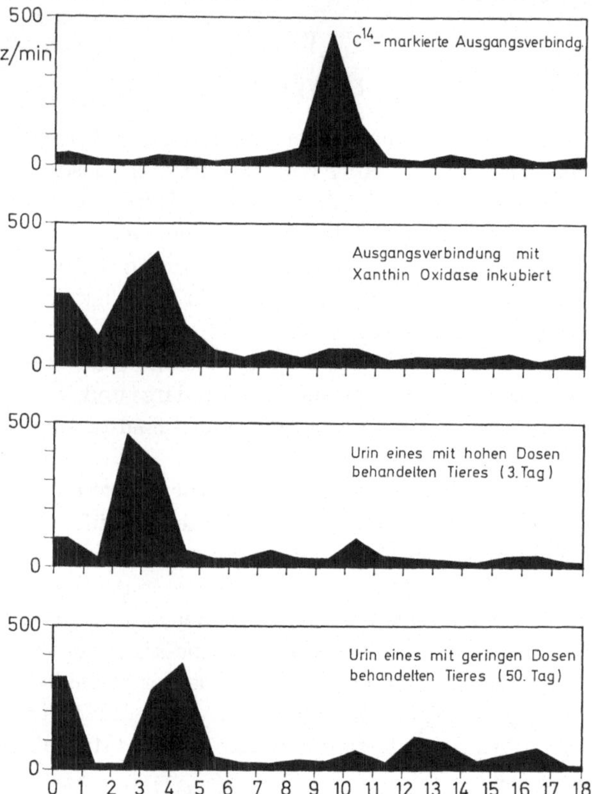

Abb. 1. Verteilung der Radioaktivität auf Papierchromatogrammen nach Chromatographie (Propanol/Wasser) von: ¹⁴C-markiertem Puryl-6-histamin; einem Inkubationsansatz von Puryl-6-histamin mit Xanthinoxidase. Urin von Mäusen, die über einen kürzeren und längeren Zeitraum mit Puryl-6-histamin gefüttert wurden

entweder mit dem Urin oder in der Atemluft ausgeschieden oder zum Aufbau biogenen Materials verwendet werden (Abb. 2).

Nach längerer Verabreichung eines in 8-Stellung des Purinrings ¹⁴C-markierten xenobiotischen Purinderivats kann man aus den Organen des Tieres (Leber) markiertes, spektral und chromatographisch reines Adenin und Guanin isolieren. Das endogen entstandene markierte Kohlendioxid wird hierbei auf bekanntem physiologisch-chemischem Weg in die 6-Stellung der beiden Purinbasen eingebaut (Abb. 2).

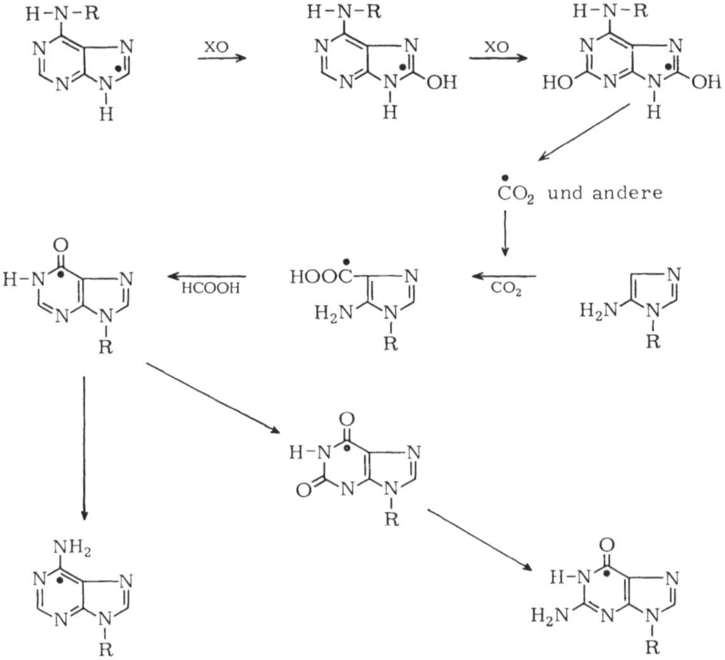

Abb. 2. Schema des Abbaus xenobiotischer Purinderivate in vivo und der Verwendung von Abbauprodukten zum Aufbau biogenen Materials

Tabelle 1. *Zusammenhang zwischen der cytotoxischen Wirkung von puryl-6-substituierten Aminen und Aminosäuren und deren Substratfähigkeit für Xanthinoxidase*

Purylderivate von	Getestet	Cytotoxisch	Davon Substrat
Primären Aminen	15	9	9
Sekundären Aminen	5	0	0
Tertiären Aminen	4	1	0
Aminosäuren	9	1	1
Cyclischen Iminen	6	3	3
	39	14	13

Das „in vitro"-Modell, bestehend aus Xanthinoxidase und Peroxidase ist so leicht zu handhaben, daß wir eine große Zahl (etwa 80) xenobiotische Purinderivate auf einen möglichen Abbau hin testen konnten. Die Ergebnisse für die puryl-6-substituierten Amine sind in der Tab. 1 zusammengefaßt.

Sieht man von einer Ausnahme ab, so scheinen alle puryl-6-substituierten Amine mit cytotoxischer Wirkung auch Substrate für das Abbaumodell zu sein. Die in Abb. 3 wiedergegebenen Ergebnisse sind weitere Stützen dieser Regel.

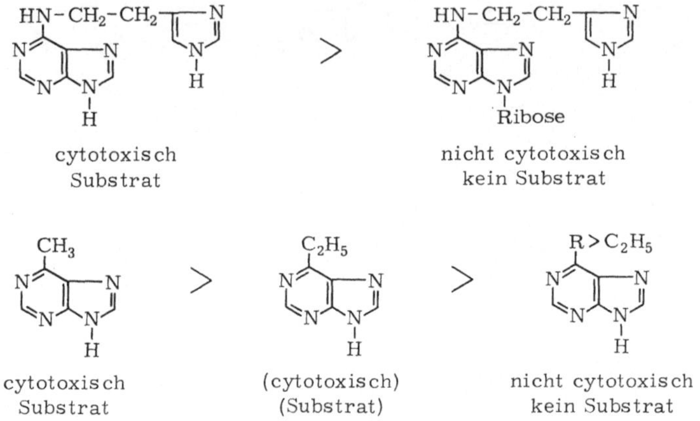

cytotoxisch
Substrat

nicht cytotoxisch
kein Substrat

cytotoxisch
Substrat

(cytotoxisch)
(Substrat)

nicht cytotoxisch
kein Substrat

Abb. 3. Zwei Beispiele für den Zusammenhang zwischen cytotoxischer Wirkung und der Substratfähigkeit für Xanthinoxidase. Derivate ursprünglich cytotoxischer Substanzen verlieren parallel die cytotoxische Wirkung und die Substratfähigkeit

Neben dieser Relation zwischen Substratfähigkeit für Xanthinoxidase und cytotoxischer Wirkung bietet dieser Abbauweg auch eine Deutung für die Spezifität cytotoxischer Purine. Es ist bekannt, daß die Xanthinoxidase-Aktivität in Tumorzellen geringer als in vergleichbaren Normalzellen ist. Man kann sich deshalb vorstellen, daß es cytotoxisch wirksame Purinderivate gibt, die von Normalzellen rasch abgebaut und damit entgiftet werden. Tumorzellen bauen hingegen langsamer oder gar nicht ab und werden geschädigt [3].

Literatur

1. Lettré, H.: Cytotoxic Agents of the Purine and Sterol Group. Progr. exp. Tumor Res. 1, 329–359 (1960).
2. —, N. K. Kapoor, and D. Werner: Catabolism of some cytotoxic Purine Derivatives by Xanthine Oxidase and Peroxidase. Biochem. Pharmacol. 16, 1747–1755 (1967).
3. — u. D. Werner: Zur spezifischen Wirkung des 6-Purylhistamins auf Krebszellen. Naturwissenschaften 55, 43 (1968).

Sachverzeichnis